REVENGE OF THE WINDIGO

The Construction of the Mind and Mental Health of North American Aboriginal Peoples

In *Revenge of the Windigo*, James Waldram looks at conceptual knowledge of Aboriginal mental health: its form and substance, its construction and dissemination, and its implications for Aboriginal peoples. Waldram shows how three disciplines – anthropology, psychology, and psychiatry – have together constructed a profoundly distorted portrait of Aboriginal peoples, based on a tangled web of theory, method, and data rife with conceptual problems, shaky assumptions, and inappropriate generalizations.

The work examines how culture has been theorized and operationalized in the study of Aboriginal mental health, and also evaluates the contribution that Aboriginal peoples have inadvertently made to theoretical and methodological developments in the three fields under discussion. Waldram finds that scholars and researchers have mostly failed to comprehend the meaning of contemporary Aboriginality in terms of mental health and illness, preferring instead to rely on their own scientific methods as the only means to properly observe, measure, assess, and treat Aboriginal peoples.

Using an interdisciplinary approach, the author critically assesses the enormous amount of information that has been generated on Aboriginal mental health, deconstructs it, and in the process, provides direction for new avenues of research.

(Anthropological Horizons)

JAMES B. WALDRAM is a medical anthropologist and professor in the Department of Psychology at the University of Saskatchewan.

ANTHROPOLOGICAL HORIZONS
Editor: Michael Lambek, University of Toronto

This series, begun in 1991, focuses on theoretically informed ethnographic works addressing issues of mind and body, knowledge and power, equality and inequality, the individual and the collective. Interdisciplinary in its perspective, the series makes a unique contribution in several other academic disciplines: women's studies, history, philosophy, psychology, political science, and sociology.

For a list of the books published in this series see p. 415.

JAMES B. WALDRAM

Revenge of the Windigo

The Construction of the
Mind and Mental Health of
North American Aboriginal Peoples

UNIVERSITY OF TORONTO PRESS
Toronto Buffalo London

© University of Toronto Press Incorporated 2004
Toronto Buffalo London
Printed in Canada

ISBN 0-8020-8826-0 (cloth)
ISBN 0-8020-8600-4 (paper)

Printed on acid-free paper

National Library of Canada Cataloguing in Publication

Waldram, James B. (James Burgess)
Revenge of the windigo : construction of the mind and mental
health of North American Aboriginal peoples / James B. Waldram.

(Anthropological horizons)
Includes index.
ISBN 0-8020-8826-0 (bound).   ISBN 0-8020-8600-4 (pbk.)

1. Indians of North America – Psychology.   2. Indians of North
America – Mental health.   3. Ethnopsychology – History.   I. Title.
II. Series.

RC451.5.I5W34 2004   155.8' 497' 009   C2003-906290-2

This book has been published with the help of a grant from the Canadian
Federation for the Humanities and Social Sciences Federation, through the Aid
to Scholarly Publications Programme, using funds provided by the Social
Sciences and Humanities Research Council of Canada.

University of Toronto Press acknowledges the financial assistance to its
publishing program of the Canada Council for the Arts and the Ontario Arts
Council.

University of Toronto Press acknowledges the financial support for its
publishing activities of the Government of Canada through the Book
Publishing Industry Development Program (BPIDP).

For Pam,
who inspires me daily

Contents

Acknowledgments xi

1 **Introduction: Monsters and Mental Health** **3**
Themes and Influences 8
Plan of the Book 14
Terminology 16
About the Title 17
Conclusion 18

PART A: CONSTRUCTING THE ABORIGINAL

2 **Constructing Aboriginal Personality: The Early Years** **21**
Ruth Benedict and the Boasian Tradition 22
The Emergence of Psychoanalytical Anthropology and the Search for
the Indians' 'Basic Personality Structure' 27
The Indian Education Research Project 29
Conclusion 42

3 **The Psychoanalyst's Aboriginal** **44**
Anthropology and the Rorschach: No Experience Required 44
The Generation of Aboriginal Personality Portraits 48
Atomism and the Northern Indian 55
Persistence of the Rorschach 60
Conclusion 67

4 **Measuring the Aboriginal** **69**
Acculturation and the Conceptualization of Aboriginality 69

Measuring Aboriginal Cultural Orientation   76
Measuring Aboriginal Personality: The Minnesota Multiphasic
Personality Inventory   84
The Confusion of Race and Culture in the Measurement of Aboriginal
Intelligence   89
Constructing the Aboriginal Variable   95
Conclusion   101

PART B: THE DISORDERED ABORIGINAL

5   The Construction of Aboriginal Psychopathology   105
'Latent Schizophrenics and Primitive People': Early Studies of
Psychopathology   105
Marginality and the 'Caught-Between-Two-Worlds' Paradigm   114
Acculturative Stress   118
Community-Based Epidemiological Studies   124
Conclusion   133

6   The Alcoholic Aboriginal   134
The Biologically Susceptible Aboriginal   135
The How and Why of Aboriginal Drinking   142
Indian Drinking and White Man Drinking   157
Emerging Epidemiological Issues   161
Conclusion   165

7   The Depressed Aboriginal   167
Conceptualizing Depression and Suicide   168
Measuring and Treating Aboriginal Depression and Suicide   176
An Ethnographic Approach to the Study of Aboriginal
Depression   185
Conclusion   188

8   The Culture-Bound Aboriginal   190
The Culture-Bound Syndromes   190
Windigo Psychosis   192
Pibloktoq   195
Ghost Sickness   199
Why the Culture-Bound Syndromes Persist   203
Conclusion   211

9   The Traumatized Aboriginal   212
Conceptualizing Trauma and PTSD   212
Trauma and Aboriginal Peoples   215
Historic, Cultural, and Collective Trauma   221
Trauma and the Construction of 'Residential School Syndrome'   228
Conclusion   234

PART C: TREATING THE ABORIGINAL

10   The Clinician's Aboriginal   239
The Anthropological Roots of Aboriginal Values Research   239
The Psychologist's Approach to Aboriginal Values   243
Delineating the Ethics, Values, and Behaviours of *the* Aboriginal   249
Essentializing the Aboriginal/Non-Aboriginal Dichotomy   256
Values and Treatment   259
Conclusion   269

11   Healing the Traditional Aboriginal   271
Aboriginal Theories of Mental Health and Illness   272
The Holistic Aboriginal   275
Re-opening the Mind/Body Debate   278
The Use of Culture and Tradition in Treatment   286
Defining 'Traditional Aboriginal Healing'   294
Conclusion   298

12   Conclusion: The Windigo's Revenge   300
Disturbed, Disordered, and Dysfunctional   301
Problems of Culture and History   306
Defining the Aboriginal   312
Contemporary Aboriginal Cultural Realities: Creolization and
Beyond   316

Notes   321

References   335

Index   393

Acknowledgments

This book has been several years in the making, during which time I have been afforded the opportunity to work through my ideas in several venues. I am particularly indebted to the Culture, Community and Health Studies program at the Centre for Addiction and Mental Health in Toronto, where I spent a sabbatical in 2000–1. While at CAMH, I was provided the opportunity to present some of my developing work in their seminar series, and received valuable feedback. The opportunity to use the CAMH library was also important in providing me with ready access to difficult-to-locate materials. While on sabbatical I was also affiliated with the Department of Anthropology at the University of Toronto, where again I was able to present some of my ideas and receive valuable feedback. The Robarts Library proved to be central to my project during that year. Presentations at McMaster, McGill, and Manitoba universities, as well as the annual meetings of the Canadian Anthropology Society, the Society for Applied Anthropology, and the American Anthropological Association, also provided me with the opportunity to gauge reaction to my work. The first draft of this book was written during that sabbatical, and I appreciate the opportunity to do so afforded me by the University of Saskatchewan. I am also indebted to the anonymous reviewers who examined the manuscript for the University of Toronto Press, and thank them for taking the time to fully engage with this project and offer some important insights and advice. The University of Toronto Press, as always, has been a delight to work with, and I especially want to acknowledge Virgil Duff, Lauren Freeman, and my copy-editor, Allyson May. Funding to undertake the research for this book was provided through a grant from the Social Sciences and Humanities Research Council of Canada.

This book has been published with the help of a grant from the Canadian Federation for the Humanities and Social Sciences, through the Aid to Scholarly Publications Programme, using funds provided by the Social Sciences and Humanities Research Council of Canada.

Finally, I want to acknowledge the valuable contribution to this book, intellectual and otherwise, of Pamela Downe, who challenged me constantly to refine my ideas, offered important criticism and, when appropriate, praise, and who shared her expertise with me on a daily basis as I struggled at times to pull all of this together.

REVENGE OF THE WINDIGO

CHAPTER ONE

Introduction:
Monsters and Mental Health

Briefly stated, our textbooks are filled with conclusions about human behavior that have been based on assumptions, methods, and subject samples that are culturally biased and do not reflect the spectrum of existing human variations, especially within a culturally pluralistic society ... (Marsella, Dubanoski, Hamada, & Morse 2000: 51)

What do we think we know about North American Aboriginal mental abilities, mental health, and mental illness, and on what basis do we think we know it? That is the central question I wish to address in this book. While this appears to be a simple, straightforward question, it leads to a tangled web of theory, method, and data, rife with conceptual problems, shaky assumptions, and inappropriate generalizations.

This book is *not*, strictly speaking, about the mental health of Aboriginal peoples. It is not my intent to present tables of epidemiological data on the rates of selected mental health problems. Rather, my subject is *knowledge* about Aboriginal mental health, who has generated that knowledge, how it has been generated and communicated, and the implications of its existence for Aboriginal peoples. The book seeks to critically assess the enormous amount of information extant on Aboriginal mental health, to deconstruct it, and, through this exercise, to provide some guidance for a new course, where warranted. While learning little here about the mental health of Aboriginal peoples, the reader will discover a great deal about the intellectual traditions that have shaped how, from the perspective of mind and culture, order and disorder, Aboriginal peoples have been portrayed.

I repeat, so that there is no confusion: I am not writing about Aboriginal peoples; I am writing about what scholars and researchers have written about Aboriginal peoples. In this sense, the book is more of a critical intellectual historiography than a text book.

This book is also not intended to be a history of my three target disciplines – anthropology, psychology, and psychiatry – although at times it may look like it is. In order to understand how knowledge about Aboriginal peoples has been generated, it is essential to anchor the present analysis in some of the historical and theoretical trends in these disciplines, to pay homage to the intellectual geneologies which have shaped thought on these matters (Kuper 1999; Darnell 2001). While I intend to draw connections between scholars and disciplines from time to time, a solid history of these disciplines would require a different approach (and such histories already exist). Thus I ask the reader's indulgence if my historical discussions fall short or fail to make the kinds of connections that they themselves feel are warranted. I am focused here on the end-product of this intellectual gaze, the images of Aboriginal peoples that have been and continue to be constructed, and how this has been done. I wish to build upon the pertinent intellectual traditions, especially over the last century, to see how these images developed, why they developed in the manner they did, and how they are interconnected. But in all instances where there have been developments of historical or contemporary scholarly interest, I return to my central concern: what, if anything, has been said about the mental capabilities and health of Aboriginal peoples? If you knew nothing of the issues of Aboriginal mental health or the intellectual traditions that informed them, and undertook to learn by reading the vast material that has been produced, in the end, what would you think you knew?

I intend to concentrate on issues of mind and mental health, and this means I cannot address some of the broader contributions that specific scholars have made to various fields. Typically, scholars' ideas develop over long careers of research and writing, but new developments in their thinking have not always been applied to the topic of Aboriginal peoples. Some readers may feel that I am emphasizing relatively minor aspects of otherwise stellar scholarship, turning our icons into straw persons by extracting some of their more dubious pronouncements from exhaustive records of solid work. But my concern is solely on what they wrote that is of relevance to an understanding of Aboriginal mental abilities and mental health issues: when they have stopped writing about these topics, for purposes of this book I have stopped being interested. Further, in the cases of individuals who have made extensive contributions to the fields under discussion, I shall feel free to nip and tuck my way through their work to support the points I feel need to be made, rather than attempting to summarize their work as a whole.

Enough of the caveats. Let me share how I have come to undertake this project, for this story explains in many ways the perspective I take on the issue.

Over the years I have spent considerable time in Algonkian communities in northern Canada, mostly Cree and Ojibwa, where I have heard time and again the stories of the windigo (or witiko), the cannibal monster familiar to students of Algonkian cultures and those interested in the culture-bound syndromes. The Cree and Ojibwa whom I encountered did not seem overly concerned with the question of windigo's reality. 'It's just a story,' I was patronizingly informed one night around the campfire. Yet I was puzzled by the literature I had read as a graduate student in the late 1970s, which made me expect to find cannibal psychotics all over the north! When I first read Lou Marano's (1985) dissection of the notion of windigo psychosis, in which he effectively argued that this disorder existed primarily in the minds of gullible explorers and anthropologists, I felt relieved that the puzzle had been solved for me, but I was also troubled. If scholars of both anthropology and psychiatry had been mistaken for so long, what other errors might we have made? Were there any more faux-cannibal-psychotic-monsters out there? It was not until I began research in prisons that this question resurfaced in my mind.

Throughout the 1990s, I undertook research in federal and provincial prisons in Canada (Waldram 1997). Several incidents in the course of that research suggested to me that many mental health professionals were clearly having trouble understanding Aboriginal inmates. My entrée into this issue began with a simple question put to me by a psychologist: 'In the treatment of Aboriginal offenders, does culture matter?' Some time later another psychologist disclosed that they were thinking of employing an old instrument to better assess Aboriginal men. The 'Indian Culturalization Test' (discussed in greater depth later in this book) was clearly designed for American Sioux peoples and had some serious flaws, yet it was being considered for use with a primarily Canadian Cree population. There are important cultural differences between the two peoples and its use in this context would have been problematic. Asking some Cree peoples if they eat dog, for instance, would have been offensive. Further, the fact that many Sioux words were used in the instrument did not seem to concern the psychologist, perhaps betraying an assumption that once characterized the view of many Westerners, that all Indian languages were essentially the same.

Another researcher showed me the results of more than a hundred statistical analyses comparing Aboriginal men with non-Aboriginal men on a variety of psychological tests. These data, which simply grouped all Aboriginals and all non-Aboriginals into two dichotomous categories, suggested very few differences, leading him to conclude that the instruments used were, by and large, culturally appropriate for the Aboriginal men. I was suspicious of this interpretation, largely because I knew the Aboriginal men tested to be from diverse cultural backgrounds. Some were from very remote areas and spoke, at best, only a little English. Was it appropriate to cluster such individuals with others who had been raised in non-Aboriginal adoptive homes? Were individuals from these two different experiential backgrounds equivalently 'Aboriginal' for purposes of understanding the cultural appropriateness of the tests in question? Did these tests even say anything about culture? As my research progressed and I was able to review the case management files of several hundred Aboriginal offenders, I found many instances of problematic racial or cultural typing, suggesting either little concern for understanding the role of culture in forensic treatment or else a view that all Aboriginals were essentially alike, making fully developed cultural profiles unnecessary. My interest was piqued: there seemed to be a prevailing and unquestioned assumption that the Aboriginal men were well understood and not really all that different from each other and from non-Aboriginals. Yet the basis for those assumptions seemed remarkably weak.

I grew increasingly frustrated at the discordance between what I was reading and hearing about Aboriginal peoples in the mental health literature, the clinics, and the prisons and my own experiences and knowledge based on more than two decades of anthropological research. Having worked in both northern and southern parts of Canada, as well as in urban areas, I have been immersed in a variety of cultural contexts that, together, span the tremendous diversity of Aboriginal cultures. As a professor in Native Studies for some seventeen years, I had witnessed, and experienced, the concern and sometime anger of Aboriginal peoples reacting to simplistic, stereotypical, and essentialist portrayals of their cultures. Aboriginal peoples are convinced that they are not well understood by the rest of North American society, and it was my sense, at the beginning of this project, that they were correct.

A sabbatical leave allowed me the time to delve more deeply into the issue of how Aboriginal mental health was conceptualized within the fields of anthropology, psychology, and psychiatry. At the outset, I expected that the literature would be scant. My interactions with psychologists and psychiatrists who worked with Aboriginal peoples certainly led me to such a conclusion. My expectation was challenged when I encountered the 1981 bibliography on American Indian and Alaska Native mental health by Kelso and Attneave (1981), which identified more than 1360 articles, and Mail and McDonald's (1980) bibliography of almost a thousand citations on alcohol among Indians. And these were two decades old! More recently, Manson (2000) had indicated that between 1980 and 1995 some 2000 journal articles and book chapters on some aspect of the mental health of American Indians had been published. As I began to follow the leads of the literature, my file boxes filled with articles. Aboriginal mental health is nothing short of a major scholarly industry. In an attempt to make sense of it all, I have tried to focus as much as possible on the more authoritative and influential works, those that seem to have pioneered a particular method or perspective, those that are cited more frequently than others, or those that allow me to make a particularly salient point. Furthermore, it has been necessary to concentrate on only a handful of mental health topics to keep the project manageable. I have not been able to look into every disorder as defined by the ever-evolving *Diagnostic and Statistical Manual* (DSM) of the American Psychiatric Association. Nevertheless, the sheer volume of material is mind-boggling, even more so when one realizes that, in the end, it seems to add up to so little.

This is a critical piece of work. I examine the efforts of individuals, some giants in their fields, who have contributed a great deal to our understanding of Aboriginal mental health. In some instances, perhaps, I have gone too far in my critique and have been too mischievous. Playing devil's advocate always carries a risk. Many of the problems I identify in this book also characterize my own past work – there are no saints here – and it was my growing unease with the accepted conceptual and methodological paradigms which, in part, led me to write this book. I also recognize that I have probably made the same errors here that I criticize in the work of others; this may demonstrate how deeply embedded these paradigms are in the scholarly discourse. But I am rattled by the fundamental problems in our knowledge base, and by pushing the analysis into underlying constructs and challenging methodological assumptions, I hope to encourage all of us to pause and rethink what we think we know. After all, what we as researchers and clinicians think we know affects people's lives, *Aboriginal* peoples' lives, in profound ways, and if we have it wrong the consequences – erroneous diagnoses, ineffective or damaging treatment, stereotyping and stigmatization of individuals and whole communities – can be dire indeed. The stakes are high: lives can be destroyed, and lives can be lost. That some Aboriginal peoples have and continue to experience real pain and suffering is beyond question. It is my hope that the work presented here will have a broadly based positive impact on this situation, even if it appears on the surface to be devoid of practical suggestions.

Themes and Influences

Several themes emerge throughout this book. My paramount interest is in how culture has been conceptualized and operationalized in the study of Aboriginal mind and mental health. Culture is implicitly at the core of scientific studies of Aboriginal peoples, for it is in their perceived cultural difference, their exoticism or 'otherness' (not to mention their convenience) that we find the reason for their attractiveness. Forcing Aboriginal peoples into a single, uniform, and implicitly homogeneous variable category to be contrasted with another, similarly homogenous category, the non-Aboriginal or 'white,' is a strong convention in comparative research. So too is the employment of static notions of culture, such as the culture area concept or the notion of the 'ethnographic present,' a timeless, changeless past which intrudes into the present. Culture is complicated. After more than a century of ruminating, theorizing, and debating anthropologists still cannot agree on what it is, and hence what we see in much research is a fairly uniform way of dealing with this fact, that is, by keeping it simple. But parsimony, in this instance, fails us. My aim here is to identify, as much as possible, the intellectual underpinnings of explicit and implicit models of culture that appear to be guiding research. In some instances, as in ethnographic studies of specific populations, this is fairly easy, but in other instances, such as broadly based epidemiological studies, sometimes only hints of a cultural model can be teased out.

A secondary theme is how Aboriginal peoples have inadvertently contributed to the development of theory and methods in the mental health and psychological, psychiatric, and anthropological professions. In 1968, famed cultural psychiatrist Alexander Leighton (1968: 217) was brought to comment that: 'the American Indian people are among the most studied in the world from an anthropological, and to some extent psychological, point of view. Much of this work has been of an exceedingly high quality and some of it has resulted in new knowledge and insight regarding the social and cultural processes of mankind.' Indeed, Aboriginal peoples were the testing ground for theoretical and methodological issues and debates that had global dimensions in many fields. When one looks at the individuals who have played key roles in the development of the knowledge discussed in this book – Franz Boas, Margaret Mead, Ruth Benedict, Sigmund Freud, Erik Erikson, Abram Kardiner, Ralph Linton, Alfred Kroeber, as well as their students and disciples – one cannot help but appreciate the significance of the amassed intellectual power. When Boasian historical particularism encountered Freudian psychoanalysis, and as the notions of culture, mind, and body were debated, the playing field became Aboriginal North America. As the Americanist tradition in both anthropology and psychiatry emerged as strong if not dominant players in the global intellectual arena, Aboriginal peoples became the sources of data through which new concepts were articulated and new methodologies refined (Darnell 2001). Looking back, it becomes clear that while the substance of these issues and debates has often been ignored or forgotten, the interpretations and conclusions, devoid of their historical context, lingered to become the building blocks of contemporary understanding. So, for example, Ruth Benedict's notion of cultures as personality types, a pioneering conceptualization in the 1930s now confined to the annals of anthropological history, surfaced in the psychological literature 1970s and 1980s with sweeping generalizations of *the* Aboriginal personality. Old studies have been treated as if they are pertinent today, as if, for instance, A.I. Hallowell's Saulteaux Rorschach protocols of the 1930s and 1940s explain some salient feature of contemporary Saulteaux alcoholism. When jumping disciplinary boundaries and leaping carelessly into each other's intellectual backyards, anthropologists, psychologists, and psychiatrists have all too frequently cut to the quick, focusing on the kinds of 'facts' one acquires from reading abstracts, ignoring the context that informed them.

Several theoretical influences also permeate the volume, some more obvious than others. First is the notion of post-coloniality, and by this I mean specifically a comprehension of how the colonizer has maintained control of indigenous populations through the production of knowledge about them, along the lines elucidated in the works of Homi Bhabha (e.g., Bhabha 1983, 1991; see also Duran and Duran 1995).[1] My interest is in understanding how knowledge about Aboriginal peoples, how the 'truth' of their mental states, has been generated by non-Aboriginal scholars, and also how this truth has been accepted uncritically by many scholars of Aboriginal heritage. All of these scholars have adopted the paradigm of an objective science, a universal truth. Since the early 1980s, considerable critical attention within anthropology has focused on the issues of ethnographic truth, the authority to determine the cultural truth of others, and the 'scientific-ness' of cultural description through ethnography (e.g., Geertz 1973; Marcus & Fischer 1986; Clifford 1988). This critique resonated with me, as it did with many anthropologists; while these views were received as too extreme by some, others were not afraid of the suggestion that we were considerably less objective than we wanted to believe. The fields of psychology and psychiatry have not as readily experienced this 'crisis of representation,' and they have been considerably less dissuaded by postmodern critiques, perhaps because of their firmer roots in positivism and the discourse of science (Greenfield 2000). As fields of study, psychology and psychiatry have certainly demonstrated very little of the existential angst, colonial guilt, and critical deconstruction that have permeated anthropology.

Much of the early writing on the Aboriginal mind and mental health is suffused with the notion of the 'primitive.' 'Primitives,' it has been suggested – and Aboriginal peoples are discursively included in this notion – are incapable of complex thought; their thought is based on intuition and superstition, whereas the Westerner's is based on positivism and empiricism. But primitivist discourse is more complicated than this, for the 'primitive' occupies two contrasting and contradictory positions within the intellectual tradition of the West. Primitiveness is not simply a sign of inferiority, a lack of cultural and intellectual development, or evidence of an earlier stage of human cognitive evolution. Primitiveness is also a metaphor for a utopian society, one uncontaminated by the pollutants of civilization. Primitiveness exemplifies what the West has lost, what it pines for and laments and, in some ways, what it hopes to recover (Clifford 1988; Kehoe 1990; Torgovnick 1990, 1996).

Only rarely have these ideas been applied to the study of psychopathology. Two scholars who did, Lucas and Barrett (1995), employed a concept they called 'psychiatric primitivism,' which, like other primitivisms, relies on a 'body of ideas, images and vocabularies about cultural others ... [that] while ostensibly about peoples from elsewhere ... is more fundamentally concerned with the way the West understands itself in contradistinction to these others' (289). The roots of this idea can be found clearly in the contrasting positions of the seventeenth century's Thomas Hobbes, with his view of the life of 'primitives' as 'solitary, poor, nasty, brutish and short,' and Jean Jacques Rousseau, who a century later, expressed the view that the 'primitive' was a 'noble savage' uncontaminated by the corruption of civilization (Lindholm 2001: 33). Lucas and Barrett labelled these two contrasting perspectives the 'Barbaric' and 'Arcadian':[2] the Barbaric 'equates primitive society with degeneration, disruption and pathogenesis,' while the Arcadian 'treats primitive societies as pristine, harmonious and therapeutic' (289). The tension that these two perspectives create plays out in the epistemologies of the West, for 'the primitive is both a stranger from an exotic land and a primal force within ourselves' (290). Madness and disorder struggle with sanity and order; the Barbarian wrestles with the Noble Savage. In both the Barbarian and Arcadian traditions, the 'primitive' is still childlike, the difference being largely a matter of spin: cognitive underdevelopment which impairs versus utopian innocence which liberates. Madmen and 'primitives' are 'free of the constraints of reason' (Lucas & Barrett 1995: 297). And, as the concept implies, much is said about the West as well; just as 'primitives' are stereotyped, essentialized, and constructed, so too are the West's views of itself. Such simple, dualistic thinking is problematic. It should not therefore be surprising that the discourse on schizophrenia, for instance, has frequently encompassed ideas of the 'primitive,' if not in the gendered persona of the cave 'man,' then at least in terms of the cognitive underdevelopment and impairment characteristic of such 'primitives.'

While psychiatry is rife with primitivist metaphors, anthropology may well be the primitivist discipline par excellance. Roger Keesing (1990: 48) has described how anthropology has such a vested interest in 'characterizing exotic otherness' that its practitioners have routinely ignored the compelling evidence of cultural change, such as the existence of radios, wage labour, churches, and schools, among the peoples they study. When faced with the evidence that 'primitives' are no longer 'primitive,' anthropologists have, in Keesing's words, retreated to a belief 'that their essential cultural-ness lives on despite the outward changes in their lives' (48). This idea will emerge as an important theme in this book.

In the deliberation that follows, the reader will occasionally see an oscillation between the Arcadian and the Barbaric, in discussions of Aboriginal order and Aboriginal disorder, in illness and in therapy. The astute reader will also discover contradictions even where they are not identified; the nature of the discourses themselves are contradictory and the notion of Arcadian and Barbaric societies exists in a dialectical relationship. 'From a Barbaric perspective,' Lucas and Barrett (1995: 314) have written, 'the disintegrated and sick society, the violent savage and schizophrenic psychosis form a single constellation.' In contrast, 'From an Arcadian perspective, the harmonious and ordered society, the natural Primitive, and the creative ritual healer go together' (314). Exaggerating group differences becomes the norm; analysis creates widely distinct categories and cements them there.

The analysis is also influenced by 'constructivist' and 'critical-interpretive' frameworks in anthropology (Gaines 1992a, 1992b; Lock & Scheper-Hughes 1996; Greenfield 2000). As Clifford Geertz (1973: 9) once wrote, 'What we call our data are really our own constructions of other people's constructions of what they and their compatriots are up to.' According to Attwood Gaines, all medical knowledge, including psychiatric and so-called ethnopsychiatric knowledge, represents culturally constructed systems, characteristically imperfect and contradictory. Culture is something that is 'constructed through invention, borrowing and recombination,' something that is not necessarily 'homogeneous and integrated' (Gaines 1992b: 6). This includes the concept of the 'West' itself, a constructed cultural entity that is more appropriately thought of as a geographical, rather than cultural, referent. Lock and Scheper-Hughes (1996: 43), adding an element of subversiveness to the idea of constructivism, have argued that medical anthropology's task should be to examine 'the way in which all knowledge relating to the body, health, and illness is culturally constructed, negotiated, and renegotiated in a dynamic process through time and space.' The 'essentializing and universalizing Western epistemological assumptions underlying the theory and practice of biomedicine' are to be the targets of this critical-interpretive approach (43–4). Science is no longer a sacred cow, and, as Foucault's (1973) work has demonstrated, once exposed to critical insight the damage caused by its hegemony often becomes apparent. Gaines (1992b), for instance, has suggested that too much medical research has been based on the use of misleading and inappropriate categories of identity, and that the 'West,' 'Indian,' 'Black,' 'Christian,' 'Jew,' and so on are essentially meaningless concepts designed primarily to facilitate research. Fish (2000) has recently pointed out that since fields such as psychology employ the individual as the unit of analysis, aggregation becomes necessary to achieve large enough sample sizes for statistical purposes. This approach, conveniently ignoring the implications of creating and reifying ethnic or racial categories as meaningful cultural groups, emerges as seriously troubling in my analysis.

While Gaines's focus has been on the critique of psychiatric classification, my aim is much broader. I am more interested in the generation and definition of key concepts and methodologies; indeed, I expend considerable energy critically examining the methods employed in various studies. I also occasionally approach my subject like a literary archaeologist, peeling away discursive layer after discursive layer to get to the point where influential work was first formulated, to establish a genealogy of ideas, tracing their interconnectedness as they have passed from scholar to scholar and even from generation to generation. The portraits that emerge are disturbing – the house of cards analogy is appropriate – and ultimately brings me to question how comfortable we should be about what we think we know about Aboriginal peoples, how they think and perceive the world, their cognitive abilities and disabilities, their mental health and their mental illness.

Finally, I am also indebted to emerging notions of creolization as expressed by Gilles Bibeau (1997) and others (e.g., Kirmayer & Minas 2000). Bibeau argues that the idea of closed, well-bounded communities may well be an artifact of a culturally constructed scientific gaze, especially within anthropology, and that at any rate processes of globalization, which began some 500 years ago, have all but obliterated a conceptualization of cultures as internally homogeneous and existing apart from the influences of other cultures. Creolization challenges us to explore the construction of self and identity within the context of cultural heterogeneity, to locate the 'multiple realities' that comprise the experience of both individuals and cultures. 'Today, more than ever,' Bibeau (1997: 32) has written, 'heterogeneity seems to be built into culture itself and cultural experts must look for the interstices, paradoxes, ambiguities and inconsistencies which have become constitutive parts of meaning systems in most societies around the world.' But this should not be the project of only *prospective* inquiries. It is important that we comprehend how existing knowledge has been constructed upon the false assumptions of cultural homogeneity and isolation, and how these knowledge artifacts have become universal truths imbedded within scientific discourse. It is important that we ask where boundaries have been drawn and why, and then challenge these constructs to see if they withstand scrutiny.

Kirmayer, Brass, and Tait (2000: 613), in a review article on the mental health of Aboriginal peoples, have recently called upon scholars to undertake 'a cultural critique of psychiatry' as a necessary step in 'open[ing] up a space for creative formulations of theory and practice.' Work on this book commenced some time before their article was published, and my thinking on this very issue obviously predates it, but I am heartened by their call. What follows is, indeed, a cultural critique of psychiatry, but also of anthropology and psychology, and of the ways in which these disciplines have been and remain interrelated in the project of constructing *the* Aboriginal. I seek to uncover the connections among them, how they have informed each other, sometimes harmoniously, at other times acrimoniously, as well as the important ways in which they have ignored each other. What makes this book somewhat unique is that I examine how these disciplines have focused on a specific population, a sometimes mythical and constructed population to be sure, but one that is indeed reified, given life, through the discourse I wish to critique. This book aims to examine what we can learn about how mental order and disorder are conceptualized by concentrating on a set of societies which are seen as a more or less integrated or homogeneous whole for purposes of research and theorizing.

Plan of the Book

In planning this book, I have tried to provide an in-depth exploration of several central themes in the mental health literature, both generally and as they pertain to the Aboriginal population. Many themes overlap, making the organization of the book difficult. Studies of personality discuss psychopathology, studies of psychopathology refer to acculturative stress and alcoholism, studies of alcoholism invoke personality. Further, in each chapter I have tried to approach the topic at hand somewhat differently, to make different points about the totality of the Aboriginal mental health knowledge base. In order to avoid redundancy, after having made a specific point about conceptual or methodological issues, I do not continually revisit it in subsequent chapters. For instance, in chapter 3, I discuss the methodological problems involved in utilizing the culture area concept as a sampling frame, so I do not continue to raise this issue elsewhere in the text when discussing studies where culture areas were employed. And, where I discuss the problems of failing to adequately define the Aboriginal population under discussion, it should be considered a problem pertinent in other areas as well without me continually flagging it. The reader should simply accept that this same critique would apply.

The book is divided into three parts. Part A examines how *the* Aboriginal has been constructed over the past century, with an emphasis on essentialized notions of culture, mind, and personality. Chapter 2, 'Constructing the Aboriginal Personality,' opens with a discussion of the work of early-twentieth-century anthropologists such as Ruth Benedict and her contemporaries, who utilized American Indian populations as important sources of data to develop theories of the relationship between culture and personality. It continues with a detailed discussion of the University of Chicago's 'Indian Education Research Project,' which involved many renowned anthropologists and psychoanalysts in various ways. Chapter 3 looks in more detail at one outgrowth of this research, the emergence of the Rorschach test and its utilization with Aboriginal North American populations, and the notion that many societies were 'atomistic' and rife with suspicion and invidiousness. In chapter 4, I look at more recent developments in the measurement of Aboriginal culture, personality, and intelligence, with case studies of the Minnesota Multiphasic Personality Inventory (MMPI) and the Wechsler series of intelligence tests.

Part B examines the ways in which Aboriginal psychopathology has been conceptualized and measured and presents several case studies. In chapter 5 some of the early studies of psychopathology are discussed, and I examine the concept of acculturative stress and review recent epidemiological work. From here I present several chapters on specific issues: chapter 6 looks at alcohol; chapter 7 at depression and suicide; chapter 8 at the culture-bound syndromes, especially windigo psychosis, *pibloktoq* (Arctic hysteria), and ghost sickness; and chapter 9 at trauma and post-traumatic stress disorder.

Part C examines issues in psychotherapy and treatment and includes discussion of both conventional psychotherapeutic approaches and 'traditional' Aboriginal approaches. Chapter 10 looks at how the Aboriginal has been packaged for consumption by therapists in an effort to achieve 'cultural competence' and provide culturally appropriate care. I also examine several conventional approaches to the treatment of Aboriginal peoples, including directive versus non-directive therapy, family therapy and group therapy, all of which build upon stereotypical and essentialized portraits. Chapter 11 is a critical examination of 'traditional Aboriginal healing,' how the notions of 'tradition' and 'healing' have been constructed by both non-Aboriginal and Aboriginal peoples to provide an alternative to conventional treatment approaches. I also question the idea that Aboriginal peoples were/are 'holistic' in their thought regarding the supposed separation of mind and body.

As noted earlier, I have not attempted to survey the breadth of disorders contained within the DSM, or to address every issue relevant to a discussion of mind and mental health. Instead, I have chosen to review those issues I believe to be of particular contemporary relevance to Aboriginal mental health. Not everyone will agree with my selection, and readers will no doubt also note the absence of discussion on several other important topics, especially gender. In a great deal of the research I have examined, gender is either total disregarded or else appears as a variable alongside many others, and with little discussion. It would be redundant to continually point out that gender was not included in a particular analysis. Readers should consider the absence of gender to be a flaw in the research to date, parallel to the general absence of social class or socio-economic status issues.

Readers will also note that I have consistantly employed the past tense to discuss research literature in the book. In the course of my research I noticed the disturbing consequence of discussing scholarly work in the present tense, that is, the propensity for old ideas to appear contemporary. Research with Aboriginal peoples in the past is often treated as if it were still pertinent to the same peoples today, as if there has been no cultural change whatsoever. Many scholars simply ignore the temporal dimension when discussing the work of others. I will not contribute to this problem with my work here.

Terminology

In my research I restricted myself to the indigenous populations of Canada and the United States (excluding Hawaii), and when speaking generally about all of them, I use the term, 'Aboriginal.' From here it gets complicated, because various terms are used, and have been used over the years, on each side of the border. When I wish to refer to Aboriginal Canadians, I will use 'Aboriginal,' the term found in the Canadian constitution; when I refer to Aboriginal peoples in the United States, I use 'American Indian,' or simply 'Indian,' which represents both those peoples in the lower forty-eight states and the Natives of Alaska. This term is employed by several scholarly journals in the United States, although it seems to compete with the term 'Native American' for predominance. All of this being said, I revert to the term employed by specific authors when discussing their work, even where it breaks with these conventions. Further, when discussing more specific groups within these broad categories, I likewise use the terms employed by respective authors. These can vary according to author preference, region, which side of the international border they are on, historical factors, and community preference. In Canada, the Aboriginal population is frequently broken down into three subcategories: the federally recognized Indians, the Inuit, and the Métis. In the United States, there are the Indians, the Eskimo, and the Alaska Natives. Some authors will refer to the Chippewa, others to the Ojibwa or Ojibway, and others still to the Saulteaux or Anishinabe (with this latter term often spelled in different ways). Many Aboriginal groups have recently rejected European nomenclature and are returning to indigenous names. The application of various terms for aboriginality will be scrutinized in this work, and its problematic nature exposed. Similarly, the terms 'white' and 'white man' will also appear in the text, admittedly in an ambiguous way because of the dearth of attention paid to their definition. Readers should assume, at the first instance, that 'white' refers euphemistically to the European settler society in North America, with the proviso that ultimately I will offer some critical comment on the term and its operationalization. While my focus is on the Aboriginal peoples of Canada and the United States, the broader lessons learned here are probably applicable to our understanding of knowledge about other cultural groups.

About the Title

As I mentioned earlier, the windigo in Algonquian folklore is a cannibal monster who roams the northern forests, preying on unsuspecting passers-by. The folklore also suggests that a human being, under the right circumstances, can transform into a windigo and feast on his or her relatives. Early historic and ethnographic reports of windigo lead to another kind of transformation, the transformation of this folk belief into a bona fide mental disorder, windigo psychosis, considered by many to be a culture-bound syndrome. But no actual cases of windigo psychosis have ever been studied, and Lou Marano's scathing critique in 1985 should have killed off the cannibal monster within the psychiatric annals. The windigo, however, continues to seek revenge for this attempted scholarly execution by periodically duping unsuspecting passers-by, like psychiatrists, into believing that windigo psychosis not only exists, but that a psychiatrist could conceivably encounter a patient suffering from this disorder in his or her practice today! Windigo psychosis may well be the most perfect example of the construction of an Aboriginal mental disorder by the scholarly professions, and its persistence dramatically underscores how constructions of the Aboriginal by these professions have, like Frankenstein's monster, taken on a life of their own.

Conclusion

I have taken some inspiration from those within my field who have used varying perspectives to turn the lens on our own sense of truth, our own construction of knowledge. We have become far too comfortable within our scholarly skins, accepting too readily the knowledge passed on to us by previous scholars. From time to time it is necessary to look back and to rethink this progression of knowledge, to at least consider the possibility that there is a need for a critical rehashing of the paradigm, if not a paradigm shift. It is with this need in mind that I offer my analysis.

PART A

Constructing the
Aboriginal

Constructing Aboriginal Personality: The Early Years

Perhaps it is not too much to expect that a number of gifted psychiatrists may take up the serious study of exotic and primitive cultures in order to learn to understand more fully than we can out of the resources of our own cultures, the development of ideas and symbols and their relevance for the problem of personality. (Sapir 1932: 521)

One Hopi is a delightful friend; two are often a problem; and more than that number are frequently a headache. (Eggan 1943: 357)

Over the years, researchers have demonstrated a profound interest in understanding *the* Aboriginal, his/her personality and intellectual abilities. This interest was due in part simply to intellectual curiosity, and a great deal of the research sought to advance theoretical developments in the field of culture and personality, to understand how personality was shaped by culture in specific ecological contexts. But much research also had more pragmatic goals. At the beginning of the twentieth century there was a deep concern that Aboriginal peoples were on the road to extinction, if not in a biological sense then certainly in a cultural sense, and a major effort was launched to describe these disappearing cultures. Efforts designed to determine the intellectual abilities and deficits of Aboriginal peoples also emerged as part of an assimilative agenda, to allow for proper and more effective educational programs and testing as a means of dealing with the 'Indian problem,' the continued existence of a 'primitive' people in a modern world. The purpose of this chapter is to critically examine some of the pioneering research on the construction of the Aboriginal personality as a necessary precursor to my discussion of more contemporary studies. While the chapter will focus primarily on the work of several renowned anthropologists, psychologists, and psychiatrists in the 'Indian Education Research' project, I begin with an examination of the work of the 'Boasian' anthropologists, and in particular, that of one of the most influential scholars of Aboriginal personality, Ruth Benedict.

Ruth Benedict and the Boasian Tradition

The 'Americanist tradition' in anthropology is grounded in the pioneering work of Franz Boas in the late nineteenth century (Darnell 2001). Boas trained so many of the first generation of North American anthropologists that his influence on the field as a whole remained strong at least until after the Second World War (Darnell 2001) and, I would argue, well into the 1960s (if only as a point of contrast for newly developing ideas). His broad project was oriented towards the discrediting of scientific racism, including the increasingly influential evolutionist ideas of psychoanalyst Sigmund Freud (more on both of these topics later). But underlying this concern was a Rousseauian predilection to believe in the existence of the 'noble savage,' a framework that sought harmony in (some might say, superimposed harmony upon) the non-industrial peoples of the world (Lindholm 2001). Boas's legacy, in many ways, is based upon his emphasis on the collection of cultural materials from North American Aboriginal cultures that were perceived to be disappearing. This emphasis resulted in the generation of an enormous body of 'salvage' ethnographic data by Boas himself and by many of his students. Boas also influenced the development of a new paradigm of inquiry, historical particularism (Harris 1968). According to Fogelson (1999: 81), 'The dominant Boasian modus operandi favoured short-term fieldwork, collaboration with key elder informants, and the co-production of texts.' For Boas, a culture was largely a patchwork of traits diffused from elsewhere, and the goal of anthropology was to reconstruct the past of cultures which lacked written records by documenting and tracing the diffusion of traits from group to group (Barrett 1984; Darnell 2001). In many ways, it was under Boas's influence that anthropologists began to speak and write of 'cultures,' as specific, explicitly bounded entities, as opposed to 'culture' more generally (Kuper 1999). Culture was also largely a mental construct for Boas (Erickson & Murphy 1998), an early nod to what would much later become known as cognitive anthropology. Ruth

Benedict, Boas's star pupil, was among the first to speak of Aboriginal North American 'cultures,' eschewing Boas's patchwork notion of culture in favour of a 'configurationist' approach which saw the components of cultures as interdependent and integrated (Barrett 1984; Darnell 2001). In so doing, Benedict extended Boas's concern with the relationship between psychology and culture and pioneered research into the personality of Aboriginal North Americans.

Benedict remains one of the most influential of all American anthropologists, and her work on American Indian cultural patterns is classic. There is no need to rehash that work in general since, like that of Boas, it has been the subject of many works on the theory and history of anthropology. My concern here is with Benedict's conclusions regarding American Indian personality, and the basis on which she reached these conclusions.

Benedict was trained directly by Franz Boas at Columbia in the early 1920s, and, along with Margaret Mead, came to believe that entire cultures could be integrated around one or two salient psychological traits (Harris 1968; Kuper 1999). Cultures, like individuals, could have 'personalities,' or at least a modal personality which shaped the culture and psychological orientation of individuals. Her work was mostly synchronic, following Boas's lead, with little attention paid to cultural changes wrought by colonialism. Her three most influential publications relevant for my purposes were 'Psychological types in the cultures of the Southwest' (1928), 'Configurations of culture in North America' (1932), and *Patterns of Culture* (1934b). In these works she developed her now infamous schema in which societies were characterized as 'Apollonian' (the Pueblo Indians), 'Dionysian' (the Plains Indians), 'Paranoid' (Dobu Islanders, a non-American Indian group), or 'Megalomaniac' (Kwakiutl).[1]

The Apollonian Pueblo Indians, she argued, distrusted individualism and suppressed it in their societies. Individuals avoided overt leadership roles and the accumulation of personal wealth. The community as a whole, according to Benedict, provided both reinforcement and sanction through ceremonies and other group activities. Emotions were also suppressed, and the expression of violence was rare. 'The Zuni,' concluded Benedict, 'are a ceremonious people, a people who value sobriety and inoffensiveness above all other virtues' (1934b: 59). Alcohol problems and suicide, therefore, were said to be infrequent.

Benedict suggested that Apollonian societies were actually quite rare, and that 'the American Indians as a whole, and including those of

Mexico, were passionately Dionysian' (1934b: 80). In fact, rejecting the broadly anti-evolutionist ideas of historical particularism, Benedict employed cultural developmental discourse to argue that Dionysian behaviour was 'a permanent possibility in individual psychology' (233), perhaps a kind of primal savagery characteristic of 'natural man' that gained expression in some cultures and was suppressed in others because of specific historic events. The Plains Indians, according to Benedict, were 'Dionysians.' Intensely hedonistic, they were described as valuing 'all violent experience' and all opportunities to express their individuality and 'break through the usual sensory routine' (80). As a result, the Plains Indians were committed to obtaining supernatural power through dreams and vision quests, and were prepared to utilize fasting and 'hideous torture' to facilitate the experience (81). This intense, individual quest for alternative experiences was enhanced by the use of drugs and alcohol, before colonization, in the case of some of the southwestern groups, and after colonization throughout most of the North American plains.

Benedict intensified her discussion of the Dionysian by turning her attention to the Kwakiutl, described as manifesting an extreme form of the Dionysian characteristics which emphasized the individual over the collective. 'The object of all Kwakiutl enterprise was to show one-self superior to one's rival,' Benedict wrote. 'It found expression in uncensored self-glorification and ridicule of all comers' (1934b: 190). The practice of potlatching was seen as particularly and characteristically Dionysian. At these massive feasts, various chiefs and their people assembled to distribute, and in some cases destroy, valuable goods as a means of impressing guests and gaining prestige and titles. It was an intensely competitive system which gave the winners bragging rights as to their superiority. As Benedict wrote, 'Judged by the standards of other cultures the speeches of their chiefs at their potlatches are unabashed megalomania' (190). There were losers, of course, as much as there were winners, and losing brought shame. Hence suicide was common among the Kwakiutl, according to Benedict.

Benedict's research was clearly part of Boas's broader agenda to document the cultural traits of vanishing Aboriginal North American societies. But she also believed that the comparison of cultures was both valid and important (Barnard 2000). This led to an emphasis on cultural description and the detailing of traits, and in particular on patterns of trait diffusion (Bock 1988).

In order to properly appreciate Benedict's work, we need to examine the sources of her data as well as her scholarly influences. Perhaps surprisingly, much of the data on the American Indian examples employed in her book, *Patterns of Culture*, came from work done by others. Her discussion of the Pueblo Indians, a culturally diverse group, was focused mostly on Zuni, and in addition to some field research of her own, she relied on the work of several other anthropologists. Boas provided the data for her case study of the Kwakiutl. These two societies were selected precisely because, in Benedict's assessment, 'knowledge of these tribes is comparatively full and satisfactory' (1934: xi). Benedict also examined the available literature, engaged in discussions with the ethnographers, and ultimately had them examine her work to verify 'as to the facts' (xi). To provide a contrast, she also introduced a lengthy discussion of the Plains Indians as a composite, with no Plains society in particular as the focus, utilizing secondary, published, ethnographic material from other Boasians such as Clark Wissler, A.L. Kroeber, and Robert Lowie. She took these works further, however, and under the influence of gestalt psychology, endeavoured to provide 'a more just psychological understanding of the data' (Benedict 1923: 7).

Since the publication of *Patterns of Culture* Benedict's work has been criticized by many anthropologists. Marvin Harris (1968: 404), for instance, argued that her work could not be 'appreciated without reference to the dubious factual foundation on which Benedict reared her psychologistic portraits.' Both Harris and Victor Barnouw (1973) in effect argued that 'Benedict's sketch of the Apollonian way of life achieved its beautiful symmetry only as a result of the omission or selective de-emphasis of nonconforming data' (Harris 1968: 405). In particular, it was suggested that Benedict ignored reports of alcohol abuse and violence at Zuni, as well as factional strife. Both Matilda Coxe Stevenson (1904) and Ruth Bunzel (1933), whose work Benedict used, had observed prevalent drinking in Zuni, and Elsie Clews Parsons (1917), another source, had described certain Zuni curing ceremonies in terms that were considerably more Dionysian than Apollonian (Barnouw 1973: 99, 101). Bunzel also documented that Zuni was actually in the throes of a major factional upheaval at the very time she and Benedict were conducting their research there in the-mid 1920s (Barnouw 1973: 101). Yet Zuni was described by Benedict as peaceful and harmonious. The ethnographic work of Stevenson, Parsons, and Bunzel on which Benedict drew, moreover, cannot itself be characterized as strong. Stevenson, for instance, worked in Zuni for only six months and, by her own admission, provided a 'restricted account' of Zuni culture (Stevenson 1904: 18), while Parsons (1917) described ceremonies and other activities that she herself did not witness.

Benedict's description of the Kwakiutl is equally problematic. Benedict did not undertake field research among them, basing her analyses entirely on the work of her mentor, Franz Boas, and selective presentation of ethnographic data is again evident. Barnouw (1973: 103–4) noted that Benedict's description of the activities of the 'Cannibal Society,' including cannibalism itself as well as other vigorous and 'wild' activities, ignored the fact that most of this behaviour was performed ceremonially and with sleight-of-hand as part of planned, organized activities and was not, therefore, the impulsive expression of frenzied participants. Furthermore, as Rohner (1969) has so vividly demonstrated, Boas's significant research was not without its own contradictions and flaws. For instance, despite his assertions that good ethnography required the use of many informants and the learning of the indigenous language, Boas worked with only a small handful of Kwakiutl and never learned that language. Similarly, rather than spending intense periods of time in single communities, as he advocated was necessary to truly learn a culture, Boas travelled frequently from village to village, often remaining for only very short periods of time (in fact, relatively short fieldwork periods came to characterize Boasian research; Murray 1999). Most of his research was undertaken during the summer when many men and women were away from the villages fishing. Boas rarely even lived in the Kwakiutl villages, preferring rental lodging in nearby non-Indian towns.

Essentially, then, a critical examination of Ruth Benedict's formulation of American Indian societies, an early exercise in culture-and-personality, demonstrates it was fundamentally flawed. The dubious quality of her data was combined with the selective presentation of data that fit her theoretical analysis and a reluctance to view Aboriginal culture within the context of the historical processes of colonization – a problem common to the broader historical particularist school. The facts, even as she understood them at the time, did not interfere with the development of broad, sweeping generalizations regarding the essential character of Aboriginal North American societies and the personalities of their members. The existence of intracultural variability, theoretically a possibility within her configurationist approach, all but disappeared in practice in her work, possibly because she had been influenced by psychoanalyst Carl Jung's notion of 'archetypes' (Lindholm 2001). Nevertheless, *Patterns of Culture* was destined to become a classic in anthropology, and it is still read in classrooms all over the continent. Marvin Harris (1968) was brought to conclude that one criticizes *Patterns of Culture* at one's peril.

The Emergence of Psychoanalytical Anthropology and the Search for the Indians' 'Basic Personality Structure'

For North American anthropology, the first half of the twentieth century was dominated by theoretical and methodological developments related to the relationship between culture and personality. North American Aboriginal societies were frequently the testing ground for these new ideas and, as importantly, for new, experimental partnerships among anthropologists, psychologists, and psychiatrists. While Ruth Benedict pioneered the way, many of her contemporaries were eager to join in. These were exciting times!

The roots of this emerging psychological anthropology are found in the ideas of psychoanalyst Sigmund Freud. Freud's evolutionary ideas, in which he saw intellectual parallels between 'primitive' peoples, children, and mentally unstable Westerners, ideas with broader Victorian roots, became pervasive, and his influential book, *Totem and Taboo: Resemblances between the Psychic Lives of Savages and Neurotics* (1950) was widely read by anthropologists of the time. His emphasis on the importance of early childhood experiences as the foundation upon which personality was laid proved to be particularly resonant with anthropologists, even where some of his other ideas were rejected. Broadly speaking, psychoanalytical anthropologists conceived of cultures as consisting of conflicting interests that required mediation, an obvious reflection of Freud's notion that the mind itself was the site of a constant struggle between the unconscious and unruly 'id' and the sensitive, anxious, and weak 'ego,' mediated by the 'superego,' that aspect of the mind that sought to impose social values. But it was the 'neo-Freudians,' especially Abram Kardiner, who developed these ideas further and came to influence more directly many of the leading anthropological scholars of this era (W.C. Manson 1988).

Kardiner, a psychoanalyst who had studied with Freud, had reservations about the extent to which Freud's theories were applicable across cultures (Erickson & Murphy 1998) and argued instead that different cultural experiences led to somewhat different personality types. Along with anthropologist Ralph Linton, Kardiner developed the idea of 'basic personality structure.' According to this 'psychodynamic' formulation, all members of a given society were assumed to share certain early childhood experiences (primary institutions), which in turn generated and maintained a basic personality. This basic personality in turn influenced, shaped, and maintained other aspects of the society, such as religious systems (secondary institutions). According to Kardiner and Linton, basic personality structure was shaped by primary institutions but then projected onto secondary institutions (Erickson & Murphy 1998; Bock 1999: 69; see also Kardiner & Linton 1939). Culture was integrated because of these shared, early experiences.

Like Benedict, Kardiner had studied anthropology with Franz Boas at Columbia, and beginning in 1933 he organized a seminar series at the New York Psychoanalytical Institute, and later at Columbia, that brought together many influential Boasians, such as Ralph Linton and Ruth Benedict. The seminars developed a well-defined modus operandi which saw ethnographers present more-or-less raw data to the group, followed by Kardiner's psychoanalytical interpretations. The series thus fostered the idea of collaboration between psychoanalysts and anthropologists, as well as the importance of 'blind' analysis of materials, in which psychoanalysts were asked to interpret data without benefit of the knowledge of the societies under consideration. Projective tests to measure personality, and especially the Rorschach, became centrally important, as did the generation of life history materials. Kardiner and his associates were well aware that there were significant gaps in the ethnographic materials they worked with, which had characteristically been gathered by anthropologists without reference to psychoanalytic frameworks (Harris 1968). Interestingly, a debate emerged in this dialogue regarding the applicability of the basic personality approach to 'Western society.' Contrasting Western society with that of 'primitive' peoples, Kardiner wrote, '"Western" society is not a single culture but a conglomeration of cultures in which the socioeconomic order has gone through a host of viscissitudes' (1945: 121). The assumption of the homogeneity of the 'primitive' cultures, however, was firmly embedded in the psychoanalytical approach from the beginning (Littlewood 2000), and Aboriginal North American cultures provided much of the raw data that fuelled the discussions.

Kardiner took issue with Benedict's characterizations of the Zuni and Pueblo Indians, describing them as too vague and even inaccurate, but not necessarily with the overall personality portraits she had painted. Freudian influences were clear in his work. The inherently peaceful existence of the Zuni, for instance, was not challenged, but

Kardiner and Linton argued that this was due to 'the formation of a powerful in-group' resulting from a strong dependence on the mother, combined with fears of mother desertion, and to the lack of sibling rivalry (Kardiner & Linton 1939: 116). The Kwakiutl were aggressive and sought to humiliate each other because of individual frustrations caused by a strict social hierarchy. The intense initiation of the Canni-bal society was interpreted by Kardiner as the product of the acting-out of Oedipal fantasies and sibling rivalries (Bock 1999: 71).

Culture-and-personality studies inevitably came under attack by the 1950s (Spindler 1978: 20), and by the 1960s few anthropologists were interested in psychoanalytical theory (W.C. Manson 1988: xiv; Marsella, Dubanoski, Hamada, & Morse 2000). Even the expression 'culture and personality' started to disappear, and became the object of considerable derision (Lindholm 2001). Key debates focused on the trait list approach to personality, which was built upon ethnocentric Western assumptions of individualism and which had led to the use of reductionist and frac-tured instruments designed to measure personality. Psychoanalysis as a theoretical paradigm also proved immune to adequate operationaliza-tion when applied to the problems of culture and personality. As Harris (1968: 448) noted somewhat sarcastically, 'what the great figures in the formative phases of the culture and personality movement were asking us to do was to trust them as we would trust an analyst, not for the dem-onstrated truth of any particular item, but for the accumulating evi-dence of coherence in a believable pattern.' Nevertheless, by the time the psychoanalytical approach fell into disfavour a considerable body of ethnographic work had been done, some of it considered classic anthro-pological literature, which established the personality baseline and notions of normality and abnormality for *the* Aboriginal American. The Indian Education Research project demonstrates the interdisciplinary influences that were brought to bear on the 'Indian problem' perhaps better than most.

The Indian Education Research Project

One of the first, and certainly most documented, examples of the use of psychological research for applied purposes was the 'Indian Education and Administration Research' project (also referred to as the 'Indian Personality and Administration Research' project), initiated in 1941. By this time, a new interest in acculturation had emerged within anthro-pology, best seen in the seminal formulation, 'Memorandum for the

Study of Acculturation' published in 1936 by anthropologists Robert Redfield, Ralph Linton, and Melville Herscovits. The concern with understanding the way in which cultures changed as a result of continuous, first-hand contact represented something of a break with the Boasian past and its preoccupation with reconstructing culture history, yet many of the emerging acculturationists were Boasians to varying degrees, and the Boasian emphasis on detailing traits and searching for patterns of diffusion was retained.[2]

Spearheaded by the Commissioner of Indian Affairs, John Collier, the Indian Education Research Project was a massive examination of five different Indian tribes that set the tone for subsequent inquiries that focused on the psychological consequences of acculturation for American Indians. Adopting the neo-Freudian view that personality and values were formed in early childhood, the ultimate goal of the research was to comprehend American Indian personality in a way that would assist government administrators in designing programs to more effectively guide their charges into the modern world.

Collier was a sociologist by training, and a firm believer in the importance of using social science research to aid in the understanding and resolution of contemporary social issues and problems. Assuming the position of commissioner in 1933, he set in motion sweeping policy changes to reverse earlier, damaging government policies that had as their goal the assimilation of the American Indian population. The Indian Reorganization Act, introduced to Congress in 1934, was the platform upon which Collier would build. The general intent of the Act was the preservation of American Indian societies as distinct cultural and social entities, and the problems of the present and future were seen as resolvable only through the mechanisms of the cultures themselves (Collier 1945).

Collier viewed the various American Indian tribes as an 'ethnic laboratory' for the development and humane application of social science principles, theories, and methods (Collier 1945: 296). He lamented that anthropology in particular had had little input into understanding 'the practical and governmental problems concerning the Indian' (272–3). These problems he described in a manner which seemed to anticipate ideas of primitivism and post-colonialism. He wrote: 'The Indian race, in any meaningful sense (since, as the Indian himself shows, biological race has little practical or heuristic significance), is a projection by the white man, the Indian's persecutor. It is a mental projection which as the generations passed brought into being actualities of inferior status, of poverty, of excessive introversion and loss of hope and loss of the will to live ...' (266). Perhaps significantly, Collier viewed these problems not as the product of inherent deficiencies among the American Indians, but rather as that of incompetent government policy guiding the peoples through the myriad social and cultural changes resulting from contact.

With the support of American Indian ethnologist/historian D'Arcy McNickle, an employee of the Indian Service, the research that would be organized under Collier's administration had a breathtakingly massive goal: 'to attempt to evaluate scientifically, if possible, policy and practice in the United States Indian Bureau' (Collier & Thompson 1946: 141). Anthropologist Clyde Kluckhohn (1943: 213) wrote with reference to this period of Indian policy development, 'In no field of administration has anthropology's master concept, culture, been so basic to planning and to action.' The more immediate problem to be addressed, however, was one of education. Collier wanted 'a realistic and radical reexamination both of the aims and of methods in Indian schooling and Indian administration' (1945: 294–5). Psychological analysis was central to this re-examination. Project Director Laura Thompson, of the University of Chicago (1951: 12), acknowledging that much was known about the 'economic status of the Indians, their natural resources, standards of living, [and] general health and schooling,' questioned 'what was happening to their personalities under the impact of modern American civilization?' The task at hand was clear: 'If we could discover, by means of the methods of science, how recent changes were affecting the Indian psychologically, in social and natural context, we would, it was hoped, be able to define his real needs and resources more precisely and help him more effectively to make a creative adjustment in the modern world' (12).

The work would proceed in two phases. The first was to focus on educational issues and was based on extensive data gathered in various communities (the 'Indian Education Research' project, sometimes referred to as the 'Indian Personality Research' project); the second phase would interpret the results of that research for use by administrators (the 'Indian Administration Research' project). Taken together, these two phases represented a new scholarly agenda focusing on research for practical purposes that became known as 'action research' (L. Thompson 1950: 5). In order to undertake this work, Collier recognized the need to bring on board research expertise.

The University of Chicago's Committee on Human Development,

and later the nascent Society for Applied Anthropology, ultimately assumed responsibility for the research. Their approach was explicitly interdisciplinary: researchers trained in anthropology, sociology, psychology, psychiatry, human geography, and history were to be involved. An examination of the project staff indicates the extent to which the brightest and best were assembled as part of this experiment. Anthropologists involved in capacities ranging from consultants to field researchers included such influential Americanists as Conrad Arensberg, Ruth Benedict, Fred Eggan, A. Irving Hallowell, Solon T. Kimball, Clyde Kluckhohn, Margaret Mead, Morris Opler, Omer C. Stewart, Edward H. Spicer, Ruth Underhill, Evan Vogt, and W. Lloyd Warner. Psychologists, psychiatrists, and psychoanalysts involved included Grace Arthur, Erik Erikson, Robert Havighurst, William Henry, Bert Kaplan, Bruno Klopfer, Alexander Leighton, and Dorothea Leighton.[3] Local administrators and other individuals, such as teachers and health staff, also became involved in executing some of the research. Under Thompson's direction, over a period of six years research was undertaken in eleven communities affiliated with five distinct Indian tribes, and over a thousand children were studied (L. Thompson 1951: xvi). The selection of the tribes to be studied were guided by several criteria, which included the following: the tribes had to be representative of Indian Service problems and have a government staff deemed sympathetic to the *project*; they had to represent culturally different and distinct American Indian societies; and there had to be an extensive, pre-existing body of ethnographic and other information on them. The six tribes eventually selected were the Hopi, Navaho, Papago, Sioux, Zia, and Zuni. An extensive publication record ultimately resulted from these studies, and some of the monographs became cornerstones of North American ethnology courses, if not classics.[4] An explosion in social science reporting on American Indians erupted at mid-century, and central to this explosion were characterizations of personality, ability, and psychopathology.

The 'Battery of Tests'

The interdisciplinary approach embraced by the Indian Education Research Project involved some fifty different scientists, some employed in the field and others analysing data in Chicago. By the 1940s, the culture and personality school had rejected the ill-defined conceptual and methodological approach characteristic of the early psychoanalytic anthropologists and begun to adopt more complex approaches involving standardized psychological tests, some new and others more seasoned (Harris 1968). A 'battery of psychological tests' was employed in the project, including the Rorschach, the Thematic Apperception Test (TAT), the Grace Arthur Point Performance Scale, the Emotional Response Test, the Moral Ideology Test, the Free Drawing Test, and the Goodenough Draw-A-Man Test (L. Thompson & Joseph 1965). The cross-cultural applicability of these tests was still an unresolved issue, and a brief overview of the key tests is in order.

Perhaps the best-known test is the Rorschach Psychodiagnostic (Ink-blot) Test, designed to provide a description of the basic personality of the respondent. The instrument was developed and first published in Switzerland by psychiatrist Hermann Rorschach in 1921. It was not specifically developed for use in cross-cultural circumstances, but one of its leading proponents, Bert Kaplan (1954: 3), argued that it was probably more 'culture-free' than other techniques employed in personality studies. At least five different approaches were developed in the United States in the 1940s and 1950s (Butcher, Nezami, & Exner 1998: 68);[5] one of these was by Bruno Klopfer, and it was Klopfer's approach that was employed in the Indian Education Research project. In fact, many of the researchers employed to administer and analyse the Rorschach were trained by Klopfer at his Rorschach Institute, and Klopfer himself served as an advisor to the research.

The Rorschach test consists of a series of ten symmetrical ink blots which are shown to the respondent, who is then asked to relate what he or she sees in the image. The responses are recorded and later scored following a fairly complex manual which, among other things, examines for the use of partial versus whole elements of the image, and whether the perception is of the black blot itself or the white background. The ink blots were considered to be random and inherently meaningless, and hence not bound by any specific cultural interpretation. They could be scored without direct reference to the culture in question, although interpretation of the scores was clearly, in my view, a cultural act. According to Laura Thompson and Alice Joseph (1965: 92), 'The test gives a complex picture of the basic personality, and includes information about mental capacities and efficiency, emotional attitudes and drives, the balance of the personality and the defense mechanism adopted against outside pressure or inner conflicts.'

The Thematic Apperception Test was developed in the 1930s by Henry Murray at Harvard University and, like the Rorschach, was a popular instrument among psychological anthropologists of the day (Bock 1988: 72). A set of cards displaying various human figures was shown to the respondent, who was asked to tell a story about what was happening in each scenario. Verbatim responses were recorded. Thompson and Joseph (1965: 92) noted, 'It is assumed that the child projects more or less of his conscious and subconscious emotions, attitudes and experiences into his stories.' The TAT would elicit data on both 'overt levels of personality' and the more 'covert' levels, 'to reveal what the subject cannot or will not say about himself' (Henry 1947: 521). The test was designed for middle-class Americans, but researchers were interested in expanding its usefulness in other societies. William Henry, a member of the Committee on Human Development, had a particular interest in testing the TAT cross-culturally, and saw the Indian Education Research project as a prime opportunity to do so. He was particularly involved in the research with the Hopi and Navajo, which employed a series of twelve line drawings designed for the study by an Indian artist. These were not simply 'Indianized' versions of standard TAT drawings, however. While two were adaptations drawn from the generic set of the Harvard Psychological Clinic, according to Henry (1947: 12) the remaining ten 'were devised to represent situations presumed to be common to the experience of every Indian child. They were all drawn using Indian clothes and surroundings.'

The TAT tests were administered by Alice Joseph for the Hopi (102 tests), and psychiatrist Dorothea Leighton for the Navajo (104 tests). Analysis, however, was done in Chicago. The TAT analyses were then presented blind to a large group of participating scientists and staff in the Indian Education Research program. Each TAT analysis was followed by the analysis of the same case using another source of data, such as the Rorschach and the Free Drawings. The purpose of this approach was to test the TAT against other tests, tests that had been predetermined to provide accurate representations of individuals. This approach lead to conclusions as to the 'correctness' of the TAT interpretation. While Henry concluded that the experiment demonstrated the usefulness of the TAT for other societies, he was nevertheless frustrated by the incongruence in language and framework brought to the conference table by the disparate group of scientists, and, inspired by colleagues Erich Fromm and Bruno Klopfer, set about formulating 'a single frame of reference' to be used by all (Henry 1947: 25).

Attempts to measure intelligence were made utilizing the Grace Arthur and Goodenough Draw-A-Man tests. The researchers acknowledged that intelligence tests in general were designed for 'white' children, and American Indian children could not be expected to perform as well (Leighton & Kluckhohn 1969: 148). It was believed that these two particular tests, less dependent on verbal capabilities, would not handicap the children. But results of the Navajo study were not entirely optimistic: Leighton and Kluckhohn concluded that the tests failed to measure 'native intelligence,' that success was too dependent on school education, and that neither test gave 'a final and convincing evaluation of "intelligence" in all cases' (1969: 155). Nevertheless, there was a clear indication that the University of Chicago team was particularly interested in developing and refining cross-cultural techniques, and that the opportunity afforded to them by John Collier presented an excellent laboratory to test out their ideas.

Testing the Hopi

Anthropologist Laura Thompson, as project director, was the central figure in all of the research undertaken in the Indian Education project and author of the final report (Thompson 1951). Her work with the Hopi was the most sophisticated of the research done and nicely serves as a state-of-the-art example of the work undertaken across the various tribes.

In a broad sense, American Indians were seen as experiencing a 'crisis,' an ill-defined diagnosis in most of the studies of the project. Thompson presented the most elaborate explanation of the crisis: the Hopi had developed a culture which existed in a delicate balance with the human and natural environment, a culture which was capable of providing the Hopi with all the psychological and social comforts needed, but which was now experiencing disruptions due to cultural encroachment and acculturative pressures. How was the Hopi personality, developed within the context of a highly rigid, structured and isolationist society, changing as a result of external social and cultural pressures, and what were the consequences of cultural and personality changes for the future viability of the Hopi people? More specifically, how could the Indian administration help the Hopi adjust while maintaining their essential, internal cultural integrity (Thompson 1950)?

Field research was undertaken in 1942 and 1943 in two Hopi communities, Walpi (First Mesa) and Oraibi. Like many of the studies in the Indian Education Research project, the focus was on children, and 190 aged six to eighteen were involved (81 from First Mesa, and 109 from

Oraibi). The sum of the results of the psychological tests was a portrait of Hopi 'personality-in-environment,' one which combined elements of ecological theory with neo-Freudian concern for the developmental stages of early childhood. The Hopi were described as a people who had survived in 'a difficult and uncertain environment,' who had maintained 'a delicate and balanced adjustment between the group and the environment,' and who, for defensive purposes, had 'crowded on Mesas' (Thompson & Joseph 1965: 128). Hopi personality must be understood within this context. Yet the overall picture of the Hopi was flattering. Regardless of the question of whether or not the tests used were appropriate for cross-cultural investigation, the Hopi emerged from the analysis as highly intelligent and complex personalities.[6] Based on the Grace Arthur, Goodenough, Rorschach, and Thematic Apperception tests, it was concluded that 'Hopi children, in contrast to all the other tribes investigated and also to most white children, are on the average very intelligent, highly observant, and capable of complex abstract thinking' (Thompson 1950: 92). The Rorschach and TAT results suggested that the 'Hopi as individuals and as a group tend to approach problems as complex, organized wholes within the various component parts in relationship' (1950: 91).

Specifically on the issue of personality, the Hopi were described as '*unusually* complex,' an observation that no doubt betrayed an underlying assumption of primitive simplicity (Thompson 1950: 95; emphasis added). They were 'deeply disciplined' and 'disinclined towards emotional outbreaks,' 'generally cautious,' and generally 'well behaved' (Thompson & Joseph 1965: 109). In a word, the Hopi appeared stoic. This was interpreted as the 'price of peace' paid by the Hopi in return for a stable, safe life, but it was a price 'paid at the level of individual personality in a certain repression of spontaneity and a tendency toward rigidity, which in some individuals may become even somewhat obsessive, and also in the generation of a certain amount of hostility which finds expression in gossip, jealousy and accusations of witchcraft' (Thompson & Joseph 1965: 133). In summarizing Hopi personality, Thompson (1950: 119) wrote that 'Analysis of the psychological findings in context suggest that Hopi personality tends to be characterized by a subtly balanced complexity within definite boundaries; an emotional, social and esthetic maturity within allowed areas; a many-sided and deep-rooted control system; a high, puzzle-solving type of intelligence; and an abstract, as well as practical, mental approach.'

All was not perfect, however. The Hopi were described as experiencing a high degree of anxiety of a vague nature, unattached to specific objects of fear (Thompson & Joseph 1965: 110). One exception to this was the anxiety caused by the 'use of malicious gossip' and accusations of witchcraft, but this did not readily lead to paranoia (120). Furthermore, a specific group was singled out as potentially problematic: young males at Oraibi. Thompson (1950) noted that they showed 'a definite trend toward personality disturbance which, if revealed among the Euro-American children, would indicate a trend toward compulsion neurosis' (97). This was due to 'an imbalance in the social system related to a breakdown in the social-ceremonial organization' caused by cultural changes in Mennonite-dominated areas, and it was concluded that this problem was likely to spread to other, more traditional areas over time (Thompson 1950: 119–20).

Keeping in mind that the ultimate goals of the research project were practical, from an administrative perspective, what solutions to the Hopi 'crisis' emanated from this analysis of their personality and intelligence? In general, administrators were again reminded of the high Hopi intelligence and capacity for abstract thought. 'In dealing with the Hopi,' wrote Thompson and Joseph (1965: 101), 'it would indeed be a grave mistake to adopt the baby-talk and the oversimplified methods which are often used toward half-witted persons and those who go under the collective name of "natives".' In the area of education, it was stressed that ' the Hopi 'maturation curve' rather than white developmental norms' should be employed (Thompson 1946: 184). The influence of John Collier was clear in some of the broader recommendations. Thompson (1950: 186) asserted that the retention of Hopi culture, especially the 'indigenous belief system,' was essential to their adjustment to the rapid changes that were occurring around them. 'Personality disorders and social breakdown characterize Hopi communities that have lost their values and their ceremonies,' she noted (Thompson 1946: 210). But the Hopi could not live in isolation; they had to change, and in a way that avoided 'crystallizing or taking refuge in tradition' (Thompson 1950: 187).

The administrator had an important role to play in helping the Hopi maintain their cultural integrity while undergoing the necessary change. Thompson in effect argued for the deliberate manipulation of Hopi leadership to ensure that leaders were put in place who were open to change, especially change influenced by the broader American society (Thompson 1946: 210–12). Coercion was to be avoided, and the enlistment of support from the Hopi was essential. The most successful approach would be change *through* Hopi culture rather than in spite of it.

While effectively essentializing Hopi culture and personality based primarily on psychological studies of children, Thompson and her colleagues approached their subject with caution, even trepidation. They noted, 'we are aware of the dangers of over-simplification, misrepresentation and omission ... We consider the results to be exploratory rather than definitive' (Thompson & Joseph 1965: 14). Despite offering the work 'humbly,' the Indian Education Research project was still about assisting administrators to guide American Indian cultural change, and the recommendations made to administrators, perhaps not surprisingly, appeared not so humble. As John Collier wrote in the forward to *The Hopi Way*, this was an exercise in 'scientific planning' (Thompson & Joseph 1965: 8), and humility was not a characteristic feature of the social sciences of this era.

The Role of Ethnography

Abram Kardiner's psychodynamic approach to research was predicated on the collection of different, largely independent data sets pertaining to primary and secondary institutions as well as basic personality structure. It was the psychiatrists' job to analyse the personality data, but they were not equipped to gather and analyse the cultural data on these various institutions. For this reason, ethnography was central to the interpretation of the psychological data collected from the Indian Education Research project. Indeed, as noted earlier, one of the criteria for selecting the cultures and communities to be involved was the existence of a substantial body of ethnographic data. It is clear that this knowledge served both to orient the researchers and to 'validate' the interpretations derived from the psychological tests. Henry (1947: 97), for instance, who had no first-hand knowledge of American Indian societies, had his TAT interpretations reviewed by anthropologists Clyde Kluckhohn, W. Lloyd Warner, and Alfred Whiting, and noted that 'they expressed a high degree of confidence' in his analysis based on 'the extent to which the details of the report check with anthropological field data' (101). Ethnographic data were also used to place the research data in context. A problem with this approach was evident in the case of the Zuni study, where the inability to find an ethnographer knowledgeable of the people delayed publication of the monograph until some twenty years after the research had been done. Ultimately, anthropologist John Adair was brought on board to 'provide the kind of tribal description that would be helpful in understanding the implications of the research findings' (Leighton & Adair 1966: v), even though his work at Zuni was undertaken some years after the Indian Education Research project and primarily involved returning war veterans. Adair did not study children, but gained access to notes taken during earlier research on child behaviour at Zuni by anthropologist Omer C. Stewart, and combined these with data from published sources and various Zuni experts (v–vi).

It seemed quite logical, and compatible with the scientific method employed by these researchers, to utilize existing knowledge in their studies. The central question, however, pertains to the extent to which the interpretations of the psychological tests were influenced by this existing knowledge. The Papago study demonstrates the way in which the ethnographic data were employed in the analysis: 'Information and observations regarding social background, life-history, and overt behavior obtained from various sources were compiled by one of the anthropologists on staff. The results of each test were scored, analyzed, and interpreted independently by other members of the research staff. In a general meeting this work was compared, discussed, and integrated' (Joseph, Spicer, & Chesky 1949: 246). Leighton and Kluckhohn (1969: 227), in the Navaho study, were even more blunt about the importance of ethnographic data. They argued that these data were integral to 'success' in analysing the psychological data, adding that had the tests been interpreted 'entirely blind, the conclusions might have been markedly skewed.' The psychological tests, 'in their present state of imperfection ... cannot be trusted implicitly to give the information desired but must be checked against, and used in conjunction with, material obtained by the time-honoured methods of observation and interview.' If, as was suggested, ethnographic data gathered prior to the testing was in fact crucial to test interpretation, then we might have a house of cards, with interpretations only as valid as the data that inform them. Here it becomes pertinent to examine the Sioux study by Macgregor.

Gordon Macgregor's (1946) monograph, *Warriors without Weapons*, was an examination of the Sioux of the Pine Ridge agency in South Dakota. Some 200 children, aged six to eighteen, were involved. Bruno Klopfer acted as a consultant, Royal Hassrick, an anthropologist at the University of Pennsylvania, conducted the Rorschach tests, and William Henry analysed the TATs. However, as in the other studies, Macgregor was heavily dependent on existing ethnographic data, in this case the work of Scudder Mekeel and Erik Erikson. Macgregor saw the Sioux personality as reflecting the disorganizing effects of the early reservation years, especially the deterioration of social institutions. The 'modern Indian way of life is one of emptiness' (121), he wrote, which caused great insecurity among these peoples and forced the individual to 'withdraw into himself and cover up his feelings,' that is, to invoke his 'stoical reserve' (153). While IQ tests demonstrated that the Sioux children scored slightly higher than 'white' children, deteriorating cultural conditions had led to anxiety and withdrawal, living under 'constant repression of their energy' (204). In adults, however, this repression occasionally led to violent outbursts, often the result of alcohol consumption. Macgregor argued that the Sioux were traditionally a society characterized by high levels of aggression that was channelled into culturally appropriate release mechanisms, such as war with other groups. The changes wrought by the implementation of the reservation system forced the men, in particular, to suppress these 'aggressive drives' (154), with only partial success. 'Psychologically defeated,' according to Macgregor, they turned upon each other and themselves in fits of violence and suicide. He noted the particularly negative consequences of increasing male aggression towards females. They were 'warriors without weapons.' Government programs, he argued, should target the men, as they 'were the keystone in the formal social structure, and the culture was organized around their careers and achievements' (212).

Macgregor noted that he 'borrowed heavily' from the studies of the Pine Ridge Dakota undertaken by anthropologist Scudder Mekeel and psychoanalyst Erik Erikson. Mekeel had an interest in both American Indian history and contemporary issues. Under John Collier's administration, Mekeel served several years as director of the Applied Anthropology Unit in the Indian Affairs office. In a critical review of Mekeel's ethnography, anthropologist Thomas Biolsi (1997) painted an unflattering portrait of a young graduate student from a privileged background (his graduate work was at Yale) encountering American Indians for the first time at Pine Ridge in 1930. The young Mekeel, according to Biolsi (1997: 135), had been trained in an anthropological tradition that led him on an intellectual search for the 'primitive.' Utilizing the paradigm of 'integrationist' cultural relativism, which presumed 'autonomous, discrete, and internally integrated primitive cultures' (137), and having trained under Edward Sapir, who believed in the idea of 'genuine' and 'spurious culture' (Sapir 1924), Mekeel was dismayed by the large number of Oglala people who were, in his estimation, 'in-between' American Indian and American cultures, and hence 'loafers, criminals, [and] delinquents' (134). In other words, they were not authentic Sioux and therefore, in Biolsi's interpretation, 'anthropological non-data' (139). Mekeel actively sought out that minority of Oglala individuals who fit his preconceived notion of authenticity. The concept of acculturation as a paradigm through which to study changing cultures was just emerging, and Mekeel represented the anthropological norm of the day in judging 'mixed cultures,' those undergoing change as a result of culture contact, as inauthentic (143). 'What interested the relativist on contemporary reservations was *survivals*,' noted Biolsi (143), 'not contemporary changes or transformed organization' [italics original]. Mekeel actively constructed Lakota culture, and then acted as tour guide for Erik Erikson and, ultimately, as an ethnographic authority shaping the ideas of Gordon Macgregor (who published Mekeel's obituary in 1948 in the *American Anthropologist*).

Erikson, who had studied with Anna Freud at the Vienna Psychoanalytic Institute, was taken into Sioux country in 1937 by Mekeel and Alfred Kroeber, although Mekeel was clearly his main guide. Mekeel, according to Erikson (1963: 113), 'took me to his favorite and best-trained informants in the field and urged them to talk to me as they would have talked to him.' His work with the Sioux was brief, nothing in comparison to the year-long study undertaken by Macgregor, and appears to have been somewhat of a guided tour by Mekeel.[7] Primarily interested in child development, Erikson's perspective on personality differed somewhat from Kardiner's notion of basic personality type. Erikson believed that while culture essentially moulded personality, there was no singular personality type characteristic of a culture. The child actively integrated the values, attitudes, and cognitive orientations of his or her culture in the process of building personality: culture provided the materials, but the individual undertook the construction (Kracke 1987). Utilizing both his own data from interviews and notes provided to him by Mekeel and Kroeber, Erikson painted a Freudian portrait of a classically 'primitive' people, whose cultures and personalities were shaped by primal needs and childhood experiences. His primitivist perspective, clearly influenced by Mekeel, was never more clear than when he described the 'old Dakotas' as the 'embodiment of the "real Indian" – a warring and hunting man, endowed with fortitude, cunning, and cruelty' (Erikson 1963: 115). His Freudian interpretation of the Sun Dance was equally primitivist, focusing (as have most non-American Indians) on the self-torture involving wooden skewers puncturing the chest. 'This ritual,' he opined, 'may be a symbolic restitution necessitated by a critical experience which once upon a time caused an intense conflict between his rage against the frustrating mother – and that part of him which forever feels dependent and in need of faith, as assured by the love of the parents in this world and the parental powers in the supernatural' (1963: 191). Erikson's concern with the *contemporary* context of impoverished reservation life, and the ongoing effects of colonialism leading to psychopathology, nevertheless represented a departure from earlier culture and personality theorists, even if his theoretical explanation lay more in individual psychology than in historical process.

Macgregor's analysis of Sioux culture and personality must be seen in a different light when the work of Mekeel and Erikson are examined. The concern with the authentic, the ethnographic 'pure products' (cf. Clifford 1988), led him logically to conclude that the main problem with these people, both psychologically and practically, in terms of government administration, was that 'the modern Indian way of life' was 'one of emptiness' (Macgregor 1946: 121). They were, indeed, 'warriors without weapons.'

Conclusion

Researchers in the first half of the twentieth century were clearly fascinated with the personality of *the* American Indian. The Indian Education Research project in particular was a testing ground for the intersection of anthropology, psychology, and psychoanalytic psychiatry. Inspired by the work of Ruth Benedict and the nascent culture-and-personality school, the project represented an opportunity to explore cross-cultural, interdisciplinary research techniques using teams of researchers from disciplines that had little experience working together. It provided a wonderful opportunity to employ various psychological tests, some relatively new, in an effort to demonstrate their cross-cultural utility. The project was also about practical concerns, the perceived need to develop humane government policy that built upon, rather than opposed, American Indian culture. However, since Indian policy changed direction somewhat after John Collier's resignation, in some ways as a result of a backlash against his approach, it is not possible to assess to what extent the policy recommendations emanating from the project actually benefited American Indians.

Certainly, the researchers discussed in this chapter never set out to present stereotypical, essentialized views of American Indian cultures and personalities. The portraits that they drew of specific Indian communities often demonstrated clear cultural differences, and, with some patience, suggestions of intracultural variability can be teased out. Although each culture was represented as a more-or-less homogeneous whole, a singular Indian did not immediately emanate from their work. Cautionary notes warned readers not to overgeneralize, often stressing that the psychological profiles were composites and should not be individualized. There was, however, a tendency to represent the findings in a positivist manner, and some of the monographs produced subsequently became ethnographic classics read by anthropology students continent-wide. Their impact on subsequent work cannot be underestimated. By focusing on the generalized conclusions rather than on the methods employed, a generation of readers may have misled themselves.

Despite the somewhat erratic and problematic nature of studies of Aboriginal personality, the idea that entire cultures could be characterized in terms of a modal, basic, or dominant personality persisted. This will become especially clear when we look at how this notion of culture became operationalized by those seeking to undertake comparative research or to provide culturally 'appropriate' psychotherapeutic services to the Aboriginal population. Efforts to measure and assess continued unabated, inspired in the first instance by an explosion in interest in Rorschach's funny pictures.

CHAPTER THREE

The Psychoanalyst's Aboriginal

Who could take playing with ink blots seriously? (Hallowell 1976: 9)

Psychoanalytical approaches to the study of personality dominated the field for decades, and the belief that the key to understanding individual and group personality was hidden in the unconscious led to the emergence of many different projective techniques. As we saw in the last chapter, the Rorschach Psychodiagnostic (Ink-blot) Test was one such technique, and was something of a revolutionary development for psychological research. Not surprisingly, it was quickly employed in the analysis of Aboriginal North American personality and psychopathology. Indeed, the question of its cross-cultural applicability dominated a great deal of this work, as researchers sought to demonstrate that the ink blots, in and of themselves, harboured no intrinsic cultural meanings yet could identify underlying personality characteristics of individuals. Many influential ethnographers tried their hand with the Rorschach despite serious methodological and conceptual problems, generating enduring portraits of *the* Aboriginal.

Anthropology and the Rorschach: No Experience Required

In many ways this story of the Rorschach begins with anthropologist A. Irving Hallowell, one of the leaders of the early culture and personality approach, and one of the first to utilize the Rorschach test in non-Western societies (Bock 1988: 59). Hallowell, influenced by the emerging psychological anthropology of Edward Sapir (Hallowell 1976: 8), studied both Freudian and gestalt psychology, worked briefly with Franz Boas at Columbia University as a student, and subsequently participated in seminars featuring both Boas and Ruth Benedict. He is best known for his extensive work with the Saulteaux (Ojibwa) of Berens River, Manitoba.[1]

Hallowell's first trip to northern Manitoba was in 1930, but it was not until 1937 that he employed the Rorschach. Like others, Hallowell (1976: 9) believed that this relatively new test was 'culture-free' and that its main advantage was that 'it was a subtle means of probing many of the complexities of personality.' Hallowell freely admitted that he was a novice in the use of the technique: 'From the scanty literature on the Rorschach, I learned enough to be able to try my hand at administering and scoring the test. On my next trip to the Berens River I stopped in Chicago hoping to see the Rorschach expert, Samuel J. Beck, but I missed him. So on my own I collected a large sample of protocols from both adults and children' (1976: 9). It was after this field trip that Hallowell met Rorschach expert Bruno Klopfer, and the two engaged in discussions of the materials Hallowell had gathered. Several presentations at the American Anthropological Association's annual conference in 1938 were met with curiosity but, to a greater extent, 'derision,' as the opening quote in this chapter suggests. Undeterred, Hallowell continued his work using the Rorschach.[2]

Hallowell believed that the Rorschach was a valid method for studying 'nonliterate' peoples, despite obvious cultural and language barriers. He even argued that it was not necessary for the person administering the technique to be an expert in its analysis; indeed, the administration of the instrument was seen to be entirely separate from the interpretation of the protocols. One advantage of the Rorschach, according to Hallowell (1941a, 1945a), was that it could be interpreted by researchers who had no knowledge of the individuals or cultures in question. While Hallowell asserted that 'adequate communication between investigator and subjects is even more important in psychological than in ethnographical projects' (1941a: 235), no such communication was apparently necessary to render interpretations of their personality and culture. Even if we accept the premise that interpretation could successfully be done blind, the actual testing conditions remain crucial to understanding the protocols. Hallowell's own description of the problems encountered in personally administering the test to Saulteaux peoples brings into question the cross-cultural validity of the technique:

> In the first place, it was necessary to motivate individuals to look at the cards. This did not prove to be such a simple task, since these Indians are

not accustomed to interviews, clinical examinations, or tests of any sort. Besides, they are not used to being isolated in order to perform any task, and isolation was a difficult practical problem to be solved. What I did was to tell my prospective subjects that I had something to show them, and I let it be known that each individual would receive a package of tobacco or a chocolate bar. I presented them with either one as a preliminary to the presentation of the cards. Nevertheless, some of the Indians refused point blank to look at the cards at all; others said that they would do so at some future time, and never showed up. On the other hand, some individuals apparently enjoyed the experience and even thanked me for letting them see the cards ... To many of these Indians I am sure there seemed something 'phoney' about sitting quietly and looking at blots one after another. It was not only a totally unfamiliar task – as it is with everyone – but in terms of their experience it was particularly strange because there is not even the vague analogy of looking at pictures and of course they do not read. At any rate, they often appeared apprehensive and tense at first, on the defensive and fearful of making a mistake ... Many of them handled the cards so cautiously that obviously they were not at ease and consequently not in a state of mind to associate freely to the blots. (Hallowell 1941a: 239–40)

Hallowell's candid assessment was supported by Jennifer Brown. Familiar with the Berens River community herself, she has related that, 'Some descendants of Chief Berens [Hallowell's main informant] remember him showing those funny pictures (the Rorschach test) and his efforts (sometimes strained, as he knew) to elicit responses' (Brown 1992: xvii). It seems that neither the Saulteaux nor Hallowell's scholarly colleagues were willing to take the test seriously.

Hallowell was not unique in experiencing problems administering the Rorschach to Aboriginal peoples, nor was he unique in his frank descriptions of these problems. Anthony F.C. Wallace, a graduate student of Hallowell's who was also trained in the Rorschach technique by Bruno Klopfer, encountered similar difficulties in the use of the test. Wallace undertook research among the Tuscarora in 1948, administering the Rorschach to seventy individuals (short of the 'standard Rorschach practice' of 100; Wallace 1952: 43), roughly 20 per cent of the Tuscarora population. Some of the Tuscarora contacted by Wallace were already familiar with the Rorschach and had internalized the popular view that the test somehow implied being 'crazy' or 'stupid.' Wallace (1952: 44) noted that some thought he was trying to prove that

Indians were, in fact, undesirable, despite his explanation that he was interested in learning about 'the Indian outlook on life.'

Another anthropologist who attempted to use the Rorschach was John Honigmann, a leading figure in psychological anthropology at mid-century, who first undertook research among the Slave of Fort Nelson, British Columbia, in the summer of 1943. His original research proved to be difficult work, and the residents were reluctant to talk with him during his seven-week stay (Honigmann 1946). In fact, he noted that he was able to generate only thirty-five to forty 'informant hours,' including a couple of Rorschach protocols for 'Métis' children. Honigmann presented a somewhat confusing view of Slave culture by including the 'Métis' and 'part-Indian' designations along with 'pure Indian,' references in part to biological heritage and in part to cultural orientation. The fact that his Rorschachs were undertaken with 'Métis' without a clear discussion of their relationship to the culture of the Slave makes interpretation difficult. In subsequent work with the Kaska, Honigmann (1949) encountered yet more difficulties using the Rorschach. 'The situation often grew so painful,' he admitted, 'that it was necessary to beg the subjects to remain for a few more minutes' to complete the exercise (1949: 240). Frances Ferguson (1962), who collaborated with Honigmann in an analysis of Rorschach protocols in a study of Great Whale River Eskimos, described similar difficulties in the testing of nine Eskimos in the community. Three of these refused to hold the cards, and two of them, children, were uneasy during the test. The Eskimo language was used, with an interpreter. 'Owing to the language limitation,' Ferguson commented, 'it was not possible to arrive at determinants with the same ease as with Indo-European speaking peoples. For this reason there must be a certain amount of speculation as to what the determinants actually were' (80). As a result, Ferguson in effect challenged the cross-cultural applicability of the technique, suggesting that while 'in European culture a high percentage of detail, particularly of animal or anatomical content, suggests insecurity and compulsiveness, these hypotheses may require alteration when applied to a culture as different as that of the Eskimo. It might be that the demands of the Eskimo environment translate what looks to us like compulsiveness into function activity designed to further the survival of the individual and the group' (81).

In retrospect, the Rorschach test appeared to be an incredibly unreliable method for assessing personality cross-culturally, but its use remained prominent in anthropology for several decades. The tests were often undertaken using translators, although the implications of this practice were rarely addressed. Aboriginal informants were often described as apprehensive and fearful of the test, and their responses were often compared, unfavourably, to those of non-Aboriginal peoples in terms of both speed and content. Notwithstanding the acknowledged methodological complications, the analysis of protocols went ahead anyway, and portraits of Aboriginal personality and psychopathology were generated. The Rorschach seemed to carry with it much of the mystique that surrounded psychoanalysis itself, frequently leading researchers to defer to it when faced with contradictory ethnographic data. While Ferguson's (1962) Rorschach protocols of Great Whale River Eskimos indicated that their personalities were characterized by inhibition, for instance, ethnographic and other qualitative descriptions of these peoples clearly suggested that they were quite affable and outgoing. Ferguson glossed over the potential problems with the Rorschach, suggesting that, because of environmental pressures and close living arrangements, emotional control was adaptive, but that 'underlying the affable, fun-loving behaviour so typical of the Great Whale River Eskimo, there is a habitual disinclination for emotional involvement, a long-standing mode of adjustment, with the smile sometimes being part of a defence system which prevents emergence of emotional forces disruptive to the harmony of the group' (85). In other words, with the Eskimo, seeing was not necessarily believing. The idea that the ethnographic portrait of a people might reflect only a contrived public personality, and that a truer portrait would emerge through the use of such projective techniques, was certainly at odds with the conventional belief of Rorschach analysts such as Klopfer, cited by Ferguson (81, n.3), that other data were essential to interpretation of the protocols. The two data sets clearly did not always agree, and when they were at odds, more often than not the Rorschach analysis appeared to carry the day.

The Generation of Aboriginal Personality Portraits

Anthropologists persevered in their use of the Rorschach, generating psychological profiles of many different Aboriginal North American groups. Unlike the early historical particularists in North America, or the structural-functionalists who were launching their own challenge to anthropological theory and method in Europe, much of the use of the Rorschach centred on issues of intracultural variability and cultural change. The test presented researchers with an opportunity to begin to devise a more realistic view of contemporary Aboriginal cultures. The Rorschach became an important tool in the ethnographers' methodological armament. But what did these Aboriginal cultures look like?

Hallowell, as the dean of psychoanalytical anthropology, provides a good starting point in answering this question. He was particularly interested in the role of the individual in culture, especially cultures undergoing change, hence his interest in nascent psychological methodologies (Bee 1974). According to Darnell (2001: 243), Hallowell produced 'a potent combination of ethnography, psychological reality, and history' which was 'virtually unique among early Boasians.' But he also entered the field with a thorough grounding in 'taken-for-granted Freudian notions of the punitive superego, emotional ambivalence, and the mechanisms of repression' (Lindholm 2001: 154). Through the combination of standard ethnography and the Rorschach, he developed a particular interest in understanding the implications of different degrees of acculturation among the Indians of the Lake Winnipeg region in Manitoba, although much of his work also focused on reconstructing the culture of those who were closest to the 'primitive' state of uncontaminated aboriginality (Hallowell 1976: 10).[3] He also generated Rorschach protocols for some Chippewa from Lac du Flambeau, Wisconsin, as representative of a related cultural group which had undergone even greater acculturation. His major analyses of Saulteaux/Ojibwa/Chippewa personality were based on 217 subjects (120 men and 97 women, between the ages of sixteen and eighty). Forty-four came from an inland group of Lake Winnipeg Saulteaux, whom Hallowell described as the least acculturated; 58 came from a more acculturated lakeside group; and 115 were drawn from the Wisconsin group (Hallowell 1955: 346; see also Hallowell 1942; Caudill 1949).

Like many anthropologists of the day, Hallowell subscribed to the idea of indigenous 'culture areas' in North America, following the work of Kroeber (1939).[4] This meant that he believed a priori that Aboriginal populations in the same region shared important cultural traits, including basic psychological features (Hallowell 1955). Further, Hallowell believed that a psychological portrait of Aboriginal societies before contact could be derived through the use of documents recorded by the earliest European arrivals: missionaries, explorers, and traders. Based on these data sources, the pre-contact aboriginal Ojibwa were described by Hallowell (1955: 349) as having a 'relatively simple and homogenous' culture lacking in 'any institutionalized development which brought organized social sanctions to bear upon the individual.' Emotional restraint and inhibition were frequently ascribed to these peoples by early Europeans, leading to 'the stereotype of the Indian as a stoical type of human being' (1955: 132). Interpersonal relations were marked by avoidance and what would later be referred to as an ethic of non-interference with others. Their society was 'atomistic' or individualistic, resulting in a 'highly introverted' personality structure which discouraged interpersonal tensions.'[5] 'On the surface they are an extremely patient, placid, and peace-loving people,' he wrote in 1941, 'but at the same time there are strong currents of hostility that exist on a covert level of expression' (1941a: 243). Hostile acts brought with them the possibility of supernatural sanction, a key component of the people's 'worldview,' and individuals were believed to be capable of invoking the supernatural to harm others. 'As the Rorschach data show,' he wrote in an early conference paper, 'the individual is so dominated by fantasies that his relations with all objects of the outside world – people and things – tends to be distorted' (Hallowell 1942: 44). This resulted in 'a surface amiability and emotional restraint, tinged with latent suspicion and anxiety' (1955: 350). He described a population of individuals unable 'to achieve a free and easy, or even satisfactory, rapport with others' (1942: 44), an intensely unsocial environment.

Hallowell believed, as did many others at the time, that the underlying tensions and anxieties characteristic of traditional Saulteaux culture were largely kept in check until the introduction of alcohol which had the effect of suppressing inhibitions and resulted in increasing conflict and violence (Hallowell 1955). The least acculturated inland group best fit this personality profile, even though they too had experienced some cultural change as a result of colonization, leading Hallowell to conclude that their modal personality structure remained intact. In fact, Hallowell argued that 'psychological continuity' ensued even among the highly acculturated Chippewa at Lac du Flambeau.[6] They were 'still Ojibwa in a psychological sense whatever their clothes, their houses, or their occupations, whether they speak English or not, and regardless of race mixture' (Hallowell 1955: 351). According to one of his researchers, William Caudill (1949: 425), commonalities between the groups included 'a detailed, practical, noncreative approach to problems, a high degree of generalized anxiety, an emphasis on restraint and control, an emotional indifference to things, a lack of warm interpersonal relations, a wariness and suspiciousness, and a great deal of aggression and hostility covertly expressed through sorcery.' Caudill was willing to admit, however, that some 'psychological modifications' had occurred, particularly as a result of the breakdown in social structure, which resulted in less inhibited aggressive tendencies.

Since Hallowell was concerned primarily with acculturation, and with testing the utility of the Rorschach, he was determined to discern at least some differences between the two Manitoba groups. His data suggested that the 'Lakeside' people, the more acculturated group, exhibited less of the 'introversive type of personality which almost all the Inlanders exhibited' and, because of their contact with non-Aboriginals, were 'much less under the fantasy influences emanating from within which characterizes the Inland people as a whole' (Hallowell 1942: 46). But the main difference between the two groups appeared to be not so much a matter of interpretation of the ink blots, but the speed with which those tested responded and the amount of content they provided. The Lakeside people were much faster, approaching 'the normal white average' (45). Hallowell explained: 'The Lakeside people are being released from many of the inhibitions consonant with the old native culture. They are less deliberate and cautious than the Inlanders in their approach to things [such as the Rorschach] because the sources of many anxieties have receded along with a change in culture' (Hallowell 1942: 45–6). He acknowledged that speed was not normally considered an important element in Rorschach analysis, but perhaps hard-pressed to find some difference, *any* difference, between the two groups, he suggested that 'it does measure a significant psychological difference in this case' (45). The difference, of course, was due to acculturation.

It is possible that there really were few meaningful cultural differences between Hallowell's two Saulteaux groups, and even with the Wisconsin group. It is also possible that the test itself failed to elicit significant psychological differences among the groups. But it is difficult today to reconcile the view that the Rorschach was believed to be 'culture-free' with its use in comprehending the role of culture in personality formation. Furthermore, both the administration and interpretation of the Rorschach among the Saulteaux was clearly an act embedded within the cultural framework of those who designed the analytic guidelines – European and European North Americans. Could the test be both 'culture-free' and capable of identifying cultural differences in personality?

Notwithstanding these methodological issues, Hallowell's analysis did lead him to conclude that the Lac du Flambeau Chippewa were suffering from apathy with 'an introversive personality structure ... pushed to the limits of its functional adequacy' and 'compelled to function with a great paucity of inner resources' (1955: 351–2). He described the 'breakdown of the old personality structure of the Ojibwa under the pressures of acculturation' (356) while at the same time arguing that 'the tendency towards a low level of psychological adjustment at [Lac du] Flambeau is not to be attributed to "acculturation" considered abstractly or as some inevitable force, but to a set of complex factors that we know too little about and which are extremely difficult to analyze' (356). He was nevertheless led to conclude that alcohol problems and juvenile delinquency at Lac du Flambeau were the result of the breakdown of the personality structure and traditional inner controls which, combined with a 'paucity of inner resources' and loss of traditional core values, had resulted in a paralysing apathy 'which they cannot overcome' (357). Simply put, the Chippewa were losing their basic Aboriginal character and traditional values without an adequate replacement, and as a result their personality structure was 'regressing' to a more childlike state (a conclusion based on the strong similarities between the protocols of adults and children) (366).[7] Hallowell, in effect, anticipated the 'caught-between-two-worlds' acculturative stress paradigm of many social psychologists, to be discussed in chapter 5, although he did not use this specific terminology.

While Hallowell was interested in comparing the psychological profiles of Aboriginal groups at various stages of acculturation, Wallace was more interested in comprehending personality differences within a specific group. His work thus represented a departure from that of precursors like Mead, Benedict, and Kardiner, all of whom seemed to ignore the existence of intracultural variability in personality in an effort to sustain their theories (Lindholm 2001). To examine this variability, Wallace began with Cora DuBois's (1944) notion of 'modal personality structure,' a variant of Kardiner's basic personality structure which highlighted diversity in personalities rather than commonalities but which still held that culture moulded personality. Modal personality structure sprang from the idea of 'national character,' meaning 'the peculiar distribution of individual personality traits or types which distinguishes a population' (Wallace 1952: 50). Wallace used the Rorschach to determine the most frequent type of personality among the Tuscarora, which did not necessarily represent the 'average' person or characterize the majority of individuals, and in so doing he is credited with refocusing psychological anthropology on the importance of intracultural diversity (Harris 1968; Darnell 2001). Given the vast range of personality types that could be statistically derived from a projective test, it was possible that the modal personality would not be the dominant one in any group. This is exactly what Wallace determined for the Tuscarora. Only 37 per cent of his sample actually fit this modal personality type, a total of just twenty-six individuals.

The primitivist discourse characteristic of the times was well represented in Wallace's description of the modal Tuscarora personality. He stated clearly that 'the Tuscarora modal personality type is less exotic to western norms than are most other Rorschach types reported in the anthropological literature' (Wallace 1952: 70), and continued in this vein: 'The writer's impression, however, secured from the casual consideration of [elements of the Rorschach] and the general "feel" of the records, is that the Tuscarora modal personality type is innately endowed with about the same degree of intelligence as the "average" white man, but is less inclined to have intellectualistic ambitions and tends to make less use of his innate capacities than the white man does. He has the same abilities but operates at lower efficiency; he lives less by his wits' (71). Wallace described the modal Tuscarora as a 'little shy' with 'a strong urge to be allowed to become passive and dependent' (75). 'The self-dependent, self-made, rationally ambitious person who takes care of himself is rarely found' (90), he concluded. This conclusion was offset by a characteristically psychoanalytic contradictory assertion of 'a compensatory drive to be hyperindependent, aggressive, self-sufficient' (75). 'A fear of rejection' was noted, along with a 'shallowness of affect expressed (if not felt) in interpersonal relationships' (88). The reason for these traits, Wallace surmised, was the existence of severe trauma in childhood dependency relationships (105). As tangible evidence of personality, Wallace described a Tuscarora picnic which exhibited little of the energy and noise levels of white picnics, leading him to conclude, 'It is as though the Indians wanted desperately to be with other people, but were very, very cautious about involving themselves in a too-intense, and therefore potentially too-frustrating, emotional relationship' (89).

Wallace also described 'an ultimate incapacity to feel, to adapt, to evaluate the environment realistically, and a concomitant dependence upon categories, stereotypes, and destructive logic' (75). In effect, Wallace concluded that the modal Tuscarora was incapable of understanding and dealing with 'real' or specific situations and therefore resorted to simplistic stereotypes to govern behaviour. An example he presented was their view that 'off the reservation' referred to a homogenous experience as if it was a singular locale, and the 'state' as an entirely negative entity (86).

Wallace concluded his monograph on the Tuscarora by comparing them with Hallowell's Ojibwa. In the following passage describing the two societies we find one of the clearest statements of an emerging, essentialized Aboriginal personality. It is important to remember as one reads this passage that, by Wallace's own admission, the modal personality was not necessarily representative of the majority of members in any society: 'To the superficial observer, both modal Tuscarora and modal Ojibwa would be "Indians." They would display somewhat similar shyness and reserve, similar crudity of emotional response; they would both fit the popular White stereotype of the sullen, taciturn Indian. The Ojibwa would appear to be somewhat more distant; there would be fewer cracks in the armour; his behavior would be more consistent, smoother in its cautious ritual. The Tuscarora would appear to be better adjusted (in relation to an absolute standard of mental health), both to himself and environment' (Wallace 1952: 106).

As noted above, Wallace's modal Tuscarora personality was demonstrated by only 37 per cent of those he tested, yet the figure of 37 per cent became a benchmark in many discussions concerning the representativeness of the modal personality approach. In a re-examination of Wallace's data, anthropologist Thomas Hay (1976) employed a different statistical technique and determined that the modal personality of the Tuscarora was actually exhibited by some 43 per cent of the population, a difference which Hay declared was 'highly significant' (523). Hay criticized other anthropologists who had accepted Wallace's figure without subjecting it to critical assessment, adding, 'it is a sad commentary on anthropological pretensions to scientific respectability that it was more than twenty years before anyone examined the statistical significance of the "magic number 37 per cent" which had attracted so much attention and debate' (522). Hay also noted that Wallace 'implicitly assumed that the personality characteristics measured by the Rorschach are those that are significantly related to the culture of any society,' and that 'this has also been implicitly assumed by many other anthropologists,' without justification (522). These are fair criticisms, given the importance of Wallace's work for subsequent research in culture and personality. However, Hay concluded not with a thorough reexamination of the appropriateness of the Rorschach, especially in cross-cultural contexts, but rather by suggesting that 'There seems to be reason to believe that *some* of these Rorschach dimensions *are* significantly related to culture' (522; emphasis in the original).

Atomism and the Northern Indian

The concept of social atomism as a characteristic of many northern Aboriginal societies was generated largely through the use of psycho-analytic techniques such as the Rorschach. The essence of the atomistic conceptualization of personality was established by Ruth Landes in two early articles entitled 'The personality of the Ojibwa' (1937) and 'The abnormal among the Ojibwa' (1938). The savage side of the primi-tivist pendulum appeared in its full glory in her description of a com-munity of Ojibwa peoples in Ontario, a description based on two summers of fieldwork. The Ojibwa personality was highly individual-ized (Landes did not initially use the term 'atomistic'), and her descrip-tion of the genesis of this personality read like something out of James Fenimore Cooper:

> From the very first days of life, the boy baby is taught that life is a battle with vast forces for the prize of a bare piece of meat and a hide blanket, a battle which he must fight alone, for everyone else is occupied with his own private desperate battle. He must not be dependent on others; by the age of three he is able to strike birds dead, a few years later he manages simple traps, soon he hunts with his father, and by twelve or fifteen years he is able to leave the family lodge for his own hunting grounds. Along with this insistence on economic individualism, the boy is taught to come to grips with the supernaturals, the very masters of his fate. Frequently, for a period of years, his elders drive him out to fast in some lonely spot and thus make himself receptive to supernatural communications. In part, this stresses their point that human beings can be of no fundamental aid to him: he must look for support to a supernatural benefactor whom he will attach to himself. People with a gift for receiving visions thus turn more or less completely away from simple, warm relations with their kind; and in extreme cases when they have acquired much power, deal with other Indians only for the purpose of injuring or killing them. (Landes 1937: 53)

This intense emphasis on individual isolation within the social group produced both vulnerability and hostility, on one hand, and a 'desire for supremacy' on the other (57). Landes described a kind of lawless, hedonistic society in which the individual's conduct was unfettered by social controls: 'The individual brooks no law laid down by his society if these clash with his whims, just as he brooks no rivals in the games and no trespasser on his grounds. Sociologically he is a lawbreaker, especially with respect to the regulations of marriage, incest, and sib. He marries in unapproved ways if these happen to be the most convenient ones, he pursues incestuous relations, even in the face of great odds if these appear desirable, and he ignores his sib obligations if these seem onerous or if by ignoring them he can injure an enemy' (57). For Landes, Ojibwa society was rife with anxiety and hostility; even friends could not be trusted. These extreme views laid the groundwork for the social atomism concept.

Among the key figures in the work on the atomistic Aboriginal were John Honigmann and Victor Barnouw. According to Honigmann (1949), the personality of the northern Aboriginal was characterized by extreme individualism, and he sweepingly suggested that 'a relatively homogeneous personality can be discerned in the vast coniferous forest zone extending from northeastern Canada to western Alaska' (334). This personality, he noted, was 'marked by strong emotional constraint and the inhibition of strong emotions in interpersonal relations. Emotional indifference is maintained through avoiding investing any great emotion in anything.' Honigmann even employed the psychoanalytic technique of dream analysis to understand the genesis of this singular atomistic personality. Within neo-Freudian psychoanalytic theory, dreams were seen as expressions of the unconscious mind, in which desires considered inappropriate by society (such as sexual desire) could be harboured (Erickson & Murphy 1998). Dream analysis, therefore, was an important element in generating psychological profiles (see, for example, Devereux 1951). In a 1961 article based entirely on the analysis of a single Cree man from Attawapiskat, Ontario (it was not uncommon within psychological anthropology to focus intensely on a very small number of subjects), Honigmann sought to show 'how dreams can be used to secure or support interpretations of socially standardized personality' (1961a: 579). 'Bob,' Honigmann's subject in this case, demonstrated a great deal of anxiety in his dreams, and two possible explanations for this anxiety were offered: Bob was 'conflicted about sex;' or Bob suffered anxiety about food, living as he did in a northern hunting society. Either way, Honigmann made it clear he was making 'hunches' about the meaning of the symbols in Bob's dreams. Perhaps more importantly, Honigmann was willing to once again provide a homogenous portrait of Attawapiskat Cree personality. We are, he explained, 'less interested in Bob qua individual than in the Attawapiskat Indian generically conceived' (582). His conclusion: 'Attawapiskat males possess a high level of generalized anxiety' (582).

This anxiety stemmed from the atomistic nature of Cree society; indeed, Honigmann viewed northern Aboriginal societies as inherently atomistic, following along the lines described earlier for Hallowell (Honigmann 1968).[8] These societies were characterized by 'strain, contention, or invidiousness' in their 'brittle' social relations (Honigmann 1968: 221), with a 'primary concern' for one's 'own individual interests and on great freedom from, or avoidance of, social constraint' (220). Honigmann specifically identified components of 'psychological atomism,' including 'covert hostility, envy, a view of social relations as fraught with danger, a desire to maximize the advantages of oneself or of one's close kin' (221), all leading to heightened states of anxiety.

Barnouw, who had studied extensively with Abram Kardiner and attended the famed Kardiner-Linton seminars, similarly described the Wisconsin Chippewa as having an atomistic social structure. Fully versed in Kardiner's 'psychocultural technique,' Barnouw was sent to Wisconsin in 1944 by his mentor to collect life histories and Rorschach protocols to supplement previously gathered data, which was to be analysed in the 'Psychological Analysis of Primitive Cultures' seminar (Barnouw 1950: 8; W.C. Manson 1988: 88). Like Hallowell, who served on his graduate committee (along with Ruth Benedict), Barnouw also had an interest in the study of acculturation, a theme which emerged in his analysis of the Chippewa of Court Oreilles and Lac du Flambeau. His work extended over two summers, although he worked primarily with just four informants, three of whom he described as 'caught between two cultures' (Barnouw 1950: 8). Rorschach experts Milton Sapirstein and Bruno Klopfer provided some analysis of the tests at the Kardiner-Linton seminars.

Barnouw (1950) had first heard of the concept of social atomism in a class with Ruth Benedict, and was aware that a handful of others, such as Hallowell and Landes, had used it in their descriptions of the Saulteaux and Ojibwa, respectively (Barnouw 1961). Barnouw (1961: 1006) explained that 'in an atomistic society it is not difficult for the component units to break away and exist apart from the larger society of which they are a part; political authority is weak, and there are not many mechanisms for reinforcing larger-group social solidarity.' The concept was inherently ecological: atomistic societies were most likely comprised of hunting peoples who were required to be very mobile and to adapt to changing economic circumstances, including periodic starvation. Built upon this ecological adaptation and atomistic social structure was a specific personality structure. Barnouw described the

Chippewa as highly individualistic peoples for whom cooperative activities were difficult. 'Partly because the individual is not incorporated, early in life, into a rewarding, interdependent social world,' he wrote, 'the average Chippewa presents a picture of considerable isolation ... This characteristic is strikingly expressed in the Rorschach protocols' (1950: 18). The isolation was physical, emotional, and spiritual. From early childhood, 'the average Chippewa child had few playmates' (p.19), and weak ties to parents who demonstrated little affection. As adults, the Chippewa were socially paralysed by the fear of sorcery which 'led to mutual suspicions' and 'inhibited the development of co-operative activities' (27). How a hunting society could be successful given this apparent disinclination to cooperate was unclear.

The effect of this atomistic structure was to make the Chippewa dependent upon, and subservient to, the European intruders. The trader adopted a 'parental' role that was so overbearing that he could beat drunken Indians without fear of reprisal (Barnouw 1950: 61). Bound to the trader 'psychologically by an undercurrent need for dependence' (62), the Chippewa experienced a much less traumatic process of acculturation than some other American Indian groups. Barnouw utilized the Dakota as a contrast, basing much of his analysis of that society on the problematic work done by Gordon Macgregor, discussed in the previous chapter. The Dakota were characterized as an aggressive society that, unlike the Chippewa, resisted European encroachment. When defeat finally came, according to this analysis, the Dakota were shattered and became psychologically demoralized. Barnouw's analysis suggested that Chippewa compliance with the exigencies of culture contact, based on their psychological and physical inability to mount effective opposition, actually served to insulate them from the devastating psychological trauma experienced by the resisting Dakota. The passive and emotionally undemonstrative nature ascribed to the Chippewa would eventually emerge as a central element of the 'basic personality structure' of most American Indians, as described through the 1990s.

The atomistic framework had its critics, of course. Anthropologist Bernard James (1954; see also 1961) argued that Hallowell's northern Saulteaux work, and especially the concept of 'atomism,' was not as readily transplanted to the Chippewa of Wisconsin as Barnouw's work suggested.[9] Indeed, James believed that Barnouw had a 'predilection' to find atomism in his southern group, and that the historical data employed to justify use of the concept were vague and open to a variety of interpretations. James expressed frustration at the lack of refinement of the concept itself. Furthermore, he argued (insightfully, I would suggest) that many of the personality traits attributed to the southern Chippewa were not due to the atomistic nature of their culture but were instead 'the social-psychological consequences of the pauper economy and socially depressed conditions of the reservations today' (1954: 285). James believed that the construction of personality required contemporary, field-based studies, as opposed to the historical reconstructions and projective tests used by Hallowell and Barnouw.

Despite these criticisms, the concept of atomism persisted for many years, culminating in a special issue of the anthropology journal *Human Organization* in 1968. 'The atomistic-type of society,' wrote editors Arthur J. Rubel and Harriet Kupferer (1968: 189), 'is a society in which the nuclear family represents the major structural unit and, indeed, almost the only formalized social entity.' 'Interpersonal relations outside of the nuclear family,' they continued, 'are characterized by contention, suspiciousness, and invidiousness. Moreover, these attitudes and behavior are normative.' In a theoretical treatment, but with specific reference to Aboriginal peoples, Honigmann (1968) developed his ideas to their fullest. In atomistic societies, he argued, people were intensely individualistic, with 'great freedom from, or avoidance of, social constraint' (220). Interpersonal relations are marked by reserve and the suppression of feeling, or 'frozen affect' (ibid.). This was not to say that these societies were so individualistic that individuals and families could not cooperate, but cooperation was characteristically short-term and devoid of more permanent commitments. 'Weak and ineffectual leadership' and a 'lack of social structures extending much beyond the range of the household or local segment of kin' were also characteristic (221). In psychological terms, according to Honigmann, atomism lead to 'covert hostility, envy, a view of social relations as fraught with danger, a desire to maximize the advantages of oneself or of one's close kin, and ... family-centered values' (221–2).[10] According to Asen Balikci, among the Vunta Kutchin such a situation cultivated 'bad friends,' in which trust was lacking between even the closest of individuals. The genesis of atomistic societies was explainable in two ways: some believed early life experiences were paramount (e.g., Barnouw), while others focused on adaptation to specific ecological (e.g., Hallowell) or political (e.g., James) situations. How individuals in such societies could generate social, economic, and political structures to allow for the cooperation necessary to ensure group survival was rarely addressed. As we shall see, many of the personality traits of the atomistic Aboriginal survived to become the cornerstones of contemporary, 'culturally sensitive' treatment.

Persistence of the Rorschach

Part of the beauty of the Rorschach test, in the eyes of its proponents, was its suitability for cross-cultural comparisons. Just as William Henry had sought to use American Indian populations to test the TAT, others did likewise with the Rorschach. And anthropologists were not the only ones to embrace this technique, even if, at least in the early years, they appeared to have had a monopoly on Aboriginal research. While in some respects the use of the Rorschach, as well as other psychoanalytic techniques, was more sophisticated in the hands of psychologists and psychiatrists, the portraits that they painted of Aboriginal peoples were not problem-free.

Bert Kaplan, a psychologist, worked closely with anthropologists such as Clyde Kluckhohn and John Adair, as well as several members of the Indian Education Research project, seeking to add further weight to the theoretical propositions that 'the influence of culture in creating modal personality trends has been greatly overstated' and that there were 'wide personality differences between cultures' (B. Kaplan 1954: vii). Kaplan, in justifying his use of the Rorschach, accepted that 'while the test is obviously not culture-free, it is probably more so than other techniques which might be used' in the study of personality (3). Using data gathered in 1947, Kaplan compared test results for four populations, Navajo, Zuni, Spanish-American, and Mormon, all in roughly the same region of the American southwest, to determine the existence and extent of personality differences between cultures. A total of 157 individuals across these four communities were tested; all were males, most were between seventeen and forty, and half were returning war veterans. Like the anthropologists, Kaplan too experienced problems in the administration of the Rorschach. At Zuni, where there was great suspicion of the tests ('the writer saw menace and hostility in every Zuni who looked his way'; Kaplan 1954: 5), all tests were conducted in English; in contrast, at the Navajo reservation, interpreters were used in most instances.

Two scorers were used by Kaplan to sort a set of twenty-four protocols into groups based on similarities. The first scorer, with no knowledge of the four communities originally tested, failed to generate meaningful groupings. The second scorer, however, was Alice Joseph. Joseph had not only been integral to the Indian Education Research Project, and had prior experience with the Navajo and Zuni in particular, but she was also informed as to the identity of the four communities involved. According to Kaplan (1954: 28), 'This changed the psychological task from one of simply looking for similarities to one of finding subgroups which would best fit a set of pre-conceived expectations, however vague they might be.' The results for Joseph were 'definitely positive,' in that thirteen of the twenty-four protocols were sorted correctly; another test, matching a subset of the protocols to their groups, was also successful, leading Kaplan to conclude, 'This success seems to us to be conclusive proof established under extremely rigorous conditions, that Rorschachs are to a degree similar within cultures and that they differ among cultures' (29). But statistical analysis demonstrated significant within-group variability and less than expected between-group variability. Alluding to Wallace's work among the Tuscarora, as well as TAT results, Kaplan concluded that the evidence clearly suggested that there was also a great deal of heterogeneity of personality in the groups studied, and that therefore 'cultural influences do not necessarily create uniformity in a group' (32). In other words, 'personality is influenced by, but not determined by, cultural forces' (32). Kaplan was critical of the anthropologists' tendency 'to underestimate individual variability within cultures' (32). Unlike the anthropologists, who admittedly had gone to some lengths to describe the cultures and personalities in question, Kaplan refrained from providing any description of the personalities of the subjects in his study (a 'severe limitation,' in his own words; B. Kaplan 1961: 241).

Criticism of the Rorschach continued, of course, especially with respect to its use in cross-cultural research, and anthropologists in particular began to lose interest. An early critic was Herman Lantz (1948), who, after a review of several prominent studies of 'pre-literate' peoples (including Hallowell's Saulteaux work), concluded that the results were too general and vague to be of value, and that use of the test should be confined to the Western populations for whom it was designed. Kaplan (1961: 249) himself admitted that tests such as the Rorschach worked better in western societies, and that work with non-Western peoples 'is not only a matter of increased uncertainty about the validity of the tests but involves the sparseness of some of the materials and the inability to obtain rich, imaginative, personal, and expressive data in contrast to brief, superficial, and stereotyped responses with a minimum of personal involvement.' He also agreed with Hallowell and Spindler that acculturation to Western society would affect, and improve, the suitability of the Rorschach for these peoples. Kaplan issued a harsh assessment of the state of the field in the use of such tests: 'I have looked for the positive values in these tests and found them very scant. I have looked at the difficulties in their use and found them to be enormous, and have concluded that as these tests are being used and interpreted at present, only a modicum of validity and value can be obtained from them (252).' Only the anthropological work of Hallowell seemed, to Kaplan, to have added anything significant to the understanding of personality, and he ranked Hallowell's work alongside that of Erik Erikson, Abram Kardiner (whom Lanz had also criticized), and Erich Fromm. But this was not the end of this type of research for Aboriginal peoples.

Psychiatrist Bryce Boyer, a proponent of the concept of basic personality structure, jumped fully into the Rorschach fray in the early 1960s. Influenced by anthropological literature (he was a research associate in anthropology at the University of New Mexico) and his own Freudian psychoanalytic training, Boyer worked closely with Rorschach expert Bruno Klopfer in longitudinal studies of the Mescalero Apache people. A clinician providing services to the Apache, his initial and most substantive work concerned the personality characteristics of Mescalero shamans, and, more broadly, research into the issue of personality disorders believed to afflict these individuals. The clinical language of psychoanalysis and psychopathology pervades Boyer's work, differentiating qualitatively it from that of the anthropologists, even if the ultimate, unflattering portrait of Aboriginal peoples exudes similarity.

According to Boyer (1961), existing anthropological literature suggested that shamans typically suffered from mental disorders (see Jilek 1971), including schizophrenia and personality disorders (an idea now discredited), and he set out to test the hypothesis that 'the typical shaman's character structure included traits of the hysterical personality disorder and of the imposter and that his main fixations lay within oral and phallic phases' (1961: 14). Hysterical personality disorder involved 'a compulsive need to be loved and admired, intense feelings of inadequacy, either conscious or unconscious, strong dependency on the approval of others for maintenance of self-esteem, a powerful capacity for dramatization and somatic compliance, and a tendency to repress aggressive feelings or attitudes or to act them out in concealed ways' (17). The 'imposter' was one who deceives, swindles, and cheats while fraudulently misrepresenting himself or herself. Boyer conducted two 'psychoanalytically oriented investigative interviews' with a single Mescalero shaman (whose Rorschach protocol was then analysed by Klopfer) (Boyer 1961; Klopfer & Boyer 1961), and also undertook dream analysis. According to Boyer, the shaman 'had intense feelings of inadequacy and strong dependency on the approval of others for maintenance of self-esteem ... there were strong hints that he struggled with a problem of latent passive homosexuality' (Boyer 1961: 27). While life history material revealed a troubled past involving alcohol and violence, a common occurrence among males of the Mescalero at the time, much of Boyer's conclusions were based on his interpretation of the shaman's beliefs and techniques:

> From boyhood he had been emotionally unstable. He was afflicted with childhood nightmares which included being eaten by wild animals. He began to have visions at twelve. He drank immoderately from his teens, with the typical Apache inability to consume alcohol and retain self-control, but only during the decade of his life preceding the time I made his acquaintance had [he] become a deteriorating drunkard. During his curing ceremonies his 'strongest' technique of removing 'pains' or 'witches' arrows' consisted of sucking procedures. He regularly used the primitive defenses of denial, introjection, and projection, and at least periodically was unable to distinguish objective and subjective reality. He employed magical gestures and was intensely narcissistic. (28)

Here Boyer was in effect describing very common characteristics of shamanism, including initiation (e.g., having visions) and technique (e.g., sucking). That he would view shamanism as inherently pathological, as evident in his hypothesis, likely clouded his assessment of this individual. Klopfer's analysis of the Rorschach supported Boyer's diagnosis of a character disorder, including a description of the shaman as having 'oral and phallic fixations' and Rorschach interpretations 'which we usually find with very young children or very infantile adults' (Klopfer & Boyer 1961: 178). Yet Klopfer was forced to admit that the shaman's 'strange formulations,' usually offered in his own language, '[made] it difficult to submit the record to the usual scoring procedures' (Klopfer & Boyer 1961: 176). Furthermore, Klopfer lauded the shaman's 'impressive efforts to *act* the role of Medicine Man' in responding to the ink blots, while suggesting that the *real* interpretations essentially came through. Not only was the shaman inherently pathological, he was seen as inherently fraudulent simply by virtue of being a shaman.

Boyer was clearly intrigued with the personalities and mental health status of shamans, and he authored several other papers on his work with the Mescalero and Chiricahua Apache peoples that came to essentially the same conclusions (Boyer 1962; Boyer, Klopfer, Brawer, & Kawai 1964). However, after including non-shamans in the research, Boyer and his colleagues were forced to rethink the relative nature of the shaman's psychopathologies. For instance, Boyer (1962) freely admitted that, while from the perspective of Western psychiatry the shamans clearly suffered from personality disorders, from the Apache perspective they were not deviant at all. Further, based primarily on the attainment of some 250 Rorschach protocols, Boyer (1962) and Boyer et al. (1964) argued that their data suggested that 'the typical Apache of the Mescalero Reservation suffers from a hysterical personality disorder with attributes of the impulse neurosis' (Boyer 1962: 248), and concluded that the shamans were in fact 'healthier than their societal comembers' (Boyer et al. 1964: 179). By painting the entire Mescalero population as suffering from psychopathology, the shamans emerged in a new, more positive (though still disordered) light!

Subsequent analysis revealed to Boyer (1964a; 1964b) that the Apache in general suffered from both a 'high occurrence of alcoholic hallucinosis among the adults and ... the prevalence of latent, passive homosexual yearnings among men' (1964b: 204). 'The psychosis of "choice" into which the Apache retreats when psychic strains become overwhelming,' he wrote, 'appears to be one of the group of schizophrenias' (246). The typical Apache was believed to suffer from several traumas which resulted in this state of affairs: a 'grossly ambivalent' attitude of their parents towards them as infants, which led to 'a basic stunting of id-ego differentiation which persists throughout the life of the average Apache' (270); the abrupt displacement of the toddler subsequent to the birth of a sibling; 'exposure to repetitive exhibitions of sexual and brutal aggressive actions perpetrated by drunken adults' – 'He incorporates the excitements of individuals of both sexes, and is unable to successfully repress and modify his archaic instinctual urges' – and the 'absence of a clearly defined adult model to emulate' (271). The essential problem, as articulated by Boyer, appeared to lie in the discrepancy between persisting pre-contact beliefs and the exigencies of post-reservation life. He suggested, for instance, that Apache religion, with its belief in 'the concepts of diffuse supernatural power and the retention of infantile notions of animation of the inanimate, requires relatively indiscriminate projection of infantile omnipotence onto sur-roundings, conditions which are consistent with confusion of ego boundaries.' This, he continued, represented a defect of ego growth and subjected individuals to 'the development of character disorders and psychoses' (247). Traditional child-rearing patterns remained after the establishment of the reservations, and Boyer noted that while these would have resulted in a functional personality a hundred years ago, this was no longer the case. Echoing Macgregor's 'warriors without weapons' argument, Boyer suggested that colonization had destroyed elements of Apache social structure without a corresponding adapta-tion in child-rearing practices, resulting in the maladaptation of per-sonality to context; this in turn led to the emergence of social and psychological pathologies, because 'culturally sanctioned outlets are only haphazardly provided for the resultant conflicts and anxieties' (269). Alcohol emerged as a problem precisely because drunkenness came to be viewed 'as a culturally ambivalently approved outlet for poorly integrated sexual and aggressive energies' (271).

Boyer, along with several colleagues, continued the psychoanalytical study of Apaches for many years (e.g., Boyer & Boyer 1972; Boyer, De Vos, & Boyer 1983; Day, Boyer & De Vos 1989), as well as shifting the analysis to other groups, including several in Alaska (Boyer, Boyer & Hippler 1974; Boyer et al.1989). The Alaska work was done in conjunc-tion with anthropologist Arthur Hippler, who had previous experience in the area, and allowed for a comparison between two groups, the Upper Tanana and the Tanaina. Utilizing the Rorschach, Boyer et al. (1974) argued that there was a link between ecological adaptation, the socialization process, and personality development. Through this adaptation, they argued, a basic personality emerged which was adap-tive under those particular ecological circumstances, particularly the exigencies of a hunting society. The portrait that was painted of the rel-atively isolated Upper Tanana was strikingly negative. Focusing once again on child-rearing practices as the foundation upon which person-ality was based, they described a system of interfamilial relations that appears to the reader to be astonishingly maladaptive. For instance, they described the attitude of parents towards young children as 'ambivalent,' adding that 'While they treasure their infants and tod-dlers, parents also consider them to be somewhat less than human, and dangerous' (Boyer, & Hippler 1974: 64). Citing Erikson's (1950) work, they argued that mothers 'were simply incapable of supplying the supportive emotional care which could lead to a child's developing sense of a basic trust' (65). Mothers had minimal contact with their infants, and as with the Mescalero, a toddler, once displaced by a new family member, 'developed murderous impulses toward the new rival which were channelized into insecure reaction formations' (65). 'At every stage of the child's development,' they concluded, 'his care produced frustration and mobilized aggression' (67). As adults, husbands feared their wives were out to poison them, and viewed women as dangerous and inherently unfaithful; sexual relationships were devoid of tenderness; living arrangements forced the children to be aware of parental sexual activity, which awakened Oedipal conflicts early on in life. It was concluded that latent homosexuality was present, clearly a theme in Boyer's work.

The Tanaina had been undergoing acculturation to the settler society for several hundred years, in contrast to the few decades experienced by the Upper Tanana. Their review of the primarily ethnographic literature lead Boyer et al. (1989) to argue that Northern Athabascans shared a basic personality structure, or modal personality, in the Kardinerian sense, which looked atomistic: 'They are suspicious, fearful, and suggestible, and tend to be aloof and impersonal. Their object relations tend to be shallow and explosively violent, especially when under the influence of alcohol' (1989: 455–6). But the Rorschach test revealed several differences between the Upper Tanana and the Tanaina. The Tanaina were found to exhibit 'more ego strength and personality development' than the Upper Tanana; the Tanaina revealed 'a greater tendency toward the inhibition of affect,' whereas the Upper Tanana 'were more inclined toward impulsive expressions of affect; and the Upper Tanana were found to 'use more primitive and less modulated expressions of hostility than do the Tanaina, and are more prone to impulsivity' (468–9). The successful acculturation of the Tanaina, rather than any pre-contact differences in adaptation of personality, was the main explanation offered for the differences between the two groups. It had rendered the Tanaina 'psychologically more sound' (472). The authors concluded with the observation that 'the effects of acculturation were psychologically beneficial to the Tanaina but have not yet had sufficient time to reduce, to a great degree, the aboriginal psychopathology of the Upper Tanana' (474). Their final sentence was perhaps the most revealing of all: 'It must be remembered that we are speaking of an incapacity to adapt to Westernization as psychopathological, knowing well that the aboriginal personality organization of these hunting, gathering and warring peoples may be viewed as highly adaptive to that form of life' (474). This idea, that cultural survivals brought forward into the modern era are the cause of maladaptation and psychopathology, will emerge as important in subsequent chapters.

Despite occasionally voiced concerns over the problems experienced in the use of the Rorschach test with Aboriginal groups (e.g., Boyer et al. 1965), which were similar to those expressed by the anthropologists, Boyer remained comfortable with its utility. As late as 1989, Boyer, along with anthropologist George De Vos, with whom he began to collaborate in the early 1980s, as well as Arthur Hippler, continued to support the use of the Rorschach test cross-culturally (Boyer et al. 1989; De Vos & Boyer 1989). Today, while the test remains an important tool in the assessment of personality, and is still considered to be 'culture-free' by many of its proponents in psychology (Ritzler 2001), few anthropologists employ it.

Conclusion

Psychoanalytical frameworks were used in the analysis of Aboriginal peoples for many years, and Freudians, neo-Freudians, and Kardinerians found fodder for their universalist ideas in North America's exotic backyard. Use of the Rorschach with Aboriginal North Americans essentially began as an experiment to test the instrument's cross-cultural validity, but the test quickly became a tool integral to the development of culture and personality theory and, more specifically, to descriptions of Aboriginal personality and psychopathology. The predominant view that the test had no cultural bias, and that the protocols could be interpreted by trained individuals with no knowledge of the people or culture in question, initially led to a bifurcation in its use: ethnographers administered the test and psychoanalysts interpreted the results. But the test was not just about individual personality. Broad, sweeping pronouncements about 'personality-in-culture' were rendered, and portraits of entire cultures were constructed. While the psychologists and psychiatrists may have added a degree of methodological sophistication to the use of the Rorschach, their work nevertheless suffered from the same conceptual flaws, the same 'category fallacy' (Kleinman 1977) of the anthropologists.

Aboriginal peoples do not emerge from the psychoanalytic research in a very flattering light, and barbarism seems to be an innate condition in these analyses. Aboriginal peoples were largely portrayed as unstable, aggressive, paranoid, superstitious, and neurotic in this work, barely able to sustain any kind of social organization. The most charitable of analyses suggested that while the Aboriginal personality, as an expression of an ecological adaptation, may have been functional in the past, it was not functional once the Europeans arrived. The accounts implied that assimilation to the ways of the settler society was required to modernize the Aboriginal personality, but, as we shall see, this process could create its own pathology.

Despite the problematic nature of studies of Aboriginal personality, the idea that entire cultures can be characterized in terms of a modal, basic, or dominant personality persists. This will become especially clear when we look at how this notion of culture is operationalized by those who seek to provide psychotherapeutic services to the Aboriginal population. Even though most personality work dealt with group-level data, presenting personality types that were not necessarily typical of any single individual, those involved in mental health service delivery ignored this obvious limitation and created recipes for counselling that stereotyped and essentialized *the* Aboriginal for purposes of treatment.

CHAPTER FOUR

Measuring the Aboriginal

How Native is Native if you're Native? ... There's a vast number of 'experts' existing in this world eager to tell you what defines a Native and more than happy to tell you whether you fit into that category. (Taylor 2000: 57, 58)

As we have seen, the use of instruments designed to measure various aspects of Aboriginal personality, ability, and psychopathology has a long history. With the relative demise of projective tests in the study of the Aboriginal came the development and deployment of new, more sophisticated techniques based on very different principles. Anthropologists, and their ethnographies, became increasingly distant to this process as psychometricians continued their search for universal ways to measure and assess. Myriad tests exist, too many to examine here with any thoroughness. However, the key points I wish to make can be advanced through the exploration of attempts to measure Aboriginality, personality and intelligence, and the use of two specific instruments, the Minnesota Multiphasic Personality Inventory (MMPI), and the Wechsler Intelligence Scales. I will also use this chapter to introduce and develop further some of the methodological considerations that become increasingly important throughout the rest of the volume, such as the use of blood quantum as a measure of culture, 'culture areas' as sampling frames, and the construction of a singular Aboriginal variable category to facilitate comparative research.

Acculturation and the Conceptualization of Aboriginality

One of the most pressing issues in cross-cultural research is the need to rethink the operationalization of culture, to ask why certain individuals are thought of as being members of a particular cultural group, and how this is determined. In Aboriginal mental health research, two questions are central to this concern: who is 'Aboriginal' for purposes of research, and what does being 'Aboriginal' mean? To date, efforts to operationalize Aboriginality have been haphazard. In the last two chapters we saw how constructions of homogeneity in *the* Aboriginal personality emerged within the scholarly discourse, often against the evidence. It was, of course, the *indigenous* Aboriginal population which was deemed to exhibit similarities, and there was considerable support among scholars for John Honigmann's (1961b: 123–4) assertion that the available evidence 'quite convincingly' suggested 'a high degree of psychological homogeneity' characteristic of '*the* American Indian' (emphasis added). But contact with Europeans, some were willing to admit, had sparked changes. Some Aboriginal individuals were thought to be in the throes of personal cultural change, and appeared to be at greater risk of developing psychopathology because of their liminal social and cultural status. While the issue of 'acculturative stress' will be taken up in chapter 5, I wish to explore here how this liminality has been conceived and measured. There have been many such approaches, some more conceptually sound than others, but all intended to answer Drew Hayden Taylor's question, 'How Native is Native if you're Native?' (Taylor 2000: 57).

The need to determine the cultural orientation of Aboriginal peoples as an essential part of the assessment and treatment process has been identified by many scholars (e.g., Dinges, Trimble, Manson, & Pasquale 1981; Dillard 1983; Trimble & Fleming 1989; Heinrich, Corbine, & Thomas 1990; LaFromboise, Trimble, & Mohatt 1990; Sue & Sue 1990; Herring 1990; Renfrey 1992; Garrett & Garrett 1994; Trimble, Fleming, Beauvais, & Jumper-Thurman 1996), and the adoption of an explicit acculturation framework, especially in psychology, certainly owes an intellectual debt to anthropological theorizing on this concept. Acculturation as an anthropological issue worthy of study emerged in the 1930s (Darnell 2001), and was given scholarly legitimacy by the 'Memorandum on the Study of Acculturation' published in 1936 by Robert Redfield, Ralph Linton and Melville Herscovits. Aboriginal North Americans were to play an important role in the study of acculturative processes, just as they had done in the development of the culture and personality school (Bee 1974).

For most anthropologists engaged in these studies, the unit of analysis was the culture or the community, not the individual, and the idea that groups could be compared along a scale of acculturation sprang from anthropological assertions that cultures in contact represented 'autonomous cultural systems' (Bee 1974: 96). Psychologically oriented research, including that carried out by anthropologists, while focused more on the individual, nevertheless adopted these ideas and gave birth to the notion that individuals, like cultures, could be ranked in terms of their degree of acculturation. Pioneers in the study of individual acculturation were George Spindler and Louise Spindler, who appeared to follow Boas's advice concerning the need to document the relationship between cultural change and personality 'types.' These two anthropologists were among the first to construct categories for the different degrees of cultural orientation hypothesized to exist among Aboriginal peoples, ranging from the 'native-oriented' to the fully acculturated. While the Spindlers' conceptualizations changed over time as they developed their ideas, a brief review of their main points is in order, given the influence they had on subsequent analysts.

In the original formulation, based on a study of Menominee males that utilized the Rorschach test, George Spindler (1955) identified five categories of adaptation to Western culture; these were subsequently employed in a study of Menominee women by Louise Spindler (1962). The key factors in distinguishing the categories were considered to be religious identification and participation. The categories were:

1 Native-oriented. These individuals were members of the Menominee Medicine Lodge or other religious groups and were the least acculturated.
2 Peyote Cult members. These individuals were active members of this religious group, considered to be a variation on the transitional group.
3 Transitional. These individuals were 'in transition,' participating in both Christian and Native-oriented religious activities but without identifying with either.
4 Lower status acculturated. These individuals were Catholic by birth, but their participation in that religion was minimal; they had no involvement with the Native-oriented religious groups.
5 Elite acculturated. These individuals were active Catholics who participated in combined Menominee-white groups.

Focusing primarily on religion greatly limited the integrity of the schema; religion is, after all, only one component of cultural orientation. While subsequent researchers quickly moved away from this focus, they did embrace the idea of 'transitional' individuals.

From this point forward, the measurement of individual Aboriginal acculturation becomes largely the domain of psychologists. How this was done, however, was no less problematic, and the influence of the work of Spindler and Spindler is evident. Joseph Trimble and Candace Fleming (1989: 196), for instance, first identified three 'acculturative styles': 'Many, regardless of age, are traditional and native-oriented; others are transitional in the sense that they reflect an understanding and appreciation of tribal-specific folkways yet recognize the value of internalizing the values and beliefs of the dominant, more progressive culture; and others, whether because of geographic isolation from their ancestral homes or personal choice, have fully internalized the folkways of modern society.' In this conceptualization, personal agency as an important factor in understanding individual acculturation is evident for all but the traditional group: 'Central to determining acculturative status is the extent to which a particular individual is engaged in acculturation. Is it an active or passive process, voluntary or involuntary, subtle or direct? Equally important is the determination of an attitude toward acculturation' (200). There was also a direction imbedded in the schema. Trimble and Fleming labelled their original three categories the 'successfully acculturated,' the 'marginally acculturated,' and the 'moderately traditional.' A fourth group, the 'culturally marginally integrated' was subsequently added and placed third in the sequence from traditional to acculturated (Trimble et al. 1996). This schema suggested that the traditional or native-oriented were anchored to their culture, unlike the others, and that cultural change was only in the direction of the 'dominant, more progressive culture' (i.e., white American society) as opposed to other cultural groups in North America. Perhaps unwittingly, they also seemed to suggest that there was no such thing as a 'successfully' traditional American Indian. Unfortunately, no clear evidence of the empirical basis for these acculturative styles, and no listing of the relevant individual characteristics expected of a member of each category, were presented. The authors stated only that 'a line of open-ended questions' should be employed to determine acculturative status in the areas of education, wage employment, urbanization, media influence, political participation, religion, language, daily life, and social relations. For specific instructions, readers were referred elsewhere (e.g., to Berry, Trimble, & Olmedo 1986). While case studies were presented, a lack of parallel discussion among the cases demonstrates that these ideas were still in their formative stages. For instance, education and employment observations were presented for a successfully acculturated client, but not for either of the moderately traditional clients, suggesting that traditional Indians had no educational or employment issues; similarly, language was referred to in only one case, a moderately traditional female, thereby suggesting that acculturated Indians had no language issues.

LaFromboise et al. (1990: 638) devised another influential acculturation schema, a revision of the original Spindler's framework. This was as follows:

1. Traditional – These individuals generally speak and think in their native [sic] language and know little English. They observe 'old-time' traditions and values.

2. Transitional – These individuals generally speak both English and the Native language in the home. They question basic traditionalism and religion, yet cannot fully accept dominant culture and values.

3. Marginal – These people might be defensively Indian, but are unable either to live the cultural heritage of their tribal group or to identify with the dominant society. This group tends to have the most difficulty in coping with social problems due to their ethnicity.

4. Assimilated – Within this group are the people who, for the most part, have been accepted by the dominant society. They generally have embraced dominant culture and values.

5. Bicultural – These people have, for the most part, been accepted by the dominant society. Yet they also know and accept their tribal traditions and culture. They can thus move in either direction, from traditional society to dominant society, with ease.

Here, language was clearly identified as the marker for traditionality, but acceptance by the dominant society, as in the assimilated category, would not mean that an individual could not speak an Indian language. An individual could meet the criteria for the assimilated category, yet still function effectively in their Indian culture if they chose to do so. This is where the question of individual agency becomes relevant once again, and it seems particularly important only for the bicultural and assimilated categories. The traditionalist is trapped by culture, and the marginal is caught in a perpetual state of maladaptation and dysfunction. In contrast, success, as seen in the cases of the assimilated and bicultural, depends primarily on acceptance by the dominant society. The traditional, assimilated, and bicultural individuals were defined by what they do, while the transitional and marginal individuals were defined by what they failed to do. The equation of the latter statuses with pathology is problematic, as will become clear later in this book. While attempting to convince readers of the utility of their schema for treatment purposes, the authors only confused the picture by presenting the case of an Ojibwa woman whom they categorized as assimilated but then treated for grief by employing traditional Ojibwa beliefs about death and grieving.

Issues of race and cultural authenticity are more prominent in the work of psychologist Laurence French. In an early article, French and Hornbuckle (1972) defined 'Indianism' as 'the degree of ethnic identity internalized by tribal members,' and stated that the majority of Indians, whether on or off the reservation, could be classified as being 'marginal.' At the poles in their 'Indianism continuum' were 'real' or 'traditional' Indians' at one end, and 'white' or 'middle-class' Indians at the other. In subsequent work, French (1979, 1981, 1989) presented a 'social continuum' with 'aboriginal traditionalism' at one pole and 'white assimilated' at the other. According to French, the traditional Indians were also referred to as 'full bloods' (a racial/biological designation), 'real Indians' (a question of authenticity perhaps?), and 'conservatives' (resistant to change?); these confusing appellations were not attributed to specific individuals, however. It was the traditional people who adhered to a 'Harmony Ethic,' and who spoke their Indian language. The 'middle-class' Indians at the other end of the pole subscribed to the 'Protestant Ethic' and were considered to be the most influential. The 'marginal Indians' existed somewhere in between, 'torn between their traditional cultural heritage and the dictates of the larger majority society' (French 1981: 147). 'Marginal Indians,' declared French (1979: 52), 'are those most likely to violate majority norms resulting in arrest, conviction and incarceration' (this idea will be explored further in chapter 5). In effect, while the traditional Indians were defined by culture/biology/political orientation, and the middle-class Indians by social class, the marginals were defined largely by their pathology. A working-class Indian, a traditional person who was middle class, or a bicultural person who was healthy and functioning, was not envisioned in this formulation.

There have been many other attempts to conceptualize Aboriginal acculturation, utilizing a variety of criteria. Zitzow and Estes (1981; cited in Sue & Sue 1990: 180–2), for instance, divided Native Americans into 'heritage consistent' and 'heritage inconsistent' groups. The heritage consistent individual had grown up on the reservation, was actively involved in the extended family and tribal organization, and accepted the values of the tribe; the heritage inconsistent individual eschewed traditional Aboriginal values, sought greater involvement in the social structures of the dominant society, and perhaps even denied his or her Aboriginality. Herring (1989), approaching the issue of acculturation from the perspective of family organization, posited the existence of three types. The first family type was the 'traditional' group, 'which adheres to culturally-defined styles of living'; the second was the 'nontraditional, bicultural group that seems to have adopted many aspects of non-American Native styles'; and the third was the 'pantribal group that overtly struggles to redefine and reconfirm previously lost cultural styles' (1989: 6). This last group is significant, for it represented an effort to categorize the increasingly larger numbers of Aboriginal peoples who were attempting to learn some aspects of Aboriginal culture, be it their own heritage culture or a broader, pan-Indian culture (see also Garrett & Pichette 2000). Locke (1992) came up with a three-group scheme based on 'reactions to white-dominated society,' distinguishing the bicultural, who accepted both cultures; the traditional, who rejected the 'dominant' culture; and the marginal, who accepted the dominant culture. Choney, Berryhill-Paapke, and Robbins (1995), employed a five-category model identifying traditional, transitional, bicultural, assimilated, and marginal individuals. A handful of researchers have developed the idea of biculturality in greater detail, emphasizing the relatively harmonious existence of the individual within two cultures (e.g., LaFromboise & Rowe 1983; Oetting & Beauvais 1990; and Trimble 1992).

What all the schemes I have discussed in this section have in common is a recognized need to explicitly acknowledge that Aboriginal peoples are culturally heterogeneous and that, within the context of the history of colonization, there has been an unequivocal shift towards the cultures of the settler society. Individuals and communities differ in terms of the extent of this shift, but it is imperative that we better comprehend it, and accommodate it in research, if we are to say anything about contemporary Aboriginal peoples. The simple, yet problematic, fact is that there are Aboriginal North American peoples who have no knowledge whatsoever of their heritage cultures or languages, perhaps because they have grown up in non-Aboriginal foster or adoptive homes. For purposes of research, are these individuals sufficiently 'Aboriginal' to be included as such? If Aboriginality is defined primarily as a cultural variable, then these individuals should probably not be included.[1] There are also individuals who are still very traditional, who do not speak English (or any other European language) in any meaningful way, and who have had very little exposure to broader North American culture. And there are, indeed, individuals who are fluent in English and their Aboriginal language, who can operate successfully in two or more distinct cultural arenas. It is also crucial to point out that the recognition of differing degrees of Aboriginality is frequently recognized by Aboriginal peoples themselves. O'Nell (1996), in her study of depression among the Flathead, found that they harbored a conceptualization of 'really Indians,' a traditional standard that no contemporary Flathead could achieve, as well as a sense of who was 'more Indian' and who was 'less Indian.' My research with Aboriginal prison inmates likewise uncovered an understanding of Aboriginality in which both inmates and the elders who worked to heal them recognized differing cultural experiences as an important ingredient in comprehending both an individual's problems and the treatment approach required (Waldram 1997). The recognition that Aboriginality has many dimensions, and that these need to be grasped, is not simply an artifact of scholarly inquiry, but the product of an acute understanding of history and differential experience at the level of both the individual and the community.

How do we account for this cultural complexity in research? 'If we do not assess people's ethnocultural identity,' according to Marsella et al. (2000: 50), 'we cannot know if we are measuring their culture or their ethnic ancestry ... Thus it is important to determine both a person's ethnicity and their degree of identification with their culture.' Schemes have often been crude and ill-conceived, frequently mixing social class, race, and culture, implying individual agency in some cases but not others, and suggesting that, while some individuals were in 'transition,' indicative of a dynamic model of culture, others were anchored to their cultural orientations, suggesting a static model. The question remains, nevertheless, if supplanting a singular, presumed homogeneous group with several sub-groups, also assumed homogeneous, is a more appropriate way of comprehending cultural diversity. If Marsella et al. (2000) are correct, and I believe they are in so far as there remains a commitment to cultural epidemiological research, then it becomes necessary to determine how best to measure individual cultural orientations if anything meaningful is to be said about the role of culture in mental health. It is to this issue I now turn.

Measuring Aboriginal Cultural Orientation

The idea that Aboriginal peoples could demonstrate a variety of cultural orientations ranging from the very traditional, in the Aboriginal sense, to the very assimilated, in the Euro-North American sense, has led to attempts to develop instruments to measure that cultural orientation.[2] The emphasis has frequently been on assessing acculturation and assimilation, although there have also been efforts to assess 'Indianness.' Unfortunately, articles reporting on the use of instruments often fail to include the instruments themselves or to discuss issues of validity and reliability, and we are frequently forced to settle for a general description of the constructs or variables employed. Nevertheless, considerable confusion in conceptualizing culture can be discerned.

Anthropologists engaged in attempts to measure Aboriginal cultural orientation were clearly influenced by the theory and method expressed by acculturation theoreticians and found not only in the 1936 Memorandum but also in a 1954 *American Anthropologist* outline which acknowledged that there could be variability in the degree of commitment to core aspects of a culture, such as values (Summer Seminar on Acculturation 1954). A desire to understand the consequences of contact between cultures guided their efforts, and these anthropologists often sought to measure just how much contact an individual had with a given culture as a kind of proxy measure of cultural orientation. Norman Chance and Nancy Foster (1962) (see also Chance 1965) developed an 'Inter-cultural contact scale' and a 'Western Identification Scale' in their study of North Alaskan Eskimos. The contact scale included items such as knowledge of English, whether the person had ever been hospitalized or employed, and their access to mass media. The identification scale included a preference for Western versus Eskimo foods, a preference for Western clothing, and participation in traditional activities, such as hunting for men or skin sewing for women. Theodore Graves (1967a, 1967b) developed a ten-item 'acculturation index' useful for both Hispanic and American Indian populations in the southwest, which 'seemed to be indicative of voluntary association with the dominant Anglo community and adoption of its symbols, rather than simply minimal accommodation to the requirements of the contact situation' (1967b: 343). In effect, rather than attempting to measure cultural orientation directly, or focusing on the internalization of values, Graves appeared to be measuring the degree of exposure to Anglo-American culture, suggesting that 'exposure, identification, and access are all required for change to occur' (345). Thus his scale included items such as 'Respondent lived in town rather than in the countryside; Respondent owned a TV set; Respondent reported a close Anglo friendship.' Language was also important, however, and two items pertained to the use of English in particular.

Psychologists John Berry and Robert Annis (1974a, 1974b) appeared to be working within a modernization and diffusionist framework when they developed a simple 'ownership scale' for use with James Bay Cree. As Bee (1974) has noted, culture change theorists once accepted that technological change always preceded changes in value systems in culture contact situations, and Berry and Annis appeared to have accepted this truism when they attempted to measure, quite literally, the extent to which a Cree person had 'bought into' Canadian society by purchasing various items and services (Berry, Trimble, & Olmedo 1986). Ranking these purchases from 'low' acculturation to 'high' or extensive acculturation, the list of items consisted of radio, outboard motor, snowmobile, washer, freezer, bank account, and life insurance. At least some of the items – for example, the outboard motor and snowmobile, and perhaps even the radio – represent links to economic activity. The Cree were (and still are) a hunting and fishing people and the purchase of these items might have meant nothing more than the acquisition of necessary, or better, technology. But how such acquisition caused or reflected acculturation was not clearly delineated. More importantly, Berry and Annis also seemed to be using as a benchmark for traditional Cree culture the period just prior to the introduction of these specific items, ignoring the fact that the Cree had been integrated within the Canadian and global economies, especially through the fur trade, for several centuries and therefore had a long history of acquiring European technology. And some of the items included in their list are curious: most Cree communities at the time of Berry and Annis's work did not have running water, making the purchase of washers somewhat problematic, and there were no banks or life insurance agents. The imposition of such externally generated criteria to mark cultural change underscores the problems in assuming that any cultural group will necessarily undergo change in the same way as a more dominant one. Nevertheless, the Aboriginal research of Berry and Annis led them to develop a widely accepted two-dimensional model of acculturation wherein the individual is faced with a decision as to how, and to what extent, to maintain the traditional culture and/ or associate and identify with the majority culture (Berry, Wintrob, Sindell, & Mawhinney 1982). Berry's work allowed scholars to escape the bonds of the earlier, uni-dimensional model that implied a corresponding cultural loss with cultural gain, and therefore facilitated the introduction of notions of biculturality and multiculturality. More recently, Berry (2003) has also emphasized the importance of ethnographic work before the construction of scales, the kind of work that would have been valuable in their early Cree studies.

While attempts to measure acculturation to non-Aboriginal society have seemed to concentrate on the acquisition of material items and services as well as participation in the non-Aboriginal cultural milieu, attempts to measure Aboriginality shifted direction somewhat, and focused more on values and beliefs. But these attempts, too, were problematic. Edwin Richardson (1981), for instance, authored an instrument which he referred to as an 'Indian Culturalization Test.' The test, consisting of twenty-five questions, was designed for Northern Plains peoples, and especially Sioux, and even included Lakota expressions. The empirical base of the test was dubious: according to one description, it 'draws on the knowledge Richardson gained through several years of experience in advising a club for Indian inpatients who met once per week to study and discuss Indian history and traditions' (Uecker, Boutilier, & Richardson 1980: 359). Since most, though not all, club members were Sioux, it was also concluded somewhat tentatively that, despite some ambiguity in questions, 'the scale probably has reasonable content validity for the Sioux and perhaps for other Northern Plains Indians; content validity for all Indians is not claimed' (359).

Uecker et al. (1980: 359) employed the Indian Culturalization Test in a study of the MMPI (to be discussed in the next section). Compatible with Richardson's view that there were many universal American Indian values, the intent appears to have been to develop an Indian Culture Quotient (ICQ) which would then be employed in 'determining how much the Indian Value System will affect scores on other tests' that they planned to use. The test attempted to assess language utilization, values and behaviours, and attitudes, but it was fraught with methodological problems that betrayed a weak understanding of Lakota Sioux culture. In item 7 for instance, subjects were requested to select the most applicable response from among these three:

a. I believe in bad medicine.
b. Bad medicine scares me.
c. Bad medicine is evil.

All three are interrelated components of the belief in bad medicine, a kind of sorcery, and it is not clear how one of these choices could somehow indicate greater Indian orientation in comparison to the others. Another question asked if the person had been pierced during the Sun Dance, but the remaining two options in the question asked if they felt or were immune to pain. A question on alcohol use only posited problem consumption as options: the subject was either a problem drinker not in AA, an alcoholic in AA, or a non-drinker. There was no middle ground, no problem-free social drinking. The ICQ developed from this instrument would have been largely meaningless even for the Lakota subjects for whom it was designed.

Joseph Westermeyer and colleagues (e.g., Westermeyer & Neider 1985) developed a ten-item 'Indian Culture Scale' for their research among American Indian alcoholic clients in Minnesota. They used a three-point scale, and the items ranged from language comprehension to contact with Indian family and friends to engagement in activities deemed to be 'Indian.' These latter included attendance at powwows, ricing, beading, and practising 'Indian' religion. This was an attempt to devise an instrument that could be used on any American Indian mental health patient, although they made specific reference to Chippewa and Sioux in their article.

A more complex attempt to measure culture was made by Hoffman, Dana, and Bolton (1985), who developed an acculturation instrument for use with Lakota individuals in order to test the validity of the MMPI-168. Working with thirty-seven male and thirty-two females from the Rosebud Lakota Sioux reservation in South Dakota, they developed their instrument after extensive examination of existing literature on the topic, the testing of a preliminary version in the community, and the use of a battery of tests to determine local norms (see Dana, Hornby, & Hoffman 1984). Several components of acculturation were identified, which once again demonstrated a mixing of racial/ biological criteria with cultural; these included 'language usage, value orientation, social behavior and customs, social interaction network, religious affiliation and practices, community of residence, occupational status, formal educational attainment, identification with traditional culture, and ancestry or blood quantum' (Hoffman et al. 1985: 245). These criteria were then reduced to 'five dimensions of Native American acculturation,' or subscales, through statistical analysis: 'social behavior, social membership, and social activities; value orientation and cultural attitudes; blood quantum; language preference and usage; and educational and occupational status.' Sack, Beiser, Clarke, and Redshirt (1987) also adopted a more complex approach by employing three measures, again for use with Sioux people. The first simply attempted to determine the language spoken in the home. The second was a 'traditionality' scale developed in consultation with a local community panel, and included, for example, the use of or preference for certain traditional Sioux items (e.g.,'I pick wild berries,' and

'I use tobacco to give thanks'). This scale was based on the two-dimensional model of Berry and Annis (1974a, 1974b). The third scale was based on what they referred to as 'Berry statements,' from the work of John Berry. Five statements were presented and respondents were asked to select the options with which they most and least agreed. As an example, consider the following options:

A. It is better for Indians to stay on their reservation/reserves, than to come to the city.
B. Indians should be able to live happily either on a reservation/reserve or in a city.
C. Indians should move off the reservation/reserve to the city to get ahead in this world. (46)

It was not made clear, however, why expressions of a kind of isolationist sentiment represented greater 'Indianness.' I have certainly known some very traditional, frequently aged, Aboriginal individuals, some of whom had never been off the reserve, who believed that the future for their children and grandchildren was best found in the city.

Mohatt and Blue (1982) also developed a scale for use with Lakota people, but these authors' innovative approach sought to categorize whole communities. Employing the Lakota concept of *tiospaye*, which describes a community's way of life, and in particular its traditionality, the researchers worked closely with Lakota 'cultural experts' to identify appropriate scale items. Once the scales were ready, community experts (mostly older individuals) were selected from the twenty-one eligible Lakota communities, who then used the instrument to score the communities. There were, in all, four, all of which employed a five-point Likert scales ranging from 'majority' to 'none.' The first scale, 'Balance,' scale included statements about family and community relations, such as: 'If conflict occurs, the persons and families involved are brought together and advised by an elder'; and 'Very commonly, people share food with relatives and others in the community.' The second scale, 'Rural,' related to an agrarian, rural subsistence economy. A representative statement was, 'Most residents have horses to ride.' The third scale, 'Spiritual,' related to spiritual and linguistic practices: 'The people speak Lakota.' The final scale was 'Interpersonal,' and included such statements as, 'In the *Tiospaye*, the people have chosen the leader.'

This was a radical approach given the individualistic nature of other research on this topic, but Mohatt and Blue believed it to be more compatible with how the Lakota viewed culture. The utilization of so-called culture experts was, of course, pioneered by ethnographers, who singled out particularly congenial 'key informants' to provide them with an insider's view of the culture under study. But the idea of a culture expert diverges from that of key informant in that the former appears to privilege the views of a kind of cultural elite and reinforces a conception of culture as official doctrine. Unlike the ethnographer who sought to record cultural material, Mohatt and Blue intended to construct a cultural baseline against which communities were to be compared and ranked. One can certainly question the very existence of culture 'experts,' as opposed to individuals with acknowledged domain-specific knowledge. The notion of 'culture expert' in fact appears from time to time elsewhere in the literature, and rarely is it clear what the term means or exactly who qualifies as such an expert. Further, not all individuals would be representative of their community's formal traditionality ranking. In other words, this approach, like so many others, sought to overgeneralize and perpetuate notions of cultural homogeneity at the expense of comprehending diversity.

Instruments that attempt to measure Aboriginal cultural orientation in terms of 'Indianness' should be firmly anchored in specific cultures; to this end, Mohatt and Blue (1982) and Sack et al. (1987) represent some of the best efforts in their utilization of Lakota cultural experts in the framing of instruments. But Morris, Crowley, and Morris's (2002) employment of Southwestern Indian community data from the Flower of Two Soils project of Sack et al. (1987) is particularly noteworthy for its statistical sophistication and underscores the point that the cultural content of any scale must be tied to a specific cultural context. The possbility of stereotyping and even essentializing Aboriginal cultures, however, remains, particularly since scale items typically include statements of official cultural knowledge determined by select individuals to represent traditionality, and in so doing erase cultural diversity. Some (especially anthropologists) suggest that any effort to 'measure' a culture is too fraught with both methodological and conceptual difficulties, and is inherently essentialist. I agree with this view up to a point, but would argue that there is a circumscribed role for such attempts. Richardson's view that the cultural orientation of an American Indian would affect scores on various psychological tests is a legitimate concern, even if his early attempt to design an instrument was misguided.

Attempts to measure the culture of Aboriginal individuals have differed substantially over the years. Some instruments have attempted to measure how 'Indian' individuals are by probing language use and traditional activities. Others have considered, if not focused on, the issue of acculturation and attempted to measure acceptance of or involvement in Euro-North American culture. Some instruments have concentrated on identifying preferences, but methodological complications are inherent in these attempts, especially since preferences are not necessarily a reflection of actual beliefs, knowledge, or practice. But the measurement of actual knowledge and practices has almost always been based on self-report, which is equally problematic. Some authors have reported the use of single, often very crude instruments, whereas others have employed several different instruments or techniques to get a sense of the cultural orientation of individuals. A multi-instrument approach is clearly the most effective. The intent of the measurement exercise also varies; some have sought to measure or assess individuals to facilitate diagnosis and treatment, whereas others have been interested in determining the cultural appropriateness of instruments such as the MMPI and Wechsler, discussed below. But the use of instruments in general promotes a view of cultures as the sum of various, specific, and easily identifiable traits, a marriage perhaps between the diffusionism of the anthropologists and the psychometrics of the psychologists. Conceptually, knowledge of a particular cultural trait (especially as it might be tested for on an instrument) is different from that trait having some personal, reified meaning for a culture member. And invoking the trait, say by practising rice harvesting, does not mean that one understands it in a culturally particular or meaningful way. One can certainly speak a language without having any personal or experiential knowledge of the cultures that speak that language. Similarly one may engage in a sweetgrass prayer ceremony in an effort to demarcate an Aboriginal identity in a predominantly non-Aboriginal environment while paying absolutely no attention to the meaning of the ceremony within its cultural context (Waldram 1997). Certainly almost all studies fall victim to a 'two cultures' model of North American society, that is, that one is either Aboriginal, Euro-North American, or somewhere in between these two, and further that these labels somehow represent intrinsically meaningful cultural groups. Invisible is any attempt to measure orientation to several different cultures, including different Aboriginal cultures as well as, say, American Hispanic cultures. And Aboriginality, in so far as it is measured in these efforts, is clearly linked to an on-reserve, ages-old, and possibly non-existent cultural orientation that conveniently ignores several centuries of cultural contact through colonization.

Measuring Aboriginal Personality: The Minnesota Multiphasic Personality Inventory

In some ways, measuring Aboriginality remained largely marginal to other, more immediate tasks, such as the assessment of personality. Many tests have been devised over the years to assess personality, and these in turn have been applied to North American Aboriginal peoples. These tests are too numerous to examine in any depth here.[3] Rather, I will focus on the most commonly used personality assessment tool, the Minnesota Multiphasic Personality Inventory (MMPI). Anthropologists, clearly uncomfortable with the use of such structured instruments, have left this field largely to the psychologists, and the fieldwork site has been replaced by the lab.

The MMPI was developed in the 1930s from research with Minnesota patients hospitalized with mental disorders and the supposedly normal people, friends and family, who came to visit them (Greene 1987; Hunt 1993). It was a large instrument, with some 550 statements, although smaller versions have often been employed (e.g., Hoffman et al. 1985). The respondent was asked to answer 'yes,' 'no,' or 'uncertain' to statements such as 'I am happy most of the time' and 'I am certainly lacking in self-confidence.' Some items are grouped into clinical subscales designed to measure more specific personality characteristics, such as depression, hysteria, schizophrenia, and psychopathic deviancy, while others are designed to assess the validity of the test (Duckworth & Anderson 1994). While the instrument appears on the surface to be more concerned with deviance and psychopathology, and indeed was originally intended for use in diagnosing psychiatric patients, it was also designed to elicit traits of normal personality. Since its inception, there has been a great deal of controversy regarding the appropriateness of the MMPI for non-whites, and much work has been done comparing scores for white respondents with those of African- and Mexican-Americans in particular (Bertelson, Marks, & May 1982; Butcher, Braswell, & Raney 1983; Hoffman et al. 1985; Greene 1987). The use of the yes/no format has proven problematic in cross-cultural research where local populations are unaccustomed to thinking in such absolute, rather than context-specific, terms (Marsella et al. 2000). While much less work has considered the appropriateness of the MMPI for

North American Aboriginal peoples, a sufficient body of data exists to support the contention that it is the most widely used assessment instrument with this population, as indeed it is with the U.S. population in general (Dana 1986; Allen 1998; Butcher, Nezami, & Exner 1998).

Conceptualizing Aboriginality has remained a consistent problem in the use of the MMPI, and the question of who is in fact 'Aboriginal' has been muddied considerably. Grace Arthur (1944), the designer of several tests employed as part of the Indian Education Research project described in chapter 2, was a pioneer in the use of the MMPI; her work inadvertently demonstrated early in MMPI history how an unproblematized understanding of the various dimensions of Aboriginality could affect the interpretation of the test results. Arthur tested eighty boys and girls from twenty-six different tribes using an unstandardized version of the instrument. Comparing their scores with those of University of Minnesota undergraduates, she was surprised at the Indian's good emotional adjustment, noting that the university students demonstrated more of a tendency towards hysteria than did the Indians, contrary to her hypothesis. While she acknowledged that the Indian participants came from many different tribal backgrounds, she did not explore the potential ramifications of this fact, nor did she discuss the possible role of culture in the administration and interpretation of the test, omissions which would become characteristic of much MMPI research (Allen 1998). Her references to culture implicitly confused it with race, thus she described some of her subjects as 'full-blood' and others as 'less than one-half Indian blood' (Arthur 1944: 245). This tendency, it seems, has also been a ubiquitous problem.

As the use of the MMPI for Aboriginal peoples accelerated in the 1960s, corresponding to a waning in the use of projective tests, conceptual problems continued.[4] Herreid and Herreid (1966), for instance, studied a group of ninety-one Eskimos, Aleuts, and Indians at the University of Alaska, and compared them with a hundred non-Aboriginal students. Although the three Alaska Native groups were examined both together as a single category and then as separate categories, there was no indication that the researchers understood the differences among them. Overall, they largely ignored the uniqueness of the three groups and concluded that '*the* Alaskan native appears more deviant than the Alaskan nonnative and considerably more deviant than the United States college population elsewhere' (196; emphasis added). The authors cautioned that differential English language skills might explain the difference and hinted that cultural differences might also be operative. Such cautions are endemic in the MMPI literature. Cross-cultural studies frequently disclose that the instrument has not been properly validated with the population under study, yet generalized comments on the Aboriginal personality, frequently negative, are offered anyway. Kline, Rozynko, Flint, and Roberts (1973: 730) stressed this very problem in a study of thirty-three unspecified 'native American' alcoholics, but still concluded that they were 'seriously disturbed.' Mandelzys and Lane (1980), in a study of ninety-five Canadian Native prison inmates, concluded that there was considerable doubt as to the validity of the MMPI for Native inmates, and that it was likely that they either did not fully understand the test items or else understood them in a different way, yet they nevertheless noted that these individuals exhibited a significant degree of psychopathology and emotional disturbance.

The problem of conceptualizing culture is clearly demonstrated in a frequently referenced work by Pollack and Shore (1980). In an attempt to determine the validity of the MMPI for Indians in the Portland area, they undertook tests with 142 mental health patients from 'three distinct cultures: Northwest Coastal, Plateau, and Plains' (947) (properly speaking, these are 'culture areas' and not 'cultures'). Overall, the group demonstrated a 'significant amount of pathology' (948). The authors were impressed with the similarity among all the profiles generated, and noted that while there were a few scale differences between individuals from the Plains culture and those from the other two, there were no significant differences between individuals from the Coastal and the Plateau cultures. They concluded that this similarity was due to 'a significant cultural influence on the results of the MMPI in this population of American Indians' and that *cultural influence overrides individual pathology and personality differences* in influencing the pattern of the MMPI' (Pollack and Shore 1980: 948; emphasis added). Manson, Walker and Kivlahan (1987: 169) agreed with Pollack and Shore, suggesting that 'cultural factors may mask psychopathological variation among American Indians.' But what specifically is this 'cultural influence' that Shore et al. mention? Is it based on uniform Aboriginal cultural traits across the three different culture areas? Does it refer to the homogenizing effects of European colonization on three distinct cultures? Or does it suggest an emerging pan-Indianism? We are not told. These authors also provided no information about the 'culture' of the patients, other than the broad cultural labels of the culture-area concept (to be discussed in detail shortly). We do not actually learn anything of the culture of the specific individuals in this study, nor do we know how they were placed within these cultural groups. It is simply not possible to assess the importance of any 'cultural influence' without some discussion of the actual culture(s) in question.

As noted in the previous section, Uecker et al. (1980) attempted to incorporate an understanding of Aboriginal culture, comparing 45 mostly Sioux alcoholics (anyone claiming at least 'one-quarter' blood quantum) with 111 white alcoholics. Using the Indian Culturalization Test to compute an Indian Culture Quotient (ICQ) (a problematic instrument, you will recall), statistical analysis determined that there were significant correlations between four MMPI scales and the ICQ and that the Indians were slightly less likely than the whites to show signs of psychiatric disorders. Furthermore, it was determined that the main disorder experienced by Indians, 'neuroticism,' was significantly related to identification with Indian heritage, that is, their scores on the Culturalization Test. Echoing early psychoanalytic perspectives, it was determined that the more Indian the subject was, the more neurotic. The authors concluded that, 'It seems quite probable that the Indians who identified most strongly with their Indian culture were exposed to non-Indian culture just as much as the other Indians were but that they experienced more conflict between their need to retain their Indian identity and their need to adjust to the dominant culture' (361). Nevertheless, like many others, they noted that the MMPI had not been validated for use with this population, describing its use in alcohol treatment as a 'questionable practice' (ibid.).

Approaching the issue of culture from somewhat different angles has not been successful either. Page and Bozlee (1982) attempted to account for culture in their comparative study of 'Caucasian,' 'Hispanic American,' and American Indian alcoholics by selecting subjects from a veterans medical centre, assuming that common military experience represented a similar process of acculturation even when the original cultures were different. Butcher et al. (1983) included American Indians in their comparative study of black and white psychiatric in-patient populations in Minnesota, to determine if the common minority status of the black and American Indian populations would result in similar MMPI profiles. In neither case were the actual tribal affiliations of the Indians noted, nor was justification provided for how 'Caucasian' or 'Black' could be considered cultural groups.

In a more sophisticated treatment of culture, Hoffman et al. (1985: 244) set out to test the hypothesis that 'adult Native Americans who

are less well-acculturated have elevated MMPI profiles.' An acculturation instrument, described in the previous section, was employed
along with the MMPI-168, an abbreviated version of the test which the
researchers suggested was ideal for a population that was 'apathetic'
towards non-Native researchers and which could have problems reading English (246). The analysis determined that the subjects had elevated F scores, possibly indicative of higher levels of psychopathology
(an observation commonly found with minorities).[5] But in a somewhat
unique effort to understand the appropriateness of the F-scale for this
population, the researchers consulted an anthropologist, who advised
that several F scale items, while suggestive of deviance, were consistent with Lakota culture, and that several other items might be
endorsed by subjects because of the difficult social and economic situation on the reservation. This consultation represented an important
step towards appreciating how local norms could distort MMPI
results. Overall, the researchers concluded that social acculturation
and blood quantum were considerably less important than the relationship between education/occupation and the MMPI clinical scales.
While the authors noted that the acculturation scale measuring values
was significantly correlated with six of the MMPI-168 scales, 'educa-
tion/occupation had the largest number of significant correlations
with clinical scales of all the acculturation dimensions' (253), lending
support to the idea that socio-economic status might be more important than the other factors in comprehending both Indian acculturation
and performance on the MMPI-168. Simply put, those Indians with
higher formal education and occupations 'endorsed fewer MMPI-168
items indicative of depression, agitation, feelings of inadequacy, withdrawal and nonparticipation, and impulsive acting out' (252–3). Language usage was correlated with five clinical scales for women (none
for men) leading to the conclusion that 'women who prefer to speak
and think in their native language are more group-oriented, sociable
and open, and naive and uninsightful, but characterized by depression, agitation, and self-derogation' (252). Their grand conclusion, that
acculturation, and especially education/occupation, affected MMPI-
168 scores represents one of the most significant findings associated
with the psychometric study of Aboriginal North Americans, even if
the method for assessing acculturation was problematic.

While it is true that the MMPI can be used in assessing 'normal' personality characteristics, in the Aboriginal health literature there is virtually no evidence of its use in this manner. Emphasis in almost every

instance has been on the identification of psychopathology, with Aboriginal study populations compared to non-Aboriginal sample norms. Only a few researchers (e.g., Greene 1987; Allen 1998) have argued that most MMPI studies (and I would say this is true of many other types of studies) employ an inadequate understanding of culture, often problematically equating self-identity or race with cultural orientation. Appeals to dubious New Age literature as sources of authority on *the* Aboriginal, as in the case of Hall and Phung's (2001) use of Jamake Highwater's much-maligned work, simply reinforce the feeling that contemporary Aboriginal cultural reality is not well understood. Allen (1998) argued that most studies are predicated on the assumption that American Indians can be viewed as culturally homogeneous unless proven otherwise, and suggested that this be reversed so that an assumption of cultural heterogeneity guides research. My review of MMPI studies to date largely supports this recommendation. Further evidence of the problem of implicit homogeneity exists in the form of the MMPI-2, revised in the early 1980s. In an effort to generate a normative sample more reflective of American society as a whole, the designers utilized the 1980 census to target subjects from five groups: 'Asian,' 'Black,' 'Hispanic,' 'White,' and 'Native American' (Hathaway and McKinley 1989). It was deemed necessary to sample Native Americans disproportionately relative to their proportion in the United States as whole; whereas they constituted just 0.5 per cent of the national population according to the census, their sample comprised roughly 3 per cent of the 1600 subjects drawn. Who were these 'Native Americans?' All seventy-seven were from Washington state, and fifty-seven came from a single, unidentified reservation near Tacoma. In so far as the MMPI-2 is culturally normative for Native Americans, they must all look like the Washington seventy-seven – yet we do not actually know what these seventy-seven individuals looked like.

The Confusion of Race and Culture in the Measurement of Aboriginal Intelligence

Notions of race and culture have been intertwined for several centuries, and the euphemistic nature of these concepts persists as a troublesome legacy of poorly conceptualized past research (Kuper 1999). Anthropology can be fully implicated in this confusion (Darnell 2001), although it is clear that the broad evolutionary ideas of race often attributed to early anthropology were in fact fuelled by Victorian sentiments and developments in other fields, and embraced within what has subsequently become known as Social Darwinism. While culture was seen as characteristic of the advanced, Western populations, within this evolutionary framework the Barbarian 'primitives' were viewed as anchored by essential biological characteristics in their behaviour; they had yet to fully escape the bonds of biology to become complete cultural humans, and remained creatures of 'nature' (Littlewood 2000). Whether they could ascend to culture and attain the same refined, intellectual capacity as Europeans was debatable in some quarters.

The measurement of intelligence has long been associated with the measurement of personality, and a belief that Aboriginal North Americans were both personality disordered and less intelligent than Europeans has existed for several centuries. Race plays a prominent role in this discourse. Some nineteenth century anthropologists espoused the idea of racial polygenism, that races were in fact separate species, and set about the task of developing the field of phrenology, the measurement of skull shape and cranial capacity (Erickson & Murphy 1998). One of these was S.G. Morton, who, in *Crania Americana*, subtitled '*or a comparative view of the skulls of various aboriginal nations of North and South America*' (1839) explored the issue of intelligence. Combining bad theory, problematic measurement, and a bias against Indians (see Gould 1996), Morton constructed data that demonstrated what he already took to be true, that the brain size, and intelligence, of Europeans was greater. His assessment of the Greenlandic 'esquimaux' was hardly flattering and exhibited a perspective that extended far beyond, but certainly reflected, his interest in cranial capacity: 'They are crafty, sensual, ungrateful. Obstinate and unfeeling, and much of their affection for their children may be traced to purely selfish motives. They devour the most disgusting aliments uncooked and uncleaned, and seem to have no ideas beyond providing for the present moment ... Their mental faculties, from infancy to old age, present a continued childhood ... In gluttony, selfishness and ingratitude, they are perhaps unequalled by any other nation of "people"' (Morton 1839: 54; cited in Gould 1996: 88). In 1922, Pearce Bailey compared African American and American Indians in equally disdainful terms: 'From the statistics which relate to the two so-called primitive races, the African and the American Indian, it appears that the primitive could not under any present circumstances attain the average intelligence of cultured races. This appears to be so, not because there is any detailed information as to the potentiality of the primitive mind, but because mental deficiency is so profusely distributed among Africans and American Indians that their average intelligence must be inferior to that of average European intelligence' (Bailey 1922: 188). The a priori judgment of Aboriginal North Americans, and indeed all 'primitive' peoples, as intellectually inferior remains central to much of the discourse.

Early tests of intelligence were often focused on the relationship between intelligence and race (a common theme which still plagues us today) and conceptualized in terms of blood quantum (e.g., Terman 1916; Garth 1921a, 1922, 1923, 1925, 1927; Fitzgerald & Ludeman 1926; Garth, Smith, & Abell 1928).[6] Simply put, some scholars hypothesized that the intelligence of Indians would improve proportionate to the amount of 'white' blood they had, a racist line of inquiry by current standards but perhaps the precursor to contemporary concern with blood quantum. The logic was simple, if convoluted, because it was not always merely a question of having white blood; the 'quality' of that white blood was also important. Issues of authenticity loom large. Hunter and Sommermier (1922: 258; emphasis added) for instance, referring to Indians attending an elite educational institute, stated 'it is probable that the full bloods [at the school] represent the best type of *pure* Indian, the lower types being content to remain at home or in res-ervation schools.' These gifted students, he suggested, demonstrated 'the presence of initiative and the desire to progress' despite their being full-blood. The 'quarter bloods' at the school, in contrast, did 'not represent the best of their grade,' since 'the more alert and ambi-tious near-whites will find their way in the world' without special schools. The problem, they suggested, was 'that the white blood present in the various hybrids is of a low grade,' although, they quali-fied, there was no evidence of 'negro blood' (259).[7] Fitzgerald and Ludeman (1926: 319) expressed both the historic and yet persistent sentiment behind the issue when they posed what to them was a genu-ine scientific question: 'Is the Indian, tested with the white man's tools, and in his language, handicapped to an appreciable extent, or is the Indian truly inferior to the white in intelligence?' Their conclusion, based on a study of just eighty-three Indian students from unspecified cultures in South Dakota and Nebraska, was that 'there seems to be a slight decrease in intelligence as the percentage of Indian blood increases' (327), although they cautioned that this might well be due to the effects of the language barrier.

The conceptualization of race in these early studies was obviously problematic. The supposed link between something as amorphic as degree of Indian blood and intelligence was never clearly spelled out. Blood quantum itself was often determined by self-declaration and genealogical work; interestingly, studies of this type tended not to challenge the contrasting 'white' category, and we are given little information as to how 'whiteness' was measured or how individuals were slotted into this category. Looking back on it now, of course, the whole concept of degree of bloodedness seems ridiculous, and it was clearly built upon racist assumptions. The focus on race, moreover, often blinded researchers to other factors that, in theory, should have been of greater interest, such as the language bias of intelligence tests.

Confusion and lack of clarity in the use of race and culture is not simply a legacy of the past, however. The very contemporary Wechsler series of intelligence tests demonstrates the persistence of that confusion quite well.[8] The Wechsler is actually several tests designed for different age groups: one for pre-schoolers (WPPSI), one for school children (WISC), and one for adults (WAIS). Perhaps the intelligence tests used most with Aboriginal peoples, and especially children, the tests are composed of both verbal and performance scales. They have also been revised over the years; for instance, the WISC has transformed into the WISC-R (revised) and, most recently, the WISC-III (third edition). The changes from version to version, while significant to psychometricians, are not terribly important to us here.[9]

Use of the WAIS and WISC has generally supported the conclusions determined from other tests that Aboriginal peoples score better on the performance aspects than on the verbal aspects of the tests, and that the verbal scores in particular are often significantly below that of the normative sample upon whom the test was originally based (the 1970 U.S. census) (Howell, Evans, & Downing 1958; Cundick 1970; Sachs 1974; Hynd, Quackenbush, Kramer, Conner, & Weed 1979; McShane 1980; McShane & Plas 1982a, 1982b; Mishra & Lord 1982; Browne 1984; McCullough, Walker, & Diessner 1985; Wilgosh, Mulcahy, & Watters 1986; Sack et al. 1987; Common & Frost 1988; Tempest & Skipper 1988; Plank 2001). One researcher, Plank (2001), has even suggested that these instruments actually deflate Aboriginal performance scores. Explanations for the difference between performance and verbal scores vary. Howell et al. (1958) supported a cultural explanation in their study of Navajo adults, surmising that either there was something in the 'cultural patterning' of the Navajo that made them good at performance tests, or that some of these tests may simply have tapped aspects of intelligence that were not affected by culture. Browne (1984:

3) suggested that the performance aspects, especially picture completion, were evidence of 'relatively greater strength in relational, holistic, right hemisphere information processing,' itself the product of cultural influences. McCullough, Walker and Diessner (1985: 27) speculated simply that the verbal scale might not be assessing verbal abilities at all, 'but rather some cultural differences in knowledge acquisition,' without offering any thoughts on what these cultural differences might be. Tempest and Skipper (1988) suggested that Navajo mothers were more likely to stimulate their children visually than auditorily. Sack et al. (1987) noted that lower functioning Sioux children demonstrated a greater gap between verbal and performance scores as measured by the WISC-R, and argued that these students tended to come from homes where the Sioux language was spoken, where the child's parents were more traditional, and where there was a greater likelihood of a single parent on welfare. McShane (1980) and Dana (1984) reiterated a theory that the environmental adaptation of American Indians resulted in less valuation of verbal ability and an emphasis on performance, although McShane (1980) also suggested that difficult life experiences, such as large family size and absence of fathers among the Navajo, might mean that parents had less time to verbally interact with children. In contrast, Gaddes, McKenzie, and Barnsley (1968), in a study of Salish and Kwakiutl children, tested the hypothesis that the Indian children would do better than White children on those WISC scales which measured spatial imagery. This hypothesis, based on the theory that these Indian children would perform better because of the unique geometric forms of art associated with northwest coastal Indians, was rejected. Cundick (1970) speculated that the failure of some school-age Indian children in the southwest to show improvements in verbal scores on the WISC and WPPSI over a two year period might have been the result of increasing difficulty in the curriculum, including language use, but concluded that it might also be the product of some 'self-fulfilling prophecy' (155). Perhaps the failure was attributed to their traditional cultures, which dampened their achievement motivation in academic endeavours, as Havighurst (1957) suggested.

Few studies have seen the sub-standard performance of Aboriginal peoples on the verbal aspects of the Wechsler as the product either of the fact that some were being tested in their second language, English, or had experienced a deficient English-language-based formal education (schools for Aboriginal peoples have been uniformly terrible for much of their history). It is indeed perplexing that verbally oriented intelligence tests have generally been assumed to be immune from the vagaries of language proficiency, especially where subjects' use of English is non-standard, or even non-existent (Bracken & McCallum 2001). The language problem experienced in assessing the intelligence of Canadian Inuit children, the majority of whom spoke their Aboriginal language, Inuktitut, as a first language, was evident in a study by Wilgosh, Mulcahy, & Walters (1986). In the 'Flower of Two Soils' project, one of the most comprehensive longitudinal studies on Aboriginal abilities and mental health yet undertaken (involving over 700 children from several different parts of Canada and the United States), the researchers were able to identify a gradient in test performance, with children from those Aboriginal communities where English-language acquisition was slower (many beginning to learn English only once they started school) scoring lower in IQ than those from areas where, for historical reasons, English was more predominant (Beiser & Gotowiec 2000). English-language ability, quite logically, was related to performance on an English language intelligence test, and Beiser and Gotowiec (2000) determined that where differences in English language skills could be accounted for, differences in IQ scores between Indian and non-Indian subjects as measured by the Wechsler became statistically insignificant, providing strong evidence as to the role of language proficiency. Hynd and Garcia (1979) pointed out that the issue was not easily addressed by translating the instrument, as American Indian languages were not directly comparable; for instance, 'alphabet,' which appears on the WISC-R, would be difficult to translate into languages which were entirely oral. These authors also suggested the possibility that the whole testing experience itself could be so foreign to American Indian children as to transgress local cultural norms, such as the emphasis placed by some cultures on reticent behaviour and on taking one's time to complete tasks (see also McShane 1980; Dana 1984).[10] Tempest (1998) appeared to touch upon these issues in research which demonstrated that urban Navajo students obtained higher verbal scores on the WISC-III than rural Navajo students, and that those proficient in English scored higher than those who were less so. Some authors (e.g., McShane 1980; McShane & Plas 1982a; Tempest & Skipper 1988) have also noted the relatively higher prevalence of middle-ear infections and hearing loss among American Indian children, which could in part explain lagging verbal ability in the use of English as a second language. Plank (2001) addressed the issue of language competence directly in describing American Indian children as 'Limited English Proficient,' and argued that the Wechsler tests seriously disadvantaged these individuals. Like many such assertions, however, an assumption that American Indians, almost by definition, were deficient in English language skills appeared to lead to a lack of problematization of language ability more broadly, specifically consideration of how to determine when an individual is *not* 'limited English proficient.'

The lack of culture 'fairness' in the test has also been suggested, as evidenced in questions such as 'who discovered America,' which McShane (1980: 5–6) noted might 'create undue levels of conflict and confusion,' (Of course, American Indian children are also likely to know the 'correct' answer because of their formal education; is this item a test of knowledge or of agreement with that knowledge?). Mishra (1982), in a statistical (not content) study of item bias in the WISC-R for a group of Navajo, concluded otherwise, suggesting that the majority of items were, in fact, free from cultural bias. The debate concerning the cross-cultural validity of scale items continues (Plank 2001).

There are, of course, indigenous understandings of intelligence and cognitive competence which do not reflect the kinds of abilities or knowledge tested by intelligence and personality instruments, notwithstanding that some researchers have taken the important step of consulting with Aboriginal peoples while designing their instruments. Cultural norms elicited for the purpose of quantification and measurement cannot help but be distorted from their in situ meaning. Indigenous conceptualizations, in contrast, tend to define what types of knowledge and behaviour are necessary to function in an acceptable manner within specific cultures (Berry & Bennett 1992; Stern 1999). Clearly, differing degrees of competency in various fields are readily acknowledged by culture members. An expert Inuit hunter will be lauded for his skills at survival and tracking animals, for instance, skills and knowledge which will not show up readily on tests. Similarly, the courtroom skills demonstrated by an Aboriginal lawyer in a land claim case will also be celebrated, a fact which confounds those who see indigenous knowledge and skills as oriented only to the past. Relatively little research has been undertaken in this area, however.

Constructing the Aboriginal Variable

The perceived need to measure Aboriginality and to employ an Aboriginal variable in comparative research highlights several ubiquitous methodological problems. A fundamental flaw in much of the MMPI and Wechsler research, as well as other research on personality and intelligence, is bound to the way in which subjects have been identified and categorized for comparative purposes. While over time blood quantum becomes less important in U.S.-based studies, it does not disappear altogether.[11] In addition to occasionally being employed as part of the assessment of cultural orientation by some researchers, it becomes a covert criteria for designation in the Aboriginal research category by virtue of the fact that many American Indian tribes and Canadian First Nations use blood quantum to determine tribal membership, and membership lists are a common sampling frame in research. Even here, tribes demonstrate very different definitions of what constitutes a sufficient amount of Indian blood for enrolment (Norton & Manson 1996), and notions of bloodedness are often submerged within discourses of heritage and genealogy.

Other, somewhat antiquated methods have also been, and continue to be, employed in generating the 'Aboriginal' variable. A good example is the use of 'culture areas' as sampling frames. The idea of culture areas emerged out of the diffusionist studies of the early Boasians, and its genesis has been linked to anthropologists Edward Sapir and Clark Wissler around 1916 or 1917 (Harris 1968; Bee 1974). It was fully developed by anthropologists such as Alfred Kroeber (1939) and, later, Harold Driver (1969), who devised schema dividing Aboriginal North America into discrete zones or areas, predicated on the assumption that individuals and groups within each area would demonstrate significant cultural similarities with other individuals and groups in the same area, and significant dissimilarities with those in other areas. In its heyday, the culture area concept was primarily trait-based, focusing on material culture and economic and social practices, but not on intellectual or cognitive abilities. At best, culture areas were an attempt to understand the ecological adaptations of Aboriginal cultures and the diffusion of cultural traits through systematic categorization, but the emphasis was on identifying *Aboriginal* traits. While Kroeber was interested in delimiting the boundaries of cultures to facilitate comparison as whole entities (Darnell 2001), Driver (1969: 17) subsequently cautioned that his seventeen North American culture areas were only a 'convenient framework' for organizing the immense cultural diversity of Aboriginal peoples, and that the boundaries between areas were not rigid markers of cultural difference, but rather zones of transition and blending. But this is not how scholars have generally seen them. The culture area concept effectively served to cement dynamic cultures into static, physically and temporally bounded categories from which there was seemingly no escape, since the categories are still in evidence today. While acknowledging that the cultures were inherently ecologically based, advocates of the culture area concept largely ignored how these cultures were constantly changing as a result of ecological alterations, such as the arrival of Europeans and European technology.

The use of culture areas in anthropological research is infrequent these days, although they occasionally appear in textbooks on Aboriginal North American peoples (e.g., McMillan 1995; Morrison & Wilson 1995; Waldram, Herring, & Young 1995). While Green (1999: 232) recently suggested that culture areas represent conceptual distinctions that are 'remembered' by contemporary American Indians and which they 'recognize and respect,' this appears to reflect a New Age pan-Indian sentiment and not an empirical observation. But mental health researchers have continued to be attracted by the relative simplicity and ease of use of culture areas, and the imperfect cross-fertilization between anthropology and psychology/psychiatry is seen clearly in the persistence of the culture area concept in the latter fields.[12] McShane and Berry (1988: 389) rendered the concept even simpler by reducing thirteen anthropological culture areas to just seven, 'reflecting the lesser interest of psychology in particular cultural variations.'

Several important studies employed culture areas to facilitate their research, and these will be addressed in due course. One major psychiatric epidemiological study deserves attention here because it introduces an additional, confounding element to the creation of the Aboriginal variable category. In the 'Flower of Two Soils' project, Beiser and Gotowiec (2000) explicitly borrowed the culture area concept from anthropology – as psychiatrists, they no doubt assumed the concept had a solid conceptual and empirical base in its founding discipline – and used it as the basis for the sampling frame in their research with one group of children each from the Plains, Northwest Coast, Northern Woodlands, and Desert culture areas. However, they added a twist by following the lead of Norton and Manson (1996) in assuming that, despite the culture areas, 'all Native groups in North America share certain characteristics such as history of displacement, the experience of oppression, and contemporary challenges to traditional ways of life' (Beiser & Gotowiec 2000: 239). In other words, while the cultures may have been different in the past, and to some extent remain so today (hence the utility of the culture area framework), it was also argued that there had been some homogenizing as a result of essentially identical historical processes. Norton and Manson (1996: 856; see also Norton 1999) have described this view succinctly: 'There is tremendous diversity in tribal cultures, but all American Indian and Alaska Natives have a shared history of loss of ancestral lands; restriction of traditional means of obtaining food, shelter, and clothing; imposition of alien forms of governance; mandated education in White schools; and the destruction of language and religion.'

Scholars who argue for both persisting cultural diversity (with or without the culture area concept) *and* post-contact cultural convergence are clearly working both sides of the issue. These scholars have generally failed to explain how each of these processes, cultural persistence and cultural change, were operationalized in their research and, perhaps more importantly, how each has a bearing on the problem under study. I would suggest that, generally speaking, neither process has been given much critical thought, and the result has been greatly overgeneralized assumptions regarding the Aboriginal experience. It is also necessary to at least question the extent to which Aboriginal peoples were subjected to uniform processes of historic displacement and oppression, a theme common to many contemporary discussions of Aboriginal mental health (e.g., Norton 1999). The experiences of northern Indians, who became involved in the fur trade and intermarried with the Europeans, and who currently have reserves in their traditional territories, seem very different from those groups who waged war with the settler society and were often relocated vast distances and essentially imprisoned, such as the Seminole, Navajo, and Cherokee.

In the Flower of Two Soils study we thus see a contradiction that bedevils much research: Beiser and Gotoweic (2000: 239) were justifiably concerned 'to take account of the intraethnic diversity frequently obscured by rubrics such as "Native American" or "First Nations People"' but nevertheless placed their subjects into categories that assumed contemporary cultural uniformity and homogeneity. Furthermore, they failed to reconcile their view of the contemporary importance of culture areas, and the idea of convergent acculturation, with their belief in the continued existence of significant 'differing social and historical influences' that have differentially affected English language acquisition, and hence, IQ test performance. While their samples were frequently taken from singular communities, thus controlling to some extent the cultural variables, in some of their analyses all Aboriginal children were assigned to a single 'Native' group for comparison with a similarly uniform 'non-Native' group in examining overall IQ scores, even though their data suggested substantial differences among Native groups, especially on verbal scores. In other words, neither cultural persistence nor cultural convergence became operative in the final analysis.

The attractiveness of grouping disparate Aboriginal populations into a single variable category is pervasive. McShane (1980), in a meta-analysis of sixteen studies involving over 600 subjects, lamented that tribal affiliation was not always reported (see, e.g., Whorton & Morgan 1990) and that American Indian norms could not be established across the studies because of the lack of comparability among groups. But, despite presenting data for individual groups such as the Chippewa, Navajo and Sioux, he concluded that there was a need to establish more universal *American Indian* norms on the tests. In subsequent work, McShane and Plas (1982a: 9) committed the same error of aggregation: their study of 142 American Indian children's performance patterns on the Wechsler grouped together an Ojibwa majority with some Sioux and 'other tribal groups' undefined. The subjects were divided into two groups, 'traditional' and 'acculturated,' for the analysis, presumably predicated on the assumption of cultural homogeneity within these two categories, that is, on the assumption that 'traditional' Ojibwa and 'traditional' Sioux were more or less culturally identical by virtue of being 'traditional.' In the discussion, however, the authors made reference to their participants as if they were all Ojibwa, and confusingly followed up in the conclusion by stating their belief that, since the sample was mostly Ojibwa it was not representative of all American Indian children, but *was* representative of Indian children in Minneapolis-St Paul, where the non-random sample was drawn.

Part of the problem here is the assumption that 'American Indian' represents an appropriate and meaningful research category despite cautions about inherent heterogeneity and differential processes of acculturation. A more fruitful approach to the issue has been the use of single community studies, which avoid the temptation to compare. Although the issue of intracommunity cultural variation remains pertinent, single communities, usually reserves, are considerably more likely to allow for better control of the cultural variables. Several studies have followed this approach, especially among the Navajo (Howell, Evans, & Downing 1958; Hynd et al. 1979; for other groups see also Gaddes et al. 1968; Sachs 1974; Tempest & Skipper 1988), and this allows for the possibility of the generation of local, community-level norms (Dana 1984).[13] Single-community studies are far preferable to studies involving a large cross-section of Aboriginal participants (a common occurrence in studies of value orientations, as we shall see in a later chapter). However, it is extremely rare for researchers to offer a comment on the nature of the cultures in question and how culture affects test performance. Simply identifying a group by its tribal name seems to represent a sufficient marker of important cultural differences for most researchers (Berry 2003; Trimble 2003). In some instances, even where community research has been undertaken, authors have not felt the need to disclose even basic data on the cultures involved, using ubiquitous labels like 'Indian' or 'Native' in a manner that renders any cultural interpretation impossible. This does not always prevent them from commenting on cultural matters in the use of the MMPI and Wechsler, or other such tests, we just do not always know to which culture they are referring (e.g., Cundick 1970). It has also been suggested that ethical research requires that specific American Indian communities remain anonymous (Norton & Manson 1996), and this creates a dilemma. Anonymity prevents an assessment of the culture-specific nature of the research results and may inadvertently fuel the faulty premise that the findings are indeed generalizable to *the* American Indian population. In the literature, however, much of the vagueness with respect to Aboriginal cultures has had nothing to do with attempts to protect their anonymity.

Overall, in looking at efforts to measure the intelligence and personality of Aboriginal peoples one cannot help but be struck by a most fundamental incongruity: in questioning the cultural appropriateness of various instruments, and in some cases arguing that they are culturally biassed and therefore not appropriate for Aboriginal peoples, researchers have rarely discussed the issue of culture in a meaningful way. As in many other studies, there is a lack of clarity as to what culture means and how culture in general, and designated cultures in particular, affect intelligence and personality test performance. Attempts to determine the actual culture of an individual are rare and, as we have seen, often flawed in fundamental ways. These are common problems not unique to the MMPI or Wechsler. In a study utilizing the California Psychological Inventory (CPI), for instance, Davis, Hoffman, and Nelson (1990) described Native American and 'white' subjects in terms of both race and ethnicity; assigned Chippewa, Sioux, and Crow Indians (plus other unregistered Indians) to a single 'Native American' category with no explanation; and failed to explain how 'whiteness' was conceptualized and determined and how it was relevant to performance on the CPI. The confusion also emerged clearly in a review of the utilization of intelligence and personality assessment tools with American Indians offered by Dauphinais and King (1992): in exploring 'environmental conditions' that can affect Indian children, they described unemployment, poverty, high drop-out rates, alcoholism, child abuse, and suicide as 'cultural influences.' As Everett (1973) argued in a study of social pathology among the Apache, there is a complex interdependence between traditional cultural elements and acculturation experience which Dauphinais and King do not address in any way. Just how 'high drop-out rates,' for example, constitute a 'cultural influence,' and if so *which* culture is at issue, is not explained.

Conclusion

In this chapter, I have moved from a discussion of measuring culture to a discussion of measuring personality and intelligence, and from conceptualizing and measuring cultures as wholes to treating culture as a variable in cross-cultural research. As quantitative and comparative research became more common, the individual emerged as the primary unit of analysis, at the expense of both community and cultural level studies. This shift towards individualism, especially within psychology and psychiatry, was facilitated by the tacit assumption of the homogeneity of Aboriginal peoples; the tendency to view the individual as representative of, or proxy for, *the* Aboriginal culture; and the utilization of self-declaration as a marker of Aboriginality, rather than actual cultural orientation. The emergence and dominance of psychometric approaches in the study of personality and intelligence led researchers to attempt to capture the essence of *the* Aboriginal in a few questions, to assign him or her a score or a ranking, and to see if he or she was different from other Aboriginals and, more importantly, from non-Aboriginals. This variabilizing of culture was pervasive and betrayed a lack of theoretical and conceptual development. Whatever culture is, it is certainly *not* simply a variable. Yet in the new millennium resort to the Aboriginal variable shows no sign of diminishing. Culture areas employed as sampling frames, cultures conceived of as trait lists, blood quantum and tribal membership used as proxies for culture – all of these and more characterize the problems with which we are faced as we assess the mental health knowledge to date. These problems will continue to plague my analysis as I move on.

PART B

The Disordered Aboriginal

The Construction of Aboriginal Psychopathology

> In so far, then, as the mentally unwell in modern advanced cultures tend to correspond to the well and the influential in ancient and retarded cultures, at least in certain situations, we can accept objective progress as having taken place. (Kroeber 1948: 300)

Anthropologist A.L. Kroeber's crude evolutionary ideas, cited above, might seem preposterous today, but these and similar views shaped much of the Aboriginal mental health discourse for over a century. The Barbaric Aboriginal presents as an inherently pathological, childlike individual, made so by a characteristically pathological and simplistic culture. This desperate situation was compounded by the arrival of Europeans, as Aboriginal peoples proved unable to cope with the concomitant cultural changes. Counter-balancing this perspective was the other prevailing view, that the psychopathology of the inherently healthy Arcadian Aboriginal developed only as a result of the disruptions caused by European colonization. In this chapter, I wish to examine several arenas of this competing discourse, to look carefully at how the pathological Aboriginal has been constructed. Both early and contemporary studies of psychopathology will be examined, and I will pay specific attention to the notion of acculturative stress.

'Latent Schizophrenics and Primitive People': Early Studies of Psychopathology

The mental health status of Aboriginal peoples was a topic of interest first to missionaries and explorers, and subsequently to scholars and government officials. In many ways, the story of psychiatry's gaze upon Aboriginal peoples is at least in part also the story of the relationship between the development of psychiatry itself and broader processes of European colonialism. I have already reviewed many early studies that touched upon the issue of psychopathology, especially within the context of personality. Early forms of diagnosis and treatment were crude, to say the least, and a great deal of attention was accorded to exotic problems and their causes. Over the years there have been two distinct types of psychopathological research. The first, to be discussed here, essentially involved the application of emerging biomedical understandings of disease, symptoms, and cause to Aboriginal populations. The second, to be discussed later in the book, involved attempts to comprehend psychopathology in Aboriginal terms, in other words, to look at problems through the lens of culture. Attention paid to the former, primarily epidemiological perspective, greatly outweighs that paid to the latter.

According to Littlewood and Lipsedge (1997: 298), while 'psychiatry was deployed extensively during the nineteenth and twentieth centuries to justify what we may term the internal colonisation of Amerindians and African-Americans,' it remains unclear if it was an instrument of colonialism or the product of the same mindset that led Europeans to believe that Aboriginal peoples were emotionally and intellectually childlike and inferior. A belief in cultures, especially indigenous cultures, as homogeneous and constituted of individuals expressing the same values and sense of social order prevailed during the period of colonial psychiatry, ignoring 'any unequal distribution of knowledge and power, of local contestation or global change' (Littlewood 2000: 82–3). And there is certainly considerable evidence that early Europeans perceived a substantive amount of psychopathology among the Aboriginal population – this is not surprising, given the ongoing debates at that time on the very question of their humanity (Erickson & Murphy 1998). The Jesuit Relations, for instance, contained many references to mental instability. Father François de Peron unflatteringly described the Huron in these terms: 'The nature of the Savage is patient, liberal, hospitable; but importunate, visionary, childish, thieving, lying, deceitful, licentious, proud, lazy; they have among them many fools, or rather lunatics, and insane people' (cited in Margetts 1975: 401). While such descriptions were commonplace, Margetts (1975) has argued that most early historical attention to health focused on the more immediate problem of the various epidemic diseases which were the cause of escalating mortality rates. Mental health morbidity was fascinating to Europeans but of secondary concern to the loss of Aboriginal labour and souls.

The interest of the state in the overall health of Aboriginal peoples resulted in a more focused and balanced attention on Aboriginal mental health, especially in the twentieth century and coincident with psychiatry's emerging professional interest in colonial peoples (Littlewood 2000). In a 1908 report, Aleš Hrdlička, a physical anthropologist with the United States National Museum, presented data that suggested insanity and suicide were actually relatively rare among American Indians. Based on an 1890 census, he determined that there were only forty-eight cases of insanity (thirty-three male and fifteen female, a reversal of the gender pattern among 'Whites'), and calculated a rate of 0.38 per 1000 for Indians, in comparison to 1.81 per 1000 for Whites. 'Idiocy' was also seen to be less prevalent among Indians (1.07 per 1000) than among Whites (1.55 per 1000). We must take these observations with a grain of salt, given the problems inherent in both census taking and the definitions, and application of these definitions, to the Indian population. But they suggest that not everyone, or every body of data, indicated that Aboriginal peoples experienced greater degrees of mental illness than non-Aboriginals. Indeed some, such as Snidecor (1947), openly speculated about why the Indian did *not* experience greater degrees of neuroses, given the destabilizing effects of colonization. This scepticism of apparently low rates of psychopathology ultimately emerges as a strong theme even in contemporary work. The concern was not always simply for the welfare of the patient, however, and Aboriginal mental health was often discussed within the context of the best interests of the white majority. In 1916, Lewis Terman, in reference to 'Indians, Mexicans and negroes' lamented that there was 'no possibility at present of convincing society that they should not be allowed to reproduce, although from a eugenic point of view they constitute a grave problem because of their unusually prolific breeding' (92). Angie Debo (1940) even suggested that in the late nineteenth and early twentieth centuries Indian mothers were sometimes declared insane and committed, thereby allowing white families to adopt their children and hence further Indian assimilation.

In the United States, the first mental hospital specifically for Indians was opened in 1903 in South Dakota (Spaulding 1986). The Canton Asylum for Insane Indians was constructed after an 1897 recommendation from the commissioner of Indian Affairs that a separate Indian facility be established. The number of reportedly insane and mentally deficient Indians was not particularly large, although national comprehensive data was not available. H.R. Hummer (1913), the psychiatrist who served as superintendent of the hospital for most of its history, wrote that of a U.S. Indian population of some 300,000 in 1911, there were fifty-eight 'insane' Indians in the asylum, fifty-two applications on file, twenty cases in various other institutions, and another twenty cases in the care of families – in other words, some 150 cases, a rate of 0.5 in 1000. Hummer speculated that there were probably twice as many cases, however. As he noted, 'Scarcely an employee or an enlightened Indian of any of the reservations visits this asylum who does not inform me that he knows of from one to five cases on that reservation who should properly be in the asylum' (1913: 615).

Sixteen patients were admitted to Canton in its first year, and the number of inmates reached a peak of ninety-three in 1926 before the institution closed in 1934 following reports of wholly inadequate care and horrible living conditions. Shoddy record keeping has made it difficult to determine authoritatively the types of diagnoses attributed to patients. According to Spaulding (1986), in the first four years 'dementia' and 'melancholia' were the most frequent diagnoses. Hummer (1913: 617) provided a detailed list of diagnoses for the first eight years, and by rank we find 'dementia praecox, 15; the epilepsies, 14; congenital imbecility, 8; intoxication psychoses, 6; manic-depressive insanity, 5; senile psychoses, 6; arterio-sclerotic dementia, 2; hysteria, 1; and paranoia, 1.' Major causes ranged from 'congenital defect' (thirteen cases), epilepsy (eleven cases), alcohol (six cases), and senility (five cases) (617). But Hummer also ventured to ascribe as a cause what he termed 'domestic difficulty, including loose marriage bonds, incest, and largely uninhibited sex drives, especially among the males (whose appetites for sex he described as 'voracious'). Clearly, in Hummer's view these Indians were immoral individuals: he even remarked that they masturbated 'openly ... without sense of shame' in the asylum (619)! In his discussion of causation he also noted, matter-of-factly, that some 66 per cent of the patients were 'full-bloods,' a clear hint that blood quantum was seen as an important predisposing factor for mental illness. While concluding that the Indians presented the same symptoms as appeared among 'whites,' he added that they were 'probably more destructive and decidedly filthier than the white insane' (621). Hummer's views of the Indians, their pathologies, and the causes of those pathologies appears in a different light, however, when one examines the 1929 inspection report of Dr Samuel Silk. Silk concluded that many of the patients were in fact free of mental disorder, had often been committed as a result of school problems or spousal conflict, and that only a minority required hospitalization (Spaulding 1986: 1009). When John Collier assumed the position of commissioner of Indian affairs, he had the hospital closed.

Sensationalist reports of insanity and mental illness among Indians were rife in the late nineteenth and early twentieth centuries, and explanations usually focused on their immature mental development, especially the existence of spirits and animated objects within their worldviews. Hummer himself noted that it was difficult to obtain patient histories, due to fears of 'witchcraft' and 'sorcery' (1913: 618). Bruner (1912: 387), in a review of the 'primitive races in America,' noted that 'Idiots were believed to be possessed of evil spirits, so usually they were killed by burning at the stake, but no attention or treatment was accorded the insane.' Diamond Jenness (1933: 19), Canada's foremost anthropologist in the mid-twentieth century, echoed a common sentiment of his day when he wrote that 'The Indians are mentally somewhat unbalanced.' The reason for this verdict, Jenness surmised, was their belief in 'supernatural beings' who constantly interfered with humans, with the result that individuals experienced periodic hysteria from fear. This view was supported by Saindon (1933: 2), who described the James Bay Cree as experiencing 'a good deal of hysteria,' in part as a result of 'undisciplined imagination [which] delivers itself up to the worst excesses, to the most foolish and most fantastic vagaries ... [which] block rational thought and judgement.'

The conviction that so-called primitive cultures were inherently psychopathological, and that belief in spirits and magic were causative of mental disorder, was widespread among scholars of the time (Ackerknecht 1943).[1] Freud's influential essays in the early part of the twentieth century had opened the door for the intellectual comparison of 'primitive peoples' and 'neurotics,' seeing in the former 'a well-preserved picture of an early stage of our own development' (Freud 1950: 1). Anthropologist A.L. Kroeber went so far as to argue that 'magic [was] the pathology of culture' and to cautiously allow that 'the abnormal primitive cultures [were] *perhaps* less numerous than the normal ones' (cited in Ackerknecht 1943: 52n116; emphasis added). This idea has been so tenacious that 'magical thinking' characteristic of 'primitive' people, children, and schizophrenics entered into the DSM-III in 1980 as a sign of mental disorder and remains today in varied form in DSM-IV-TR.

Environmental stress was also seen as causative of mental disorder, especially among northern Aboriginal groups which experienced harsh winter conditions. Ruth Landes (1937: 56) suggested that insanity was both recognized and comparatively common among the Ojibwa of southern Ontario. To her view of Ojibwa life as exceedingly stressful due to environmental pressures, she added that 'Insanities break out often in the winter, when the despondent hunter sees himself at the last wall, parrying the evil forces of the universe with faint hope of success' (57). Working from the reports of Landes, as well as Hallowell, Parker (1962) noted that both described depression, anorexia, and obsessive and paranoid ideation as the most common forms of mental disturbance among the Ojibwa in general.

The dangers inherent in the study of Aboriginal mental health without any consideration of historical or cultural grounding are evident in much of the research of this era. Anderson (1936; cited in Shore 1974), in a study of mental health and illness among Oklahoma Indian children, lamented the errors that haunted the diagnostic process. 'The most outstanding finding,' he wrote of his research, 'was the relatively large number of children who have come to be considered as mental defectives, whereas their real difficulty is a lack of opportunity' (61). Slotkin's (1953) analysis of Menomini psychopathology is an example of this misguided diagnostic approach. After undertaking field work in a small Menomini community between 1949 and 1951, Slotkin brought his Freudian theoretical perspective to bear on the issue of the relationship between culture and inhibited drives. In particular, he hypothesized that the Menomini would be experiencing 'cultural inadequacy,' in that the customary forms of expression of social opposition were inadequate, as indicated by increased nonconformity, the breakdown of social controls, and social and personality disorganization. Personality disorganization was very common, according to Slotkin, who presented the following evidence to support this claim:

There are three cases of institutionalized psychotics, and, significantly enough, all were diagnosed as paranoid schizophrenics. Two other cases of the same type are known to me. From conversations, I gathered that at least a half dozen others have had psychotic episodes in the past and, with one exception, these also seem to have been cases of paranoid schizophrenia. Neurotics seem to be common; mere observation made me suspect that there are at least two dozens. I tried to make case studies of the psychotics and neurotics, but there is a traditional reluctance to discuss one's private affairs with anyone (which is itself a symptom), and I could not find any way of motivating most people to violate this custom. Therefore there is a serious gap in my data, for I do not know the specific etiology producing most Menomini neurotics and psychotics. (Slotkin 1953: 15–16)

The tentative language employed, which betrays an overwhelming lack of data, points to some serious problems with the validity of Slotkin's conclusions. The admission of a 'serious gap' in his data notwithstanding, Slotkin seemed content to leave us with a picture of these 168 Menomini as suffering from 'cultural inadequacy' based primarily on casual observation. Their 'traditional' reluctance to discuss personal matters was seen as both a cultural trait and a symptom of psychosis and neurosis, in effect leaving us to equate the Menomini culture with psychopathology.

Sometimes, commentators simply could not hold themselves back, and essentially pathologized all Aboriginal cultures on the basis of their perceived primitiveness. James Baker, a medical doctor who studied a handful of Indians incarcerated for homicide, expressed the common, Freudian-inspired viewpoint of his day:

Psychiatrically it is felt that undifferentiated or latent schizophrenics and primitive people have the following elements and reactions in common. First, sublimation of basic emotional drives is weak or incomplete. Poor or unstable defense mechanisms are used in attempts to defend against disturbing basic emotional conflicts, such as occur in certain sex drives and with hostile aggressive reactions. Too often the defense used is the unstable one of reaction in opposite, i.e. reaction formation. Under the effects of drugs such as alcohol which weaken superego control, basic emotional drives that have been suppressed or repressed reacted to in opposite now appear in their raw undiluted form in an overwhelming outburst of emotional dissipation. This proposition of weak ego defenses and release from superego control is offered as the explanation as to why this group, as well as many schizophrenics and other primitive people, tolerate alcohol poorly and present marked behavior reactions when under the influence of alcohol. (1959: 275)

One of the most influential researchers in this early period was George Devereux, a Freudian psychoanalyst with an anthropological inclination. Much of his work focused on what he termed 'ethnopsychiatry,' an attempt to comprehend indigenous perspectives on mental health and illness; this work will be discussed in a subsequent chapter. However, as a clinician he also offered his views on the mental status of those with whom he worked. Devereux (1942: 71) unabashedly argued that American Indians constituted a laboratory of sorts, 'an exceptionally favourable testing ground for the basic tenets of the environmentalist approach in mental hygiene,' and 'a field of action for the mental-hygiene movement that promises to yield significant returns on a relatively small investment.' He is best known for his work with the Mohave beginning in the late 1930s. Devereux, like Bryce Boyer (discussed in the previous chapter) was keenly interested in the personality of shamans in particular. Perhaps misinterpreting Ruth Benedict's (1934a) observations that shamans would most likely be seen as disordered only within the context of (White) North American society, and that concepts of normality and abnormality were culturally contingent, Devereux (1969: 12) first wrote that the Mohave shaman was 'a psychotic in partial remission,' and later adopted the uncompromising position that 'the shaman is mentally deranged' (Devereux 1971: 28).[2] This view was common among scholars at the time, and, as Lucas and Barrett (1995: 310) have noted, 'The shaman, as representative of Barbaric society, is the quintessential figure representing its ill-health.'

Devereux's (1969) view of general Mohave psychopathology was more charitable. He found no evidence of schizophrenia, for instance, which he attributed to 'the basic structure of primitive culture, which, by its very nature, seems to play a role in preventing the occurrence of genuine (chronic) forms of schizophrenia, at least until a primitive society is subjected to massive and oppressive acculturation' (1969: 222). His statement that 'one may say that a schizophrenic is simply someone who dreams even when he is awake' (1969: 494) was rather bold for its time in asserting the cultural basis and biases in diagnosing disorder. Suicide was not uncommon among the Mohave, however, and its increasing frequency was tied to the processes of cultural change.

Devereux also openly questioned the appropriateness of Western psychiatric diagnosis for American Indian peoples, and in this he clearly echoed the views of Ruth Benedict. He presented an interesting case study that demonstrated the problems inherent in cultural misunderstandings. Two brothers from the Acoma pueblo were on death row, convicted of murder. The prison psychiatrist was, in Devereux's words, 'sufficiently sophisticated not to mistake Indianness for psychosis,' but being unable to find any 'culturally neutral evidence of real mental derangement,' declared them legally sane and hence executable (1971: 43). Upon interview, Devereux learned that the man they had killed had, in their view, been using witchcraft against them. Witchcraft was a pervasive element of Acoma culture, but Devereux was concerned about the ease with which the brothers began to talk about it. This struck him as deviant, since such phenomena were only rarely and reluctantly discussed. Further, in killing the witch themselves, rather than using an intermediary and invoking ritual, they had engaged in a second culturally deviant act. They were, in Devereux's opinion, delusional. In the original diagnosis an uninformed reading of its content resulted in the delusion being mistaken for an acceptable or normative cultural belief by the psychiatrist, and therefore suggestive of sanity. Devereux diagnosed one brother as suffering from paranoid schizophrenia and the other as having 'psychotically tinged psychopathy' (44). The original examining psychiatrist accepted Devereux's diagnosis, and the two were spared execution.

In a similar vein, Jewell (1952), in an examination of a 'psychotic' Navajo displaying withdrawal, also asked whether a Navajo or Anglo perspective should be used in understanding this individual's problems. Utilizing the culture and personality work of Kluckhohn and Leighton (1948), Jewell described the Navajo's apparent passivity and 'quiet unmovingness' in the face of fear (1952: 32), as well as depression, as a form of withdrawal, all of which he noted were 'salient aspects of the typical Navajo personality' (33). A previous survey of Navajo patients in regional mental hospitals had revealed an 'unusually high incidence of catatonic schizophrenia,' suggestive of a Navajo predisposition and leading to speculation that, in these cases, the Navajo personality traits of withdrawal and depression had been taken to an extreme (33). Jewell's case study brought this explanation into considerable doubt. He noted, for instance, that Navajos had a morbid fear of hospitals, and that apathetic and withdrawn behaviour was normal for Navajos in these circumstances. This explanation was supported by a Navajo medical interpreter, and after several interviews with the patient, Jewell, a psychologist, concluded that the apparent catatonic behaviour was not a symptom of schizophrenia, but rather the expression of a behaviour the patient thought was expected of him. As a result of the actions of both Jewell and the interpreter, the patient was rediagnosed and released to a less restrictive educational institute, where he thrived.

Much of the data utilized in some of these early studies are clearly problematic, a fact that was occasionally recognized by commentators. In a review of psychiatric epidemiology in the Arctic and subarctic, Hippler (1975) was critical of the essentially shoddy work that had been done to date, citing problems of under-reporting and the failure to take alcoholism into account in the diagnosis of psychotic disorders. But the approach taken by Vallee (1968) was perhaps all too typical. After describing the existence of manic-depression and hysteria among the Eskimos, he noted that his statements were 'not based on carefully conducted systematic research, but rather on data and observations culled from a variety of reports, most of them impressionistic' (566). Poor, impressionistic data, it seems, did not greatly limit the inclination of scientists to proffer viewpoints on the state of the Aboriginal mind.

Marginality and the 'Caught-Between-Two-Worlds' Paradigm

The first half of the twentieth century can be characterized by the conflict between the view that Aboriginal peoples experienced better mental health than the European settlers and the view that their mental health was worse, although in each case the condition was seen as inherent, linked to the essential character of Aboriginal peoples. This perspective eventually began to lose ground to a new one. It has long been argued that cultural changes can bring with them the potential for social and personal disorganization and a concomitant increase in psychopathology (Ackerknecht 1943; Leighton 1959a, 1959b; Bock 1999). As a result of colonization, and directed programs of assimilation in particular, within this framework Arcadian Aboriginal peoples appeared ripe for the generation of various disorders related to cultural changes. Edward Sapir (1924) referred to cultures such as those found in North America as 'genuine,' meaning they were harmonious and balanced, capable of meeting all of the needs of their members. Genuine culture was contrasted with 'spurious' culture, a Durkheimian dystopia wracked by anomie and disharmony. For Sapir, the 'well-rounded life of the average participant in the civilization of a typical American Indian tribe' had been challenged by contact with Europeans, which created a 'bewildering vacuity ... an uneasy sense of the loss of some vague and great good' (1924; cited in Darnell 2001: 119).

While Sapir's notion of genuine and spurious cultures was never widely accepted by others, its underlying premise of the contaminating effects of contact with Europeans was widely embraced. Hallowell (1945b: 193), for instance, suggested that culture contact among the Ojibwa and other Indians created 'a large variety of anxiety-arousing situations,' including those caused by disease. James (1961) argued further that among the Ojibwa, this anxiety was the result of the deprivations of reserve life and their inferior social status. Devereux (1969) explained a dramatic increase in Mohave suicide as the result of a breakdown in culture. Phillips and Inui (1986) similarly argued that Native Alaskan criminal behaviour, drug abuse, and psychiatric treatment were indicators of acculturative stress among those living in larger communities. Kraus and Buffler (1979) believed the breakdown of traditional relationships caused by culture contact damaged the psychological integrity of Alaska Natives, resulting in loneliness, anxiety, frustration, stress, and despair.[3]

As we saw in the previous chapter, several authors have generated acculturation models characterized by the hypothesized existence of cultural orientation categories, often ranging from the 'traditional' to the fully acculturated. While it has often been suggested that there was a positive relationship between Indianness and psychopathology (e.g., Uecker et al. 1980), contradictory evidence has also suggested that Indianness was positively correlated with fewer mental health problems (e.g., Westermeyer & Neider 1985). Particular attention has been paid to a certain type of transitional or marginal individual who, analysts have surmised, is most at risk of developing problems. Spindler and Spindler (1972: 511) described transitional people in almost schizophrenic terms, as 'unpredictable,' at one moment 'capable of great generosity and hospitality,' and at another 'dangerous violence, particularly when drinking – and they drink frequently.' LaFromboise et al. (1990: 638) defined 'marginal' Indians as those 'unable to either live the cultural heritage of their tribal group or to identify with the dominant society.' 'This group,' they continued, 'tends to have the most difficulty in coping with social problems due to their ethnicity.' French (1981: 147) described these marginal individuals as 'torn between their traditional cultural heritage and the dictates of the larger society,' and therefore 'those most likely to violate majority norms resulting in arrest, conviction and incarceration' (French 1979: 52). A special type of marginality was described as the 'apple syndrome' by Westermeyer (1979), exhibited by individuals who were raised in non-Aboriginal families and hence had no Aboriginal cultural knowledge or experience (they were seen as 'red' on the outside and 'white' on the inside). As young adults they attempted to express their non-Aboriginality but met with racism, yet having no Aboriginal background they were viewed disfavourably by other Aboriginals, leading to problems such as alcoholism, drug abuse, depression, and suicide.

The problematic nature of this marginality best finds expression in the phenomenon of being 'caught between two worlds.' The idea appears to have been borrowed from work on marginality and the 'marginal man' as discussed by E.V. Stonequist (1937: 8), who described this individual as 'poised in psychological uncertainty between two (or more) social worlds; reflecting in his soul the discords and harmonies, repulsions and attractions of these worlds, one of which is often "dominant" over the other; within which membership is implicitly based upon birth or ancestry (race or nationality); and where exclusion removes the individual from a system of group relations.' The fragility of this situation was stressed some years later by American Indian scholar D'Arcy McNickle (1968: 219), who wrote that the Indian was 'a man caught between two worlds, a man who must break free of the past in order to find his place in the future – everyone realizing that his hold on the present is precarious.' The marginal man may have internalized the norms of the dominant group, but he was prevented from actively participating in that group (Kerckhoff & McCormick 1955). According to Topper and Curtis (1987), this dilemma becomes the source of anomic depression, in the sense of the concept as used by sociologists Émile Durkheim and Robert Merton. The individual so trapped experiences 'means-goals disjunctions,' that is, he or she lacks the means to achieve the goals identified as desirable, and these are invariably goals associated with the broader society. Kerckhoff and McCormick (1955) identified this phenomenon among Wisconsin Chippewa children, who were unable to transcend an 'impermeable barrier' (54) between themselves as Indians and the non-Indian community, resulting in the expression of 'marginal personality characteristics' including uncertainty in social situations and a fear of rejection, painful self-consciousness in the company of others, loneliness, hypersensitivity, and worry about the future. It was further surmised that the 'disorganized state of the Indian group' led to identification with the white society, access to which was largely denied to Aboriginals (55). Vallee (1968: 566) described the phenomenon clearly with respect to Eskimos (without using the terminology), when he wrote that 'Behavioral disorders such as alcoholism and chronic hitting-out are most common among men who aspire to white-dominated positions and status without adequate means to fulfill these aspirations.'

Garrett and Garrett (1994: 135–6) used the term 'cultural discontinuity' to describe the situation which results from the conflict caused by the 'chasm' between 'mainstream expectations and the cultural values of Native American Indians.' Sage (1997: 45) suggested that Native Americans choosing to accept and orient themselves to the dominant culture might be alienated from their Native American culture. Renfrey (1992: 330) made the point that 'individuals seeking a bicultural lifestyle could be stranded between the two cultures, left ineffective in either.' Several other authors referred either specifically or generally to this idea (Heinrich, Corbine, & Thomas 1990; Herring 1990; Dufrene & Coleman 1992). French (1979, 1980, 1989, 1997) took a particularly pessimistic view of the problem, suggesting that the 'marginal Indian' was 'caught between [his or her] traditional heritage and the demands of the majority society,' 'torn between two diverse, and often contravening, cultural orientations, with little chance of belonging to either' (French 1979: 51). Such an individual suffered from 'cultural and personal ambiguity,' according to French (1997: 7), with a resulting 'identity confusion,' and was the most likely of all Native Americans to engage in pathological behaviour. To this we can add Phillips and Inui's (1986: 124) view that acculturative stress was often accompanied by 'deculturative stress,' that is, 'the stress of losing traditional beliefs and values.'

Acculturation theory, with its emphasis on trait diffusion and replacement, is clearly the driving force behind the caught-between-two-worlds paradigm. Trimble et al. (1996: 204–5) critiqued the standard view of the paradigm, which posited that 'there is an assumed inherent conflict between values, beliefs, and behaviors.' They continued: 'Furthermore, there is an assumption that whatever new is adopted must automatically replace something of the old. In other words, a person only has so much capacity for "culture." According to this view, conflict will exist until the individual has made a complete transition to the new culture and all of the old is replaced. Within this framework, the ultimate goal of counseling would seem to be to assist in making this transition as rapidly as possible, or in helping the client tolerate the effects of the conflict' (204–5).

Another problem with the caught-between-two-worlds argument (as with much of the acculturation discourse) is the persistent implication that there are two, and only two, contradictory and conflicting cultures, two solitudes, each largely impenetrable. Implicit too is the notion that an individual can be without culture, having experienced cultural loss without a corresponding cultural gain. Echoing Sapir's notion of genuine and spurious culture, Phillips and Inui (1986: 141) presented just such an interpretation in a study of mental illness among Native Alaskan criminal offenders:

> In order to have a 'culture' that gives meaning to individuals' experience, however, it is necessary to have an integrated set of beliefs and values. To achieve this Native Alaskans must either artificially maintain the old beliefs and values in the new environment or acquire the alien beliefs and values of the dominant White culture. But acquiring new beliefs and values is a difficult and protracted process. Many Native Americans are stalemated in an intermediate 'a-cultural' (that is, meaningless) state; they have given up traditional beliefs and values but are not yet able to adopt the 'modern' beliefs and values of the dominant culture. These rapid changes are thus associated with deculturative and acculturative stresses that can cause psychosocial maladaptation of individuals.

There seems to be little room for either individual agency or multicultural adaptation in this formulation.

Acculturative Stress

Many have argued that the Arcadian paradise in North America was disrupted by the arrival of European settlers, and the notion of 'acculturative stress' best captures the view that culture contact and change has played an important role in the creation of psychopathology. This topic has been dominated by psychologist John Berry, and merits detailed examination. Berry's ideas sprang from the now-classic anthropological definition of acculturation (see Redfield, Linton & Herskovits 1936; Berry 2003), that is, culture change which results from continuous contact between two distinct cultures, and in particular the notion of 'psychological acculturation' which, following Graves (1967b), can be experienced not only at the group level but also at the level of the individual. Over many years and in a series of closely related articles, Berry developed his theories about acculturative stress, becoming arguably the leading international authority on this issue (Berry 1970, 1975, 1985, 2003; Berry & Annis 1974a, 1974b; Berry, Wintrob, Sindell, & Mawhinney 1982; Berry, Kim, Minde, & Mok 1987; Berry & Kim 1988; Berry 1991). According to Berry et al. (1987: 492–493), 'The concept of acculturative stress refers to one kind of stress, that in which stressors are identified as having their source in the process of acculturation; in addition, there is often a particular set of stress behaviors which occurs during acculturation, such as lowered mental health status (specifically confusion, anxiety, depression), feelings of marginality and alienation, heightened psychosomatic symptom level, and identity confusion. Acculturative stress is thus a reduction in the health status of individuals, and may include physical, psychological and social aspects; to qualify as acculturative stress, these changes should be related in a systematic way to known features of the acculturation process, as experienced by the individual.' While mental health problems could arise from acculturation, this was not seen as inevitable; rather, both group and individual characteristics had a moderating influence on the outcome, as did the degree of voluntariness of the contact. Of greatest concern were those experiencing 'marginalization.' Marginalized individuals expressed little interest in maintaining their original cultural identities and characteristics yet remained aloof from the culture of the more dominant group. According to Berry and Kim (1988: 212), the state of marginality was 'characterized by having lost essential features of one's culture, but not having replaced them by entering the larger society,' leading to 'feelings of alienation, marginality, and a loss of identity.' Sounding suspiciously like the 'caught-between-two-worlds' notion, the marginalized individual was said to be 'suspended between the two cultures, often in a state of personal and social conflict' (Berry 1991: 222). Berry and Kim (1988: 212) hastened to add, however, that this did not mean that they lacked culture, but rather that, like Sapir's spurious culture, their culture 'may be disorganized and may not be supportive of the individual and his or her needs during the process of acculturation.' Marginalized individuals were seen to be at greatest risk for developing psychopathology.

Aboriginal North American samples were of predominant interest in Berry's work on acculturative stress, work that spanned more than two decades and included studies of several other populations, including immigrants and refugees, in Canada (Berry et al. 1987). It was crucial that he utilize Aboriginal groups representing differing degrees of acculturation. However, the Aboriginal populations employed in his comparative analysis, Cree, Ojibwa, Carrier, and Tsimshian, were confusingly presented in rank order which changed in both label and meaning throughout his publications. The researchers were clearly trying to understand how these societies differed, and they borrowed from a variety of primarily anthropological concepts. This inadvertently projected a strong need to find differences. Thus the first ranking was said to represent different eco-cultural adaptations, based initially on food accumulation (e.g., the Tsimshian were 'high food accumulating,' the Cree were 'low food accumulating') (Berry & Annis 1974a), then on degrees of sociocultural integration (e.g., the Cree were 'loose' and unstratified, whereas the Tsimshian were 'relatively tight' and stratified) (Berry et al. 1987: 500), and still later on levels of 'cultural congruity with Eurocanadian society' (e.g., the Cree were least congruous, the Tsimshian the most; Berry & Kim 1988: 227). Some problems in characterizing each of the four Aboriginal groups were also evident. The Cree, for instance, were seen as less congruous with Eurocanadian society than the Ojibwa, even though both inhabited a relatively remote, contiguous part of the continent, spoke related languages, had similar environmental and economic adaptations and histories of contact with Europeans, and similar contemporary lifestyles. Specific details, either cultural or historical, to support the distinctions made were not offered.

There was also an a historical dimension to the acculturative stress model. Suspicions are first aroused by the system of ranking societies, wherein interpretations of pre-contact ecological adaptations were applied to late-twentieth century populations, an ironic suggestion of the lack of cultural change given that the focus was on acculturation. The Cree at the time of Berry's research, for instance, could no longer be thought of as 'migratory,' as they lived for major portions of the year in settlements, and their food accumulation had been augmented by the introduction of grocery stores and sources of cash (e.g., trapping, wage employment, and government transfer payments).[4] Since the Cree in the late twentieth century had just as much access to food as the Tsimshian if we include contemporary food stores and factor in government transfer payments, the distinction between these two groups is blurred. Admittedly, there was some acknowledgment in earlier work that there had been significant changes over the past several centuries due to culture contact (Berry & Annis 1974a; Berry et al. 1982), including noting that the descriptions of social structure were, indeed, for the pre-contact period (Berry et al. 1987), yet the overall formulation assumed cultural congruence with the past, an assumption which should have been an empirical question. Further, Berry, Kim, Minde, and Mok (1987) described the Aboriginal populations as continuing to experience involuntary acculturation today, grouping them with refugees in this regard, and thereby implying that Aboriginal peoples remained as culturally different from Eurocanadians as, say, newly arrived Asian refugees, despite centuries of contact experience. When Berry and Annis (1974a: 399) described the Cree's 'traditional migratory life style' as being the most 'discrepant from the cultural lifestyle of the Eurocanadian larger society' they were effectively cementing the Cree in the past and denying them the contemporary culture acceded to the Eurocanadians. The Cree hunter of the sixteenth century was not compared to the Scottish trader of the same era, but rather with the Scottish trader's descendant some 500 years later!

What conclusions emanated from the work of Berry and his associates? Levels of acculturative stress were found to be higher for Aboriginal peoples than for a non-Aboriginal control group and the other groups analysed in the comparative work: immigrants, refugees, landed ethnic groups, and sojourners. Those Aboriginal individuals who were most discrepant culturally from Eurocanadian society experienced the highest levels of stress. The James Bay Cree exhibited the highest degrees of acculturative stress in the early years of Berry's work. Individual agency was a factor in understanding how an individual reacted to a culture change situation, and according to Berry et al. (1987), those Aboriginal individuals who favoured an acculturation outcome described as 'integration,' meaning the incorporation of elements of Eurocanadian culture while retaining elements of the original culture, experienced less stress than those who expressed a resistance to any further contact with the larger society. Further, those who had the greatest contact with, and participation in, Eurocanadian society experienced less stress. Berry et al. (1987: 506) noted that the conclusion that more participation means less stress was at odds with the conventional view that stress should increase with contact and change, and they believed that the decreased stress might be the result of active involvement in the educational system of the larger society. Hence, it was not the changes themselves that were seen to be the source of stress, but rather the *resistance* to acculturation, perhaps the most profound conclusion to emanate from the work. In the case of the James Bay Cree, it was concluded that changes brought about by the massive James Bay hydroelectric project (beginning in the late 1960s and accelerating in the 1980s), including the development of new, Cree-based institutions, actually resulted in a decline in stress scores (Berry et al. 1982). The Cree were seen to be actively engaged in achieving a cultural synthesis of Cree and Eurocanadian elements, which Berry, Kim, Minde, and Mok (1987) argued was conducive to good mental health.

Some of the work of Berry and his colleagues was, in retrospect, conceptually flawed, demonstrating a propensity towards a materialist and evolutionary framework in which Aboriginal societies were conceived as having experienced very little cultural change until the studies themselves began. It is clear that Berry, the pioneer of acculturation studies in psychology, was working through his ideas, in part through his studies with Aboriginal peoples, and the sophistication of his work increased at each stage. Looking back on this work, Berry (2003: 33) noted the propensity to 'pathologize' the acculturation process, a product of the over-emphasis of acculturation theory in psychology and psychiatry. Key questions remained unaddressed, however. What were the relative roles of the individual versus society in forcing or allowing for cultural change? While Berry and Kim (1988) acknowledged that the prestige of the minority group in question, that is, how it was viewed by the dominant group, might affect the extent to which minorities were allowed to integrate or were blocked from integrating more closely, this important variable was not seriously addressed. The authors merely concluded that Canada promotes a multicultural environment and therefore should be relatively friendly to the culturally different. Also, how can one explain the fact that Vietnamese refugees, individuals forced to evacuate their homelands under duress, scored lower in acculturative stress than many Aboriginal individuals who remained in their homelands and who had already acculturated to a significant extent?[5] The framework presented by Berry et al. (1987) contained the seeds of the explanation, wherein Aboriginal peoples were categorized as 'sedentary' – that is, the cultural change process had come to them in their homelands – and correspondingly engaged in 'involuntary' cultural change. This framework only makes sense for groups in the early stages of cultural contact, however, and lends considerably less explanatory power to a contact situation that has ensued for several centuries. The results for the James Bay Cree were tantalizing, nevertheless, and if Berry was able to tap into some aspect of culture change that was, indeed, valid, then the observation that cultural change has the most positive outcome when the people involved are active in the process of change looms as an important finding that might explain, among other things, the negative consequences of residential schools (see chapter 9).

Another, perhaps more significant, problem in studies of acculturative stress pertains to the lack of attention paid to the pre-contact cultures themselves. The stresses associated with culture change resulting from contact with another culture are inherently related to pre-contact formations, as Berry's work implied, yet studies of acculturative stress have rarely given us the cultural baseline. Acculturation studies frequently sprang from an implicit, and sometimes explicit, generalized view of utopian, 'genuine' Aboriginal cultures characterized by internal harmony and mental well-being prior to the arrival of Europeans. Cultural change has invariably been seen as new and wholly negative, and Berry's observations among the James Bay Cree have been largely ignored, perhaps because they were not compatible with the tenacious Arcadian model. It has also frequently been assumed that cultural change for Aboriginal peoples has solely meant becoming more Euro–North American (the two cultures model again). The ways in which elements of the various European, and even African, cultures have been adopted as part of a more positive process of cultural change, a process compatible with the adaptive mechanisms of the pre-contact Aboriginal societies, have been neglected. That there may be other explanations for current states of mental illness are rarely considered. As Levy and Kunitz (1971: 100) reminded us three decades ago, it has been 'all too easy to attribute the pathologies we can see today to the only cultural reality we are able to observe, that of contact and acculturation.' Berry (2003) himself has recently stressed the importance of ethnographic, community-level research to establish the cultural baseline from which acculturation studies can ensue, an approach that should alleviate some of the problems inherent in the early studies where the baseline was assumed rather than empirically demonstrated.

In recent years some important strides have been made in the conceptualization of acculturation. In particular, there has been a movement away from linear models in which it was assumed that cultural traits were gained and lost in a one-to-one relational way, and that the adoption of a new cultural element meant the loss of a traditional counterpart. Instead, a multicultural model has been advanced in which the individual is assumed to be capable of acquiring elements of several different cultures without incurring any loss of original elements, without confusion or stress, and can learn the context-specific nature of these new elements such that he or she can effectively operate in several cultures (Azar 1999). Acculturation is now more properly viewed as bidimensional, if not multidimensional; that is, many options are available to individuals faced with the prospect of cultural change (Berry 2003; Trimble 2003). Oetting and Beauvais (1991) have referred to this as an 'orthogonal' model of acculturation. Many of the psychologists whose work I have examined, including Joseph Trimble and John Berry (Berry's incorporation of an 'integration/biculturalism' category was a forerunner of this approach), have been leading proponents in this movement.

Community-Based Epidemiological Studies

Epidemiological studies of the prevalence of psychopathology in Aboriginal communities have become increasingly common in recent years and several warrant critical attention, in part because of their pioneering nature but also because of their ongoing influence and importance in retrospective studies of the field (e.g., S.M. Manson & Shore 1981; S.M. Manson 1986, 2000; Manson et al. 1987; O'Nell 1989; Kinzie et al. 1992; Kirmayer, Boothroyd, Tanner, Adelson, & Robinson 2000). As prevalence studies, they have characteristically forsworn the reliance on a traditional, pre-contact cultural baseline that defined much of the work of the acculturative stress theorists. Overall, these studies have painted a portrait of Aboriginal individuals as comparatively more disordered than non-Aboriginals.

The Cornell Medical Index (CMI) was a popular epidemiological tool several decades ago. Its generic nature and self-report procedure allowed for its use by individuals lacking in medical training who nevertheless wished to obtain a snapshot of health status.[6] Anthropologist Norman Chance used a scaled-down version of the CMI in his research among the Eskimo in a coastal Alaskan village in 1960 (Chance & Foster 1962). Significantly, Chance and Foster recognized that there were many questions in the index that simply made no sense to the Eskimos or which were culturally inappropriate, underscoring the importance of combining fieldwork with surveys of any kind. Questions such as 'Have you ever had jaundice' or 'Has a doctor told you your blood pressure is too low' would not make sense to an individual who had rarely even seen a physician. There are several sections to the CMI, similar to subscales, which allow the researcher to attain both a total score for an individual and a score for the separate sections (such as moods and feelings, fatigue and frequency of illness). In a survey of over 90 per cent of the adults, Chance and Foster (1962) reported that there appeared to be no age differences in CMI scores but that women scored significantly higher than men in both overall score and the subscale scores, indicating greater medical distress. In terms of frequency of responses, women scored higher than men in all sections, with the exception of reports of unhealthy habits, such as smoking and drinking. The largest gap between men and women was on the fatigue scale, with women scoring higher. All of these observations have a vague feel about them, a product of the employment of the CMI combined with the lack of other medical data, a problem which Chance and Foster acknowledged. However, the use of other sources of data, such as psychiatric interviews, would not necessarily have resulted in a clearer picture of psychiatric epidemiology, since the CMI at this time was considered a powerful tool which could not be easily discounted. In a study of Indians in Eastern Oklahoma, for instance, Martin, Sutker, Leon, and Hales (1968) found a significant discrepancy between CMI scores and the results of psychiatric interviews. However, rather than concluding that one or both techniques was simply producing artifacts, they chose to cling to the techniques: 'we are inclined to think that many [CMI] high scorers reflect an internal disquietude resulting from sociocultural stress and inadequacy which does not, from a clinical point of view, constitute psychopathology in the traditional sense' (312).

Let me turn next to several Canadian studies published in the early and mid-1970s which, collectively, proved extremely influential and yet which clearly suffered from a problem all too common with epidemiological studies – the inability to properly define cultural groups. The first of these, by Roy, Choudhuri, and Irvine (1970) involved the analysis of first admission statistics (based on clinical case notes) at a Saskatchewan psychiatric hospital between 1961 and 1966. Fifty-one Treaty Indians were distinguished from 2,607 others, and statistics on sex, age, marital status, and diagnosis were recorded. In Saskatchewan, as in Canada generally, federally recognized Indians, including those with treaty status, are readily identifiable because of a unique form of health insurance (that allows provinces to bill back to the federal government for services provided to Indians.) This system is considered to be reliable for identifying members of the Indian population with federal recognition. The other individuals in this study represented 'a wide variety of ethnic groups' (384), according to the authors, which could well have included Métis and non-recognized (i.e., non-status) Indians. The statistical analysis revealed that the Indian admissions were much younger than others, and that a significantly higher proportion of the diagnoses were for schizophrenia compared to non-Indian diagnoses. In contrast, the non-Indians had a significantly higher proportion of the diagnosis of organic psychosis. In an attempt to understand the situation further, the researchers undertook a comparative study of active psychiatric cases 'in a large Indian community' (actually ten Cree and Saulteaux reserves) and those in a neighbouring non-Indian community (again, some eighteen primarily European rural municipalities). After a six-month period of data gathering, the researchers estimated the non-Indian prevalence rate for active psychiatric disorder to be just over half that of the Indians (15.2 per 1000, compared to the Indian rate of 27.3 per 1000). More specifically, they determined that the proportion of Indians suffering from two particular disorders, schizophrenia and mental deficiency, was significantly higher than the rate for non-Indians but that there were no Indian cases of organic psychosis. They noted in particular that the elderly Indian population was 'remarkable healthy' (389). Several important biases are evident in the study, however. For instance, there was little difference between the two populations on the prevalence of alcoholism, a finding they rejected because it was 'common knowledge' that excessive alcohol consumption was greater among the Indians (389). None of the other findings were balanced against this 'common knowledge.' And the explanation of the higher prevalence of severe mental deficiency among the Indians was 'not altogether surprising;' as with the Hutterites, they suggested, 'inbreeding' could be at fault (389). Finally, after lumping the Cree and Saulteaux together to create an 'Indian' category, and placing the rest into a non-Indian category, they summarily declared the two populations to be 'culturally different' and their research to be 'cross-cultural,' despite the fact that they never actually addressed the issue of culture.

   In another study, Hendrie and Hanson (1972) undertook a comparison of psychiatric care for Indian, Métis, and other non-Aboriginal patients in a Winnipeg psychiatric hospital. They utilized what they termed a 'social' definition of Aboriginal status, and explicitly acknowledged the Métis as a distinct Aboriginal population. An Indian was defined as a person who identified as one or was so identified by relatives, or who was registered as an Indian by the federal government; a Métis was someone who so identified or was identified as such by relatives. Tellingly, while at least some examples were given of the backgrounds of those included in the non-Native category (e.g., English, Scottish, German), the tribal or cultural affiliation of the other two groups, and in particular, the Indians, was not mentioned. The size of the sample was small (twenty-five Indians, thirty-nine Métis, and seventy-two others) and the study focused on treatment rather than the identification of disorder. Nevertheless, the researchers did determine that the Métis population had a significantly lower proportion of schizophrenia compared to the Indians and the non-Aboriginals, and that the Indians and the Métis had a higher proportion of personality disorders and drug and alcohol addiction. Perhaps the most noteworthy aspect of the study was the inclusion of a social class variable. Unfortunately, the authors did not describe how class was operationalized and measured,[7] nor did they present data correlating class with diagnosis.

In 1976, Fritz published another Saskatchewan study involving a much larger data base: 140 Indians, 149 Métis, and 305 non-Natives. In this study, an attempt was also made to distinguish among the Aboriginal population, to separately identify the Indians (i.e., those who self-identified and were registered) and the Métis (again, determined on the basis of self-identification), but the latter category was problematic in that it also included non-registered Indians. And similar to the Hendrie and Hanson (1972) study, no mention was made of the specific cultural, community, or tribal affiliation of the Indian subjects. All subjects were patients in psychiatric treatment centres in Saskatchewan. Fritz determined that Indian and Métis inpatients were diagnosed as having psychiatric disorders less frequently than the non-Natives, due primarily to a much lower rate of schizophrenia among female Natives (i.e., Indians and Métis), but also due to a lower overall rate of psychotic disorders. Natives, however, received more frequent diagnoses of psychoneurotic disorders, especially depressive neurosis. Further, the largest difference between the two populations was in the category of personality/behaviour disorders, where the Indians and Métis had much higher rates of diagnosis than the non-Natives. Drug and alcohol problems were the most frequently noted for all three groups, and the overall incidence of psychiatric hospitalization was essentially the same.

In another oft-cited study, Sampath (1974, 1976) was able to undertake formal interviews with some 93 per cent ($N = 214$) of the adults in a Canadian Eskimo community in the eastern Arctic in 1970. The research involved the use of both a mental status examination (utilizing DSM-II) and the Health Opinion Survey (HOS), an instrument popular with several other researchers at the time which had as its focus the intent to discriminate between a known ill group, such as institutionalized patients, and a healthy population (Beiser 1981). The HOS results in a gradient from 'sickness' to 'wellness,' with four diagnostic categories: severe, moderate, mild, and minimal. Sampath's (1974) research led him to categorize his Eskimo subjects as follows: severe, 10 per cent; moderate, 27 per cent; mild, 58 per cent; and minimal, 7 per cent. From the mental health status examination Sampath (1974: 365) determined that 37 per cent were suffering from some form of mental disorder, a rate which 'at first glance, appear[ed] to be very high when compared to some North American studies.' However, in the absence of prevalence studies of other cultural groups, and especially Eskimo studies, he appeared content to leave this figure unchallenged and certainly did not question whether the unusually high rate could be the artifact of the methods employed. In fact, he noted that the strong correlation between the HOS and the mental health status exam demonstrated the utility of the HOS for this population. The reason for the high prevalence rate, according to Sampath, was to be found in the changes in social organization caused by 'modernization,' following contact with Europeans. In terms of individual diagnoses, he determined that the highest prevalence rate was for personality disorders, followed by neuroses, affective psychoses, and schizophrenia. Sampath noted the prevailing view that affective psychoses 'did not occur in primitive societies,' whereas schizophrenia did, and offered that the high prevalence rate of affective psychoses relative to schizophrenia among these Eskimos was reminiscent of Hutterite populations, once again trotting out this odd comparison mentioned earlier (see Roy et al. 1970). Sampath (1974) also found that 70 per cent of the females diagnosed with a personality disorder were suffering from the hysterical form with histories of dissociative reactions, which he explained as evidence of the persistence of 'a great deal of the so-called "arctic hysteria" or "pibloktoq"' (to be discussed in chapter 8).

From Canada we move now to a set of studies undertaken in the northwest coastal area of the United States. In 1968, psychiatrist James Shore, a central figure in much of the research on American Indian mental health, led a team to a small, isolated fishing community on the Pacific northwest coast for a study of psychiatric epidemiology. From a population of only 500, Shore and his colleagues (Shore, Kinzie, Hampson, & Pattison 1973; Shore 1974) generated a quota sample of 100, roughly half the total adult population. Employing the comprehensive method for psychiatric epidemiology pioneered by Alexander Leighton and Dorothea Leighton in their study of largely non-Aboriginal Stirling County in Nova Scotia,[8] two psychiatrists employed a structured seventy-item questionnaire and conducted mental health examinations over a six-month period. In addition to basic socio-economic and demographic data, they collected, among other things, a medical history, a health opinion survey, an antisocial inventory, and a psychotic scale (using items similar to those in the MMPI). 'Outside information' was also collected on the 'degree of Indian descent' (72), although it is not clear what was meant by this or how these data were incorporated. Importantly, the actual village, and even the specific culture of the people, was kept anonymous.

Based on these various sources of data, the probability of psychiatric disturbance, severity of impairment, and psychiatric diagnosis was determined (Shore et al. 1973). 'Definite' psychiatric disturbance was found for 54 per cent of the subjects, the highest category; 15 per cent were diagnosed with 'probable' disturbance. In terms of severity of impairment, 17 per cent were considered severe and a further 15 per cent moderate. In a sample of 100 adults, that is, an astounding 69 per cent were judged to be experiencing some psychiatric disturbance, and almost a third were experiencing moderate to severe psychiatric impairment! This was almost double the rate Sampath had found among the Eskimo, and which had struck him as remarkably high. The significance of what the researchers were saying seemed to elude them: while they agreed that there was 'an overall high prevalence of impairment rate for psychiatric morbidity among the members of this Indian village' (79), their data seemed to be pointing towards a profoundly dysfunctional community, at least in a psychiatric sense. Rather than questioning the methods which led to this result, the researchers offered the explanation that one segment of the community in particular, comprising the younger age groups, was experiencing a high degree of social disorganization, as evidenced by their relative lack of knowledge of 'traditional Indian values,' their knowledge of the language, and their increasing contact with non-Indians. This was as close as they came to discussing culture and its role in understanding the situation in this community. The main problem, they determined, was alcoholism, and the majority of those afflicted with this problem were men. Although they noted that alcoholism was a major concern among Indians throughout the country, they cautioned that 'It is impossible to compare these current figures with prior studies on Indian alcoholism rates because distinctions between culturally approved norms of drinking and nonnormative drinking have not been clearly made' (Shore et al. 1973: 77). And yet these researchers did not disclose anything about the culture of the people they were studying, let alone discuss the issue of cultural norms.

This study is noteworthy for two other reasons. First, the researchers attempted to measure social class, in a manner similar to that employed by Hendrie and Hanson (1972).[9] The method involved the identification of five social class groups on the basis of occupation and education. However, when they discovered that 92 per cent of their subjects fell into the lowest two groups, they reformatted the data to create an 'Indian social class' variable containing three of the five groups, and then found that there was a significant correlation between high degrees of psychiatric disturbance and lowest socioeconomic status. Second, some of the same researchers, joined by several new individuals, were able to undertake a restudy of this village nineteen years later (Kinzie et al. 1992; Boehnlein et al. 1993). New instruments were used to gather data (e.g., the Schedule for Affective Disorders and Schizophrenia Lifetime Version, or SADS-L, to be discussed in the next chapter), and the 1969 data, which had been categorized using DSM-III, was recategorized into the more current DSM-IIIR to be compatible with the system used in the 1988 study. Forty-six of the original 100 subjects were included and others were added to achieve a sample size of 131. Overall, the results demonstrated some improvement in the mental health of the community. For instance, only 31 per cent of the 1988 sample, compared to 59 per cent of the 1969 sample, were considered to have a DSM-IIIR diagnosis. But this is still quite high. An overall decline in alcoholism was also noted, and in the intervening nineteen years there had been no deaths from suicide, homicide, or traffic accidents. Yet the point prevalence rate for alcoholism remained high at 21 per cent, as did the lifetime prevalence for men (76 per cent) and women (39 per cent). The authors nevertheless saw these results as positive, suggesting that participation in organized religions as well as traditional cultural activities, combined with higher educational levels, more effective tribal government, and other positive changes to village life, were likely the most significant explanatory factors.[10] The 1988 study utilized a new technique for assessing socioeconomic status; the data correlating that status with psychiatric disturbance were, at best, ambiguous, in contrast to the more positive finding in the 1969 study.

In a review of many of the population studies discussed above, Manson and Shore (1981: 50) wrote that, while they 'may be open to various methodological criticisms ... they do each provide a broad and divergent picture of the nature and pattern of disorder in Indian and Native communities.' The results were acceptable, in other words, despite the methodological problems. Years later, these authors, along with a third, commented again on the methodological issues, focusing on the problems inherent in the use of relatively small non-probability samples, and especially those drawn from clinical or treatment populations (Somervell, Manson, & Shore 1995). They asked, for instance, what should be made 'of the apparently very high rate of schizophrenia of 4.4 percent in Kinzie et al.'s sample of 131 persons' (319). But in concentrating on the admittedly important issue of sampling, they failed to consider other aspects of the methods, in particular, especially, the theoretical and epistemological underpinnings that led many researchers to accept as valid extremely high rates of disorder. Are Aboriginal peoples so wracked with psychopathology that the methodology employed, and the limitations thereof, is not really an issue?

Attempts to undertake broad-based, community-wide or regional studies of psychopathology have become considerably less frequent in recent years. A recently published study demonstrates a different approach to community or regional studies, something of a throwback to the days when self-reported health status, using instruments such as the Cornell Medical Index, were the primary research tools. Kirmayer and Boothroyd et al. (2000) utilized an existing database from a 1991 Santé Quebéc health survey in the James Bay Cree region. A survey of 354 households, totalling almost 2000 individuals, had been undertaken using stratified and systematic sampling procedures. From this data set, the researchers derived data for 1136 Cree adults (aged fifteen to eighty-five) who had completed an interviewer-assisted confidential questionnaire on 'psychological distress.' Data were also gathered through the use of individual and household questionnaires. The instruments were administered face-to-face by Cree interviewers in either Cree or English. Kirmayer and Boothroyd et al. (2000) obtained access to these data and performed the statistical analyses reported in this paper.

The psychological distress instrument is of particular importance here. This was a fourteen-item index adapted from another instrument used by Santé Quebéc for a non-Aboriginal population. The instrument contained fourteen statements about psychological symptoms that may have been experienced in the week preceding the survey. The survey was subjected to focus group discussion with Cree people to ascertain content validity, with the result that one question was changed. Following the opening statement, 'In the past week, did you ...' the survey included items such as 'feel hopeless about the future;' 'feel down or blue;' 'lose your temper;' 'feel easily annoyed or irritated.' Respondents then selected from a Likert-style scale to respond 'never,' 'once in a while,' 'fairly often,' or 'very often.' After a detailed statistical analysis, the researchers reported that several factors were associated with a report of greater psychological distress in the past week: 'younger age, female gender, having more than elementary education, residing in an inland region [as opposed to the coastal area], residing in an isolated region, having a drinking problem in the past year, ever having used cannabis, early loss of a close relative, not having a good relationship with the community, having fewer than five close friends/relatives, having had more significant life events in the year before the survey and spending less time in the bush in the past year' (Kirmayer & Boothroyd et al. 2000: 48–9). Kirmayer and Boothroyd et al. (2000) then noted that the association of female gender, early loss, life events, and the lack of social support was consistent with research on these factors in other populations. In noting that, among the Cree as well as other North American populations, females were more likely to report distress than males, as separate from actually experiencing it, they touched upon an important confounding factor in any study based on self-reporting. However, they did not delve deeply enough into the issue of the relationship between psychological distress and higher educational attainment for both males and females, speculating only that education may increase expectations for young people that cannot be met, or that with increased education comes higher stress employment. I think another explanation is possible as well: being younger and possessed of higher education may increase the ability and willingness of Cree people to complete the questionnaires in a manner compatible with the expectations of the research designers. In other words, what was being measured may not have been psychological distress but rather willingness and ability to report that distress in a manner that would be identified by the instruments used and the researchers who used them. The researchers acknowledged some of the serious limitations of the study resulting from the fact that they were dependent upon a secondary database, and that the measure of psychological distress provided only an indirect measure of psychiatric disorder, adding that 'the measure of distress was not culturally adapted and its sensitivity to the range of expression of distress across gender and age cohorts is unknown' (52). This is an important admission, in effect saying that while the instrument was *linguistically* appropriate, in so far as it was translatable into Cree, the constructs behind it may not have been appropriate.

Conclusion

What emerges from the various studies of Aboriginal peoples discussed in this chapter is a profound willingness to accept that Aboriginal populations are, relatively speaking, rife with psychiatric disorder.
Two factors working together can explain this propensity. The first factor is a confidence in the methodological techniques employed and
their conceptual underpinnings, and especially their cross-cultural
validity, such that rigorous methodological critique is almost nonexist-
ent. The second factor betrays the two deeply rooted beliefs that comprise primitivist discourse and which are not entirely compatible.
Indigenous peoples, 'primitives,' were considered by many to be inherently disordered prior to colonization, with European contact simply
bringing to the forefront many underlying and pre-existing pathologies. Yet much research has been guided by an implicit assumption that
Aboriginal North Americans had lived a utopian, changeless existence
prior to colonization, with the subsequent emergence of psychopathology viewed as the logical consequence of too rapid or destructive cultural change. Both perspectives suggest a contemporary inability of
Aboriginal peoples to deal with their problems. To quote Seltzer (1980:
174), 'acculturation, then, is a system under strain with a *limited* range
of solutions to resolve the culture conflict facing the native' (emphasis
added). But also imbedded within both perspectives has been a tendency to search for psychopathology at the expense of comprehending
what makes for a healthy community and individual (Beiser 1981). This
tendency remains evident when we examine the research on specific
disorders.

CHAPTER SIX

The Alcoholic Aboriginal

Nothing earthly could better deserve the epithet infernal than an Indian town in the height of a drunken debauch. The orgies never ceased till the bottom of the barrel was reached. (Parkman 1909: 388)

In almost every Indian group that I know about, the initial response to alcoholic beverages was the same – a drunken orgy. When the first White man opened the first keg of liquor, nearly every Indian in proximity proceeded to get uproariously drunk and continued drinking as long as the liquor held out. (R.K. Thomas 1981)

These passages, written seventy years apart by two scholars, explain, in a nutshell, why I have included a chapter on alcohol in this book. No single Aboriginal mental health topic has dominated the research and discourse as much as alcohol, and none has generated such a combination of perverse curiosity, genuine concern, and outright absurdity, not to mention racism. How Aboriginal peoples drink, where they drink, why they drink, with whom they drink, how much they drink, what happens to them when they drink – the study of Aboriginal peoples and alcohol is an industry unto itself. And both the Arcadian and the Barbarian have fallen prey to the demon rum.

Make no mistake about it: to try to cover the literature on Aboriginal peoples and alcohol adequately is a monumental task. If there is any one topic which best epitomizes the European fascination with Aboriginal peoples, this is it. As we have seen so far in this book, alcohol enters into many other issues of physical and mental health, personality, and treatment, and it is not easy to detach it from these other topics. Co-morbidity is the norm if one takes the literature seriously. Consequently, I will not attempt to survey the field as a whole; rather, I will attack alcohol in the same way I have attacked other issues so far, strategically, focusing on issues of culture, concept, and methodology. I am particularly interested in how scholars and researchers have thought about alcohol and Aboriginal peoples, and why they have thought this way. As in the other chapters, I focus on work that I think has been the most influential. And, although there is a strong and growing parallel literature on other forms of substance abuse, it would be somewhat redundant from the point of view of the goals of this book to expand into these other areas as well.

In this chapter, I look first at the issue of biological susceptibility, primarily because of the parallels it has with the problems inherent in category and boundary construction. I then examine some of the major works on Aboriginal alcoholism, those works which have established the main explanations for how and why Aboriginal peoples consume alcohol. Issues of incidence and prevalence will be addressed only briefly, since many of the critiques appropriate to epidemiological studies of Aboriginal peoples and alcohol have already been covered in the chapter on psychopathology.

The Biologically Susceptible Aboriginal

A great deal has been written about the biological susceptibility of North American Aboriginal peoples to alcohol. Indeed, it has been suggested that the belief that Aboriginal peoples metabolize alcohol differently, and that this explains how they drink, why they drink, and the problems that drinking causes, has led to the 'myth of the drunken Indian' (Westermeyer 1974a), or 'firewater myths' as Leland (1976) calls them (see also MacAndrew & Edgerton 1969). Westermeyer and Baker (1986) have even suggested that Aboriginal peoples often faked drunkenness after consumption of only a small amount of alcohol, resulting in the interpretation that they could not 'hold their liquor.' The pervasiveness of the biological explanation is impressive; not only do many non-Aboriginal North Americans believe in it, but it has been argued that many Aboriginal peoples have bought into the explanation as well (e.g., Boyer 1964b; Lurie 1971; May 1986, 1992a; Savishinsky 1991; Kunitz & Levy 1994; May 1999).[1] As May (1992a, 1992b) has pointed out, among Aboriginal peoples such a view is fatalistic and interferes with the development of programs to reduce the damage caused by alcohol.

The scientific interest in biological explanations has followed logically from historic reports of Aboriginal drinking patterns that seemed wildly *different* from non-Aboriginal norms. These norms were anchored in a very European, class-based conceptualization of what was considered an appropriate way to drink, and how to behave while under the influence (which is not to say that Europeans actually drank this way). Evolutionary theory, which postulated the existence not only of separate biological races but also of biologically inferior 'grades of humanity' (Harris 1968: 162), also played a part in explaining European observations of Aboriginal drinking. Researchers, concentrating on singular Aboriginal communities, have clearly been attracted to the exoticism of the 'drinking party' as an ethnographic subject, leading to a common image of individuals engaged in raucous bouts of binge drinking lasting days. These studies have reinforced the implicit view that, because their approach to alcohol has been deemed different, Aboriginal peoples must somehow be reacting to its chemical properties differently.

It is not my intent to provide a detailed biological critique of studies of ethanol metabolism. My interest, in keeping with the general theme of this volume, is in the construction of the categories employed in these experiments, and in teasing out the assumptions that underlie both the categories and the broader concern that biological susceptibility is, indeed, an issue which should be studied. I shall argue that, just as there is a kind of cultural essentialism in the conceptualization of Aboriginal peoples, there is a parallel biological essentialism, a view in which the 'primitive,' either Arcadian or Barbarian, naturally succumbs to the demands of the inner savage when under the influence.

The lightning rod for the issue of biological susceptibility was research, more than three decades ago, by Fenna, Mix, Schaefer, and Gilbert (1971), who undertook a very opportunistic study of Eskimos, Indians, and whites in Inuvik and Edmonton. Limited in size, as these studies characteristically were, the study involved the controlled administration of alcohol to twenty-one Eskimos, twenty-six Indians, and seventeen whites; many of the Eskimos and Indians were actually hospital patients, and the whites were drawn from the staff of the same Edmonton hospital. Using a breathalyzer, blood alcohol levels were measured at intervals to determine the rate at which they decreased. The overall conclusion was that the Indians and Eskimos metabolized alcohol at a slower rate than the whites, likely due to genetic differences.

Critics of this famous study focused on problems with the sample, the different body weights of the Aboriginals in comparison to the whites, the existence of a proportionately higher number of heavy drinkers among the Aboriginal group, and the unreliability of the breathalyzer. Interestingly, there was little critique of the way in which the categories of Indian, Eskimo, and white were generated. These were taken to be intrinsically meaningful categories, perhaps as a result of the a priori observation which sparked the study, that in jail intoxicated Aboriginals seemed to take longer to sober up than whites. Of course, there was a whole host of potential explanations for this observation, including differences in quantity consumed and differential prison treatment of the two populations, as well as the possibility that the whites 'sobered up' in a manner more noticeable and acceptable to the European jailers and others who made these judgments. We were also not provided with any detail about the subjects themselves, about how Eskimoness or Indianness or whiteness were determined. No data were provided on cultural or biological background. Were these indeed separate 'racial' groups?

Shortly after the publication of the Fenna et al. (1971) study, other research emerged (e.g., Lieber 1972), most of which argued that Indians metabolized alcohol *faster* than whites. The majority of these studies committed the same conceptual and methodological errors of the Fenna study. Bennion and Li (1976), for instance, presented data on thirty 'full-blood' American Indians and thirty whites in a Phoenix study. The degree of Indian bloodedness was determined through self-reported geneologies; interestingly, the degree of bloodedness of the whites was not addressed. The cultural background of the Indians was also not identified. The researchers clearly assumed that they were dealing with two distinct and internally homogeneous populations. They did allow for the possibility that the Indians studied by Fenna et al. 'were from a single tribe with a genetic disposition to metabolize alcohol more slowly than whites' (Bennion & Li 1976: 12), missing the point that there were also Eskimos in the Fenna study. But then they added 'that such a disposition is not characteristic of North American Indians in general,' as demonstrated by their own study. In other words, North American Indians *in general* were represented by their sample of thirty from an unnamed tribe or tribes!

In two related studies, Farris and Jones examined the issue of ethanol metabolization for a group of American Indian males (1978a) and females (1978b). The total number of Indian and white study participants was again small (thirty-four males, thirty females), and it was concluded that the Indians metabolized alcohol faster. Some data were presented on tribal affiliation of the Indian subjects, ranging from Cherokee to Sioux to Navajo; each of the seventeen Indian male subjects had a different tribal affiliation. Whites, in contrast, were not defined other than through a declaration that they did not have Indian ancestry. I think the problem here is fairly clear: the researchers assumed that, despite the fact that their Indian subjects were drawn from so many different regions and language families, they all somehow exhibited a biological integrity that allowed them to be grouped together. To their credit, however, in their study of women, Farris and Jones (1978b) went one step further to ask whether the differences in metabolism of ethanol had any real behavioural consequences, and in one experiment, they determined that there was no difference in the performance of the Indians and whites engaged in verbal memory tasks while under the influence of ethanol.

Comparisons of the Aboriginal population with Asian populations have also been popular, the result of a hypothesized biological connection between the two continents. Wolff's (1973: 193) research is a good example of this line of thinking (see also Rex, Bosron, Smialek, & Li 1985). Wolff tested the assumption that 'North American Indians, commonly classified as members of the Mongoloid major mating populations, would show the same alcohol sensitivity as native Chinese and Japanese.' Comparing a sample of thirty Eastern Cree Indians with both 'pure' and mixed heritage Japanese and Chinese, he determined that there was little difference between them in the incidence and intensity of flushing to orally introduced alcohol, with an incidence rate of about 80 per cent, in comparison to a Caucasian rate of only 5 per cent. Prior experience with alcohol did not account for the differences between groups. The sample of Cree was not homogeneous, however; only half of the thirty subjects considered themselves to be 'pure Indian' (whatever that means), and many more indicated at least some non-Cree ancestry. The boundaries of this population, biologically speaking, appear fuzzy even if there was some degree of cultural homogeneity. In a review of Wolff's work, Brod (1975) insightfully noted the complications that the extensive 'hybridization' of the Indian population caused, and also questioned the assumption that all American Indians, and in particular the Eastern Cree, were Mongoloid. This assumption stems from acceptance of the Bering Strait theory of the populating of the Western hemisphere, but the available evidence suggests that very different biological populations migrated at different times over many thousands of years. Wolff did admit that, regardless of the results of the study, the relevance of the findings to the question of alcoholism remained unclear, given that, in his view, Indians have considerably higher rates of alcoholism than the Chinese. He insisted that there must be a biological explanation for alcoholism, but added that biology likely works in conjunction with 'sociocultural forces' (198). 'When the social cohesion of a culture is destroyed as it has been in the case of the American Indians,' he explained, 'a greater suscepti-bility to alcohol intoxication may act as one of several predisposing factors for alcoholism' (ibid.). Note how the Eastern Cree had become 'American Indians' more generically, and that Wolff concluded that a uniform destruction of Aboriginal culture had ensued. Separate from the issue of equating the experiences of these Cree with all Aboriginal North Americans, it may also be misleading to suggest that there had been a destruction of the 'social cohesion' of Cree society. Wolff does not tell us precisely where he obtained these Cree subjects, and this hampers our examination of his claims. But there is ample evidence that the Cree of Quebec, usually considered the 'eastern' branch of the Cree, were living relatively intact social lives until at least the early 1970s, when the Quebec government commenced a series of hydro-electric developments; certainly that was the view of the Cree them-selves (Richardson 1975; Adelson 2001). Wolff, it seems, uncritically accepted the historical fallacy of the uniform destruction of all Aborig-inal societies.

Recognition that Aboriginal populations were not necessarily 'pure' in a biological sense led to a concern for measuring blood quantum. Weisner, Weibel-Orlando, and Long (1984), for example, measured both percentage of Indian ancestry (or blood quantum) and drinking levels. Both measures were fraught with problems, but they neverthe-less concluded that individuals with '50%' Indian ancestry drank more than individuals with both greater and less Indian ancestry (referred to as the inverted 'U' pattern, to be discussed in the next chapter), sug-gesting that the problem was not biological but rather one of accultura-tive stress. In a similar and more recent study, Garcia-Andrade, Wall, and Ehlers (1997) divided a small group of Mission Indians into two groups, those with more than 25 per cent but less than 50 per cent Indian blood quantum, and those with 50 per cent or more Indian blood quantum, according to self-reports. An alcoholic drink was pro-vided to some, a placebo to others, and both subjective responses to the effects of alcohol and objective measures of blood pressure, pulse rate, plasma cortisol levels, and blood alcohol levels were taken after varying periods of time. They determined that overall the Indian men proved not to be overly sensitive to the effects of alcohol and that those with 50 per cent or more Indian blood reported feeling fewer effects of intoxication than those with less Indian blood. They concluded from this that, compatible with other studies, 'groups at higher risk for alcoholism have a less intense subjective response to alcohol and that groups at lower genetic risk for alcoholism have a more intense subjective response to alcohol' (986). In other words, individuals with greater Indian blood were at higher risk for alcoholism because of the genetic nature of this disease. But their study did not provide any data to the effect that degree of Indian blood was in any way a factor, and indeed there are no reputable studies that support this supposition. In fact, their data demonstrated no significant differences in blood alcohol concentration, pulse rate, or plasma cortisol levels between the two Indian groups, only that their subjective reporting of the effects differed. While they posited a possible cultural explanation, they were forced to reject the explanation that blood quantum had something to do with the expectations individuals had concerning their response to alcohol.

Over the years, there have been many reviews of the issue of alcohol sensitivity and differential rates of ethanol metabolism among Aboriginal North Americans, virtually all of which have justifiably criticized the problematic methodologies and, to a lesser extent, the underlying assumptions of race and biology. Fisher (1987) argued that the concept of race employed in these studies was faulty and that researchers characteristically failed to examine the extent to which subjects in their race categories were genetically homogeneous. His position, that 'understanding alcohol problems among Amerindians or other socially identifiable groups is best approached by examining that group's social life, rather than the genes of individual group members' was enlightened (Fisher 1987: 90). Lewis (1982: 319; see also Dozier 1966) reminded researchers that American Indians were a 'social entity rather than a biological one,' largely created by federal legislation and characteristically of mixed 'Caucasian' and 'Negroid' ancestry. Other studies have documented that intermarriage with Europeans and Africans was extensive (Snipp 1997), and that this has affected the genetic structure of Aboriginal populations (Szathmary & Reed 1972). Snipp (1997: 678) has also argued that issues of biological heritage and cultural self-identity have become 'decoupled' as a result of changing ethnic currency and federal and tribal regulations regarding tribe and band membership; in other words, simple declarations of Indian heritage, or enlistment in a tribe or band, are inadequate as biological markers. The significant attention paid to the issue of blood quantum in the United States is a particularly good example of the contradictions found in many studies that purport to enlist subjects who are biologically homogeneous while accepting various levels of 'Indian blood' as sufficient. Many years ago, Reed (1978) argued that genetic variation was much greater within 'races' than among them, and that it was logical that there would be differences in ethanol metabolism among Indian groups. He also argued insightfully that 'the concept of "the" American Indian should disappear along with the concepts of "the" white man and "the" white mouse or rat' (87). Heath (1983: 347; emphasis in the original) similarly argued that 'use of the term *Whites* is even less justified, in scientific terms, than *Indians*' (see also Heath 1987). These cautions went largely unheard.

In recent years, interest in the alleged biological susceptibility of Aboriginal peoples to alcohol has generally waned, perhaps because of both the methodological complications and the racist overtones of the older research. In the only lengthy discussion of its kind in the alcohol literature, Reed, Kalant, Gibbins, Kapur, and Rankin (1976) hypothesized that there was extensive evidence for confounding genetic diversity among the Aboriginal population, in part because of genetic drift, and indicated by linguistic evidence of very different language families. 'It would be helpful,' they added somewhat laconically, 'if future studies of native [sic] peoples included tribal or linguistic details' (855). In a review of alcohol issues, Westermeyer (1996) did not even mention the biological debate. Caetano, Clark, and Tam (1998: 237) argued straightforwardly that 'no evidence exists to demonstrate increased physiological or psychological reactivity to alcohol among Native Americans compared with other ethnic groups'; May (1996, 1999) concurred, and added that even if biological susceptibility could be demonstrated, it would have very little effect on the development of solutions to the problem of alcohol abuse (May 1982). 'Both the causes of and solutions to alcohol abuse problems in an Indian community,' May (1992a: 7) has written, 'lie in the social and cultural realm of the community itself, the subcultures within it, and the social structures in the surrounding region.' But Mail (1989: 20) postulated that at least 'some individuals may have a degree of genetic susceptibility,' and Young (1993), not entirely convinced, has suggested a need for further research. Beauvais (1998) noted that more general research on the heritability of alcoholism has continued, that it is a common area of research for all populations and not one that targets Aboriginal peoples (see, G.C. Brown et al. 1993). The difference today, it seems, is the emphasis on individual, as opposed to population, genetic traits that may allow us to predict with some certainty which individuals are at risk. To some extent, this approach avoids the tricky and scientifically indefensible issue of biologically susceptible populations.

Why has so much attention been paid to the question of biological susceptibility? I think the answer is multifaceted, and it begins with the broad assumption by many, both historically and even today, that Aboriginal peoples are inferior biologically (as well as culturally, morally, intellectually, and so on). The search for a biological explanation for what was seen as either problematic behaviour or moral failing at least got the racists off the hook, for it is not necessarily racist if one can demonstrate that populations do indeed differ biologically in some tangible and measurable, that is, scientific, way. But extending this further, and going back to the Fenna at al. (1971) study that seemed to start the modern-day debate, it appears the problem also lies in the assumption of Europeans that there was only one way to drink, to behave while drunk, and to sober up, and that any deviation from this was, well, deviant. A focus on the *patterns* and *consequences* of drinking led to erroneous assumptions regarding the people doing the drinking. I now turn to the issue of how and why Aboriginal peoples drink.

The How and Why of Aboriginal Drinking

The interest in biological differences between whites, Aboriginals, and others is reflected in studies examining drinking patterns. Early ethnographers played an important role in the development of literature on Aboriginal drinking, and often made observations on drinking behaviour, but alcohol was rarely the focus of their investigations (Heath 1987). Much of the work was opportunistic, leading to jokes about anthropologists doing 'bar ethnography' that persist to this day (see Leland 1979a). It was the ethnographers who attempted to understand how alcohol fit into Aboriginal societies, and they were frequently less concerned with delineating social pathology or alcoholism. In some instances this led to accusations that their work was irrelevant, while in others the work was summarily dismissed as little more than descriptions of quaint customs, lacking scientific rigour. There was definitely something exotic and unique about Aboriginal drinking (May 1982), and combined with the pervasive 'firewater' myths of drunken savagery, it satisfied the anthropological demand for bizarre cultural material. As it is difficult to separate out from the literature explanations of how Aboriginal peoples drink from explanations of why they drink, I propose to discuss the two topics more or less simultaneously. Generally, explanations for Aboriginal drinking express two basic themes: that drinking is best understood as a product of historical forces including culture loss and social disintegration, as well as economic deprivation, what I call the 'acculturation/anomie/social disorganization paradigm'; and that drinking should be seen as a cultural phenomenon related to pre-contact social organization and culture as well as behaviours learned from Europeans, or the 'cultural continuity/integration paradigm.' As one might expect, some work plays at the borders of these two paradigms, integrating elements of each in the kind of omnibus explanations discussed earlier.[2] I will focus here on the more distinct aspects of the two.

The Acculturation/Anomie/Social Disorganization Paradigm

The argument that has proven to have the greatest resilience, and perhaps the greatest emotional appeal, has been that Aboriginal peoples drink because they have experienced anomie and sociocultural disorganization as a result of colonization, including acculturative stress (hereafter the 'disorganization' paradigm). Many believed that rapid sociocultural change, especially that resulting from increased contact with more cosmopolitan Western influences, led to increasing rates of mental illness (Leighton 1959a, 1959b). The idea that contact with the West resulted in disintegration and mental illness is a keystone of the Arcadian tradition as described by Lucas and Barrett (1995); it heightens the fall from Eden, so to speak, and implicitly suggests that there was no mental illness in these societies prior to the intrusion of Western influences.

Edwin Lemert (1954) was one of the first to articulate this perspective, arguing that Northwest Coast Indians had suffered 'deculturation' along with a collapse in opportunities to engage in meaningful sociocultural and economic activities. 'The inebriation of the Indian,' he wrote, 'tends to be a symptom of mental disorder or emotional conflicts related to acculturation and family disorganization' (362). These peoples drank because they were bored, to 'break up the monotony of an unrewarding daily existence,' in Lemert's words (336). But they also drank as an act of 'aggression,' resistance, or protest against white authority. Anthropologist John Honigmann (1965) applied the concept of social disintegration as developed by Leighton to his work in northern Canada, and indeed Leighton's formulation, especially the idea of a malfunctioning social system which leads to psychiatric distress, influenced much of the work in this area. Berreman (1956) for the Aleut, Hamer (1965) for the Pottawotami, Kraus and Buffler (1979) for Alaska Natives, and Mail (1989) more generally argued that anxiety caused by acculturative stress resulted in drinking, and here we see early evidence of the weaving of innate psychological factors, in this case a model of personality, with sociocultural factors, all mediated by historical processes. Aboriginal peoples were 'frustrated' with their marginal existence (Topper 1974: 115), grappling with 'feelings of inadequacy' (Thomas 1981: 35), and alcohol developed into a metaphor 'of hopelessness, helplessness, defeat, and escape from historic circumstances' (Mail & Johnson 1993: 17; see also Jilek-Aall 1981). Alcohol was deemed to serve an important social function in an otherwise empty existence. Hamer (1965) suggested that the Pottawotami were suffering from an 'extreme loss of self-respect' and that 'the only dependable and satisfying social relations are to be obtained through drinking' (299). This view was echoed by Curley (1967), who likewise argued that, for the Mescalero Apache, alcohol was literally the 'behavioral glue' that united adolescent boys into meaningful social groups, while the adults lived in a 'decultured state.' Alcohol for these peoples, and especially its consequences of occasional fighting and sexual activity, added 'spice' to their lives. Littman (1970: 1784) suggested that for Indians in Chicago, many of whom suffered from some mental illness, alcohol played an important role 'in promoting psychological and social integration for those who are unable to function otherwise, and where the Anglo-American culture does not provide substitute outlets.'

Men in particular seemed to be at greatest risk of alcohol-related problems. Curley (1967) and Mohatt (1972), like many other theorists, argued that alcohol hit men hardest because historical and cultural changes had dramatically reduced their status and productive roles in society, a theme which emerges continuously in the alcohol discourse (recalling Gordon Macgregor's Sioux 'warriors without weapons'). Mohatt (1972: 266) suggested that the 'feelings of euphoria and strength reminiscent of the successful theft, hunt, or battle,' inducing 'temporary states of euphoric assertiveness,' may have 'served a positive function in preventing total despair and self-destruction' among the Sioux. Pedigo (1983) likewise argued that alcohol may have contributed to cultural survival by easing the pain and suffering associated with cultural change and degradation. Edward Dozier (1966), one of the leading proponents of the disorganization thesis, suggested that the American Indian had fallen 'from a proud existence in an earlier time,' and had been subjected to the 'pathetic revelation of his worthlessness' as a result of a number of 'degrading experiences,' including confinement to reservations, the failed attempt to turn him into a farmer, and the prohibitions placed on alcohol use (76). He had developed a 'deep sense of inferiority and inadequacy' (76) as a result, and suffered from low economic status, poor housing, lack of education, and discrimination. But alcohol was not nearly as destructive as it could have been, according to Hamer (1965: 300), because there were so few 'institutionalized norms' remaining after colonization with which alcohol could interfere.

While most saw acculturation as the cause of alcohol abuse, Graves (1967b) argued that acculturation in and of itself was not necessarily bad; problems arose when the avenues to success were thwarted upon acculturation. Acculturation in the southwest had not only resulted in the breakdown of the means for attaining traditional goals, it had created frustrations in attempting to achieve the new goals. Both unacculturated Indians and those attempting to acculturate experienced deprivation and alienation, but in different ways. Members of both groups drank, while successful acculturation greatly reduced alcohol consumption. This pattern has been reported by others as well. Maynard (1969), for instance, defined an 'alcohol adjustment syndrome' among the Oglala Sioux, in which she noted that alcohol consumption was most problematic among those who were least acculturated, those who were blocked in their process of acculturation or, those who, having acculturated, were unable to achieve their goals. The implication of these studies was that the only healthy lifestyle was one attainable through successful acculturation, a result almost too convenient for policy makers intent on just such a process. But successful acculturation was inhibited by a lack of self-confidence. Jilek-Aall (1981: 147–8; see also Jilek 1981, 1982; Jilek & Jilek-Aall 1971) described the Coast Salish individual as so in awe of the white man, so intimidated by him, and so wrought with feelings of inadequacy and doubt, that alcohol was necessary to establish the kind of self-confidence that would allow for interaction. 'Only when the Indian people can regain their cultural identity and self-respect,' she has written, 'will they have the inner strength necessary to fight alcoholism' (Jilek-Aall 1981: 157).

Generally, the social disorganization and anomie theorists focused on explaining why Aboriginal peoples drank, and not so much on how they drank. But at least one aspect of the deprivation Aboriginal peoples experienced was considered a factor in explaining drinking patterns: binge drinking, a commonly described pattern, was sometimes thought to be a reaction to the prohibition on Indian drinking in both the United States and Canada, which required individuals to consume quickly to avoid detection (Kemnitzer 1972; J.A. Price 1975; Mail & Johnson 1993). A focus on social pathology, especially interactions with the justice system, underscored the prevailing view among many scholars that the *consequences* of drinking for Indians were not only measurable but also markers of serious disorder.

Many scholars have continued to assert that the disorganization paradigm provides the best explanation for Aboriginal drinking (French 1980; Westermeyer & Baker 1986; T.J. Young 1989). Some, such as French and Hornbuckle (1980), have couched their explanations in dramatic terms, speaking not simply of acculturation but of physical and cultural genocide. The caught-between-two-worlds perspective rises again as well. May (1986: 189) argued that 'those with the highest risk for misuse are marginal to both Indian traditional and modern cultures,' while Nofz (1988: 68) suggested that 'culturally marginal' individuals, those who experience 'inner conflict' because of the existence of 'two distinct, and often contradictory, cultural milieus,' neither one of which they can meaningfully enjoy, were prime candidates for alcohol abuse. American Indian scholar Vine Deloria, Jr (1969: 86), poking fun at anthropologists, chided them for the 'between two worlds' paradigm. 'People between two worlds ... DRANK,' he mimicked, and 'for the anthropologists, it was a valid explanation of drinking on the reservation.' 'Real Indians ... drank,' he added, and according to his interpretation of the anthropologists' argument, only by drinking could young Indians 're-create the glories of the past.' While Deloria's critique rattled many anthropologists, it did not lessen the atttractiveness of the liminality perspective.

In general, the existence of *any* alcohol consumption, and not necessarily abuse, has frequently been taken as a sign of social and cultural disorganization, and few researchers have ever felt the need to demonstrate empirically that such disorganization existed or that it was causative of alcohol use and abuse. O'Nell (1993: 447) is one of the few who have challenged the assumption that alcohol abuse (and other problems such as suicide) are singular signs of the 'supposedly ubiquitous demoralization affecting American Indians.' Not all Flathead drinking was pathological, she argued. Many other scholars have frequently made the same observation with respect to particular Aboriginal groups, yet the alcohol-consumption-means-social-disorganization model has persisted. But why have so many scholars assumed that disorganization results in drinking problems, rather than that drinking problems result in disorganization? There is certainly just as much evidence for the latter proposition as for the former. Aboriginal societies have their own notions of deviant drinking, and this would suggest that those who misuse according to local cultural standards become marginal, rather than the other way around. At the very least, this alternative hypothesis requires some investigation.

The Cultural Continuity/Integration Paradigm

Let me turn now to those who have argued that alcohol is best understood within the context of pre-contact cultural formations and post-contact learned behaviours. Several themes emerge in this examination.

The first theme relates to the question of the personality structure of Aboriginal societies and individuals and how alcohol was accepted, or rejected, in accordance with inherent strengths or weaknesses in personality. Once again we return to the influential work of A.I. Hallowell. The reader will recall that Hallowell believed that the Saulteaux people he studied exhibited great reserve in their personality formation and exhibition, with suppression of emotion and aggression being the norm. Culturally approved outlets for the expression of anger and hostility existed in the form of witchcraft and gossip, but these rarely caused significant disruption in group functioning. How did alcohol intersect with this view of the Indian's personality? According to Hallowell (1941b, 1955), alcohol functioned to release inhibitions and therefore was particularly attractive to those living in societies such as the Saulteaux, who experienced a characteristic suppression of affect in their daily lives. This is the essence of the 'disinhibition' theory of alcohol use that remains influential to this day. Hallowell (1955: 141), in a frequently cited passage, defined an essential Indian character which existed beneath the surface of barely controlled anxiety: 'Since there also appears to be a connection between personality organization, culture pattern and behavior under the influence of alcohol, the conduct of the Indian when drunk was, in a sense, a natural experiment, a cue to his character. If his basic emotional structure was one that led to the suppression of a great deal of affect, in particular aggressive impulses, then we would expect that these might be released in a notably violent form under the influence of alcohol. This seems to have been what happened.' The real Indian, then, was a violent and murderous individual, and these horrible tendencies were kept tenuously in check, only to be released as the result of alcohol. This is a somewhat surprising observation, given that Hallowell also noted that, when sober, Saulteaux interpersonal relations were remarkably amiable! When faced with this apparent contradiction, Hallowell chose to represent the essence of the Indian as that of the savage. This viewpoint was hardly an exception in this era. James Baker (1959: 275), for instance, the chief medical officer at the famous Leavenworth penitentiary in Kansas, argued that alcohol and Indians were an 'explosive mix' first recognized by early settlers, and he noted that most of the Indians incarcerated in Leavenworth had engaged in 'very primitive' forms of homicide while intoxicated (as opposed to 'civilized' ways to kill).

These views were both reinforced and perpetuated by Donald Horton (1943), in what for decades was thought to be the seminal work on alcohol and 'primitive' peoples. Inspired by Hallowell's early work among the Saulteaux, Horton argued that the primary function of alcohol was, indeed, to reduce anxiety. He attempted a comparative study of dozens of 'primitive' societies throughout the world, categorizing those societies according to the levels of subsistence anxiety and belief in sorcery and witchcraft. Horton accepted Hallowell's essentialist ideas of the character of the Saulteaux and other 'primitives' as one in which social and cultural mechanisms were largely inadequate to the task of constraining behaviour once alcohol was consumed; the inner Indian invariably escaped these feeble constraints to reveal its ugly self.[3] For both Hallowell and Horton, the disinhibition theory meant that the Indians actively sought out alcohol specifically for its anxiety-releasing properties. In a review of Horton's data, Field (1962) came to a different conclusion, arguing that anxiety was not the issue at all. Rather, Field believed the data set demonstrated that drunkenness in 'primitive' societies was determined by the presence or absence of corporate kin groups which were stable and more or less permanent and which had well-defined structures. Where stable, structured kin groups existed, alcohol problems were more infrequent. Heath (1983) has suggested that Field's hypothesis was largely supported by existing data. This argument later developed into the view that levels of sociocultural integration explained alcohol behaviours, as discussed below.

The disinhibition idea, in various forms, was widely accepted. Scholars argued that alcohol reduced or eliminated cultural mechanisms deigned to maintain order, with violence and debauchery the frequent result. It has also often been suggested that Aboriginal peoples drank because they sought an acceptable vehicle to unleash their pent-up hostilities and as a means to facilitate social interaction (e.g., Foulks 1980; Honigmann & Honigmann 1945; Lemert 1958; Boyer 1964b; Hamer 1969). Were Aboriginal peoples pathologically introverted? Honigmann and Honigmann (1945), influenced by Horton and their own developing ideas of social atomism, described the northern Indian personality 'as an individualistic atom floating in the social sea, with only a minimum of social dependence,' and suggested that the Indian in a small northern Athapaskan community was indeed so introverted that alcohol provided a 'bridge whereby he can cross the culturally patterned social distance between himself and his neighbours' (599). One wonders how these people were ever able to construct a socially meaningful life prior to the arrival of alcohol, as they were apparently incapable of meaningful interaction when sober *or* drunk.

A connection between social and cultural patterns and contemporary alcohol use also characterizes the cultural integration paradigm, but collective and individual personality is considerably less central to these arguments. One of the seminal studies is that of Craig MacAndrew, a psychiatrist, and Robert Edgerton, an anthropologist (1969), who, in a volume about 'drunken comportment,' or how people behave under the influence, sought to challenge the popular view that alcohol affects the ability of individuals to 'perform customary directive and inhibitory functions' (14).They expressed dissatisfaction with the formulation of Hallowell (1955) and the others mentioned above, that alcohol releases inhibitions and undermines the emotional restraint characteristic of sober Indians. They also criticized the 'conventional wisdom' that Indians craved alcohol and that, when drunk, the result was 'horrible changes-for-the-worse' (101). They further heaped scorn on the romantic notion of the 'noble savage,' the idea that alcohol shattered an otherwise 'pristine continence' (137); slavery, torture, prostitution, and murder had existed in various forms before the introduction of alcohol. In fact, alcohol itself was known to several Aboriginal societies, particularly but not exclusively in the southwest, prior to the arrival of Europeans (see also Abbott 1998). According to their argument, how one behaved while intoxicated was, in effect, guided by cultural rules regarding what was acceptable and what was not, and how that behaviour would be judged by others. The major evidence for this argument was provided by the North American Indians. Utilizing selected, and primarily published, historical documents, such as the journals of traders, explorers, and missionaries, they argued that the initial reaction of Indians to alcohol appeared to have been restrained, often avoidant, and that when they drank, very little in the way of problem behaviour resulted. Simply put, since the vast majority of Indians had no experience with alcohol prior to its introduction by Europeans, there were no rules in place for how to drink or how to behave when drinking.

This situation changed over time, however, as the Indians 'learned' how to drink by watching Europeans. And those Europeans were an unruly bunch! The 'frontier' drinking described by MacAndrew and Edgerton (1969) looks quite a bit like the pattern of drinking that allegedly becomes characteristic of Indians, involving binge drinking of large quantities until supplies are depleted, quarrelling, debauchery, and violence. But this is not the full story, for the authors also suggested that alcohol was integrated into the existing social and cultural patterns of the Indian populations. Some Indians, for instance, concluded that alcohol was an 'evil supernatural agent' (148) which possessed the individual and was responsible for any bad behaviour, and since it was the agent, and not the individual, that was responsible, actions when drunk were largely excused. MacAndrew and Edgerton suggested that this toleration represented a cultural 'time-out,' compatible with pre-contact indigenous forms of possession and the like, in which the individual was seen, on special occasion, to be operating outside the normal social bounds that restrained and guided individual behaviour. Some individuals even pretended to be drunk, they argued, so that they could commit a reprehensible act without liability. But this cultural time-out had at least theoretically the potential to cause considerable disruption, and they suggested that other cultural factors acted to prevent 'self-inflicted genocide' (156). Despite the widespread belief that extensive violent behaviour routinely followed bouts of drinking, that alcohol transformed the Indians 'into mindless perpetrators of wanton slaughter' (ibid.), they argued that few alcohol-induced murders actually occurred and that certain individuals, such as children and Europeans, were usually off-limits as targets. Behaviour, while intoxicated, was still controlled, and the reason, again, was cultural: there were pre-existing cultural mechanisms at work, such as the existence of retaliation, which served to control the behaviour of drunk individuals. Hence, even while drunk, individuals behaved within culturally constructed parameters. 'Societies,' they concluded, 'get the sorts of drunken comportment that they allow' (173).

Also influential were Jerrold Levy, an anthropologist, and Stephen Kunitz, a medical scientist, who in a series of monographs and studies, extended MacAndrew and Edgerton's argument that pre-contact cultural formations played a role in the reaction of Aboriginal peoples to alcohol and in their behaviour while intoxicated. Collectively, these works probably represent the most detailed studies of Indian drinking to date. In contrast to MacAndrew and Edgerton, however, these authors (Levy & Kunitz 1971, 1974; Kunitz & Levy 1974, 1994, 2000a, 2000b) were concerned with refuting both the theory that alcohol released pent-up inhibitions among Indians and elements of the disorganization theory mentioned above. They were unhappy with the 'anthropological conventional wisdom stemming from a sentimental view of Indian life' (Levy & Kunitz 1974: 19) and criticized the view that prior to contact Aboriginal societies were harmonious and that subsequent deviant behaviour could be solely attributed to the effects of contact with Europeans. In their initial study, focused on the Navajo, they set out to 'explore the degree to which aboriginal [i.e., pre-contact] social organization may explain contemporary drinking patterns, the degree to which acculturation changes these patterns, and in what manner' (Levy & Kunitz 1974: 4). They argued that these societies had developed their own kinds of deviancy and their own social controls which, logically, would continue to be pertinent after contact.

With seven years of fieldwork behind them, including extensive analysis of data on mental health and social pathology, they presented a compelling argument that while the Indians in the southwest had learned how to drink from Europeans, alcohol was integrated into pre-existing social patterns, including indigenous forms of deviance and social control. They found that the 'traditional' Navajos drank the most, while the more acculturated Navajos, who in theory should have been experiencing significantly more acculturative stress, tended to drink like white people.[4] The traditional people engaged in 'peer group drinking' on the reservation, a normative form of social activity which, when the group relocated to a neighbouring non-Indian town, was then viewed as pathological. But a key issue was the definition of alcoholism, a problem that confounds many cross-cultural studies of alcohol. As applied to the Navajo, the diagnosis of alcoholism had often been based on observations of their behaviour while drinking, and their patterns of drinking, which were seen as deviant by the white population, rather than on the basis of any psychological problems or evidence of addiction, and without reference to Aboriginal normative standards (see Hill 1980; Waddell 1980; Weisner et al. 1984 for examples). According to the authors, 'In an Indian society where divorce was common in aboriginal times, where economic opportunities are limited for drinkers and nondrinkers alike, and where arrests are made for breaches of white rather than aboriginal norms and laws, it is difficult to determine whether these behaviours are caused by drinking, whether they cause drinking, or whether they are fortuitously associated because they occur frequently in many Indian communities' (Levy & Kunitz 1974: 24). Insightfully, they concluded that 'The changed definition of alcoholism from vice to disease, and of the alcoholic from culprit to patient, parallels the changed view of the Indian from ignoble savage to pathetic victim' (24). Quite simply, even heavy drinking was not necessarily evidence of alcoholism or social disorganization.

Levy and Kunitz (1974) also argued that there was no singular pattern of drinking among American Indians, and no singular cause or explanation, an argument which they sustained in more recent work (Kunitz & Levy 2000a, 2000b). Rather, they presented the intriguing thesis that drinking practices are a reflection of social organization, and hence as social organization differs, so too do these practices. They compared the Hopi, Navajo, and White Mountain Apache on various indicators of social pathology, arguing that the three groups represented differing levels of sociocultural integration from highest (Hopi) to lowest (Apache). The notion of levels of sociocultural integration owes its genesis to the cultural evolutionists, scholars such as Julian Steward and Elman Service (Harris 1968; Barrett 1984), according to whom, not surprisingly, societies such as those found in North America were relatively open and loosely integrated (in contrast to the zenith of the European 'state' society).[5] It was Levy and Kunitz's theory that, as suggested in the literature, drunkenness is greater in societies emphasizing individual independence and achievement, and hence the Hopi should have the lowest levels of drunkenness and related social pathology. While recognizing the limitations of their data, they nevertheless felt confident to conclude that it supported their theory: the Hopi had generally lower rates of homicide and suicide than the Apache, with the Navajo rates in between. Further, these rates had not changed appreciably for many years, despite increasing access to alcohol and increasing acculturation over the same time period (see also Heath 1964). Surprisingly, however, they also found that the Hopi had a significantly greater mortality rate from cirrhosis than the other two groups. These data, taken together, led them to speculate that at issue was the patterns of drinking: the Navajo and Apache engaged in more public, but occasional, drinking that drew the attention of whites and law enforcement agents, whereas the Hopi, it seemed, engaged in more private, and likely sustained, consumption.[6]

Levy and Kunitz (1974) also looked at the relationship between different degrees of acculturation and alcohol consumption. They did not attempt to measure acculturation via a single index, but rather employed several measures, such as education, employment, and involvement in religious life, to categorize four distinct Navajo communities on a continuum from least to most acculturated. They then employed a variety of scales and instruments to measure the quantity, frequency, patterns, and consequences of drinking. They determined that those individuals who were the most acculturated were most similar in these dimensions to white people, whereas the least acculturated engaged in alcohol consumption in a manner that attracted attention because of its deviance from the white norm. It was heavy, it was public, but it was also intermittent. The view that the Navajo had high rates of alcoholism, then, was mostly the result of the adoption of alcohol consumption patterns which, in the white society, signalled alcoholism. 'Whether these Navajos are really alcoholic,' they concluded, 'is still open to question if, by alcoholic, we are referring to some psychopathology of which the observed behavior is only a symptom' (Levy & Kunitz 1974: 150). The inappropriateness of the Western definition of alcoholism as an addiction was also challenged by their data that suggested the majority of Navajo quit drinking altogether in their mid-forties, with no apparent ill-effects. They simply outgrew the need for the social component that was the centre of drinking activity. The problem was not biological susceptibility, nor was it seen to be acculturative pressures and social disintegration.

Two decades after this initial work, Kunitz and Levy (1994) published a follow-up study in which they re-interviewed many of the Navajo from their earlier research. Their data reinforced the previous finding that individuals were able to stop drinking in middle age despite the fact that on several measures found in DSM-III-R they were indistinguishable from alcoholics. The pattern of binge drinking had continued among the Navajo, but a form of solitary drinking had also emerged and this was seen by the Navajo as a sign of problem drinking. Further, it was this measure of alcohol consumption that most strongly correlated with negative outcomes, such as death from alcohol-related causes, than any of the measures within DSM-III-R. Solitary drinkers suffered more from depression as well. They also discovered that the vast majority of Navajo males were abstinent, some 80 per cent in 1990. In comparing Navajos to surrounding whites, they determined that there was little difference in rates of social pathology, leading them to suggest that it was more appropriate to compare Indians and non-Indians within similar geographic contexts than it was to group all Indians together and compare them with national-level data. The researchers were also somewhat surprised to discover a wide array of drinking patterns, leading them to emphasize the need to focus on this heterogeneity rather than stereotypical views of a predominant, pan-Indian form of drinking. 'The very ambiguity of the situation,' they concluded, 'demands that we reject the notion that Navajo, or indeed all Indian, drinking is a single phenomenon ascribable to one or a few identifiable causes calling for a specific type of treatment' (239). Looking back at both the cultural integration and the acculturation explanations, they recently argued that one difficulty has been the use of 'ecological' levels or categories for analysis – entire tribes, the entire American Indian population, or whole counties – which has served to homogenize our understanding of how individuals react to alcohol. Tellingly, they added that historical differences between populations are also important to comprehend (Kunitz & Levy 2000b).

The ideas of MacAndrew and Edgerton, and Levy and Kunitz, have had considerable influence. Robbins (1973), for instance, argued that injuries resulting from alcohol consumption were actually rare among the Naskapi, and that drunken comportment was based on the social position of the actor and not the quantity consumed. Specifically, Robbins (1973: 118) concluded that 'those persons experiencing success at wage earning attempt to gain confirmation of what they see to be their increased status through the use of the friendly reaction to alcohol, while those who have been less successful manifest assertive or aggressive behavior when drinking to defend an identity threatened by their lack of access to identity-maintaining goods.' Topper (1981: 78) noted that 'every drinker has a culture, and when he is living among his people, he drinks in a manner which conforms to cultural or sometimes subcultural norms. It does not matter if his drinking is considered to be culturally appropriate or deviant, it will still be performed in a manner which is culturally patterned.' O'Nell and Mitchell (1996: 568) specifically rejected the biological and 'stress' models when they argued that drinking among Northern Plains Indian adolescents was clearly linked 'to important aspects of ... [their] history and culture,' especially 'the cultural values of courage, modesty, humor, generosity and family honor' (575). Escalante (1980: 184) has argued that drinking behaviour is best understood as a result of group pressures within Aboriginal communities, asserting that 'social control and group norms of American Indians influence excessive alcohol consumption and deviant behavior to a greater degree than do American Indian individual personality characteristics having to do with anxieties, fears, frustrations, conflicts, tensions, insecurities, dependencies, and immaturities.'

One of the more controversial cultural integration arguments was made by anthropologist Nancy Lurie, who described Indian drinking as 'the world's oldest on-going protest demonstration' (1971: 311). She accepted the premise that Indian drinking needed to be seen within the context of pre-contact and persevering cultural patterns, and rejected the idea that drinking could be related to 'identity crisis, low self-esteem, feelings of rejection, and the effects of prejudice and material deprivation vis-à-vis White, middle-class culture and society' (312). Lurie also rejected the primitivist notion that 'Indians get drunk to escape into a glorified, romanticized past and try to regain a sense of identity as Indians, at least temporarily, because they encounter so many difficulties in assimilating into and being accepted by the dominant group and its culture' (312). Indians do not drink to recapture the 'noble Red Man' within, so to speak, because that is a construction of white society and, indeed, of certain 'cold-sober Indians who lecture and engage in theatrical performances' (313). Lurie argued that Indians want success as Indians, on their own terms, and simply borrow freely from the settler society those things that appeal to them. Hence, she argued, 'Indian drinking is an established means of asserting and validating Indianness and will be either a managed and culturally patterned recreational activity or else not engaged in at all in direct proportion to the availability of other effective means of validating Indianness' (315). But this argument is tricky: how can one argue that consuming alcohol is a means of asserting Indianness without supporting the drunken Indian stereotype which so infuriates Lurie? Her observations led her to conclude that Indians are most likely to get drunk when 'they feel thwarted in achieving Indian rather than white goals or when their success as Indians or simply individuals apart from Indian-white comparisons is interpreted as success in achieving status as whites' (317). So, while the Indians originally learned to drink from traders and the like, they revised these patterns in a way compatible with their own cultures but, it would seem, also in reaction to white culture. 'Getting drunk remains a very Indian thing to do when all else fails to maintain the Indian-white boundary,' according to Lurie (325), and the fact that white people disapproved of Indian drinking and applied legal and other sanctions has been incorporated as a kind of boundary-maintaining mechanism, a form of protest. Lurie admitted that she did not provide extensive supportive material from her work with the Dogrib and Winnebago for this assertion. This is unfortunate, given its controversial nature. In the end, it is difficult to determine how this perspective is ultimately different from the drunken Indian stereotype. However, whereas the stereotype is based on the belief that Indians are simply biologically incapable of responsible drinking, or at least that they drink because white people expect them to, as Hamer (1965) suggested for the Potawaotami, Lurie argues that drinking is a deliberate act designed to offend the whites, an act of resistence in the face of power and oppression. The idea that Aboriginal drinking is a boundary-maintaining mechanism, designed to keep whites at bay, has been accepted by others (e.g., Savishinsky 1991).

The final element of the cultural intergation paradigm postulates that the attractiveness of alcohol for Aboriginal individuals was, at least in part, due to a consonance with indigenous beliefs of spirituality and power. Lemert (1954), for instance, argued that the Salish people integrated the use of alcohol not only in feasts but also in the tradition of 'spirit dancing,' in which 'intoxification was sanctioned as a means of facilitating the expression of the dancer's power' (352).[7] He also suggested that the lack of strong public opinion against drinking 'in some part ... must be attributed to the positive value placed upon ecstatic experience in the cultures of this area' (353). Dailey (1968: 57), in a study of alcohol consumption among Indians as detailed in the Jesuit Relations, argued that 'liquor greatly facilitated the attainment of dreams which was for the Indian his most valued experience. Through alcohol he was able to achieve a degree of ecstacy [sic] never possible in prehistoric times.' Hamer and Steinbring (1980) also cited several historical examples of alcohol associated with the dreaming and visioning processes. Kemnitzer (1972) and others have suggested that the Sioux word for alcohol, *mni wakan*, translates into 'holy water,' a reference to alcohol's ability to induce states of euphoria and reduce pain and suffering (see also Mohatt 1972; Hornby & Dana 1984). According to Mohatt (1972: 264), 'liquor in general created a sense of strength similar to that associated with battle or the vision.' Ackerman (1971) believed that Nez Perce individuals were attracted to alcohol as a substitute for the vision quest; Carpenter (1960) presented a similar argument for the Iroquois. Jilek-Aall (1981: 147) suggested that 'drunkeness' among the Coast Salish allowed the individual to 'again experience visions taking him back to the world of his ancestors.'[8] But not all views of alcohol's spiritual nature were revered. The Passamaquoddy, according to Stevens (1981), saw alcohol as the agent of the devil, and consequently believed that evil acts committed while drunk were not the responsibility of the individual. In general, most references to the spiritual importance of alcohol were related to earlier historic periods; contemporary evidence suggests that alcohol is generally not a part of Aboriginal spiritual traditions and that, in many cases, there are strong prohibitions against it (Waldram 1997).

Indian Drinking and White Man Drinking

Aboriginal drinking has not been examined in isolation, but rather almost always in comparison to that of non-Aboriginals, the normative baseline for this activity. But the idea that Aboriginal peoples learned to drink from the white people who lived near them has been a pervasive theme in the alcohol research (e.g., Beauvais 1998). Edwin Lemert (1958: 96) described the characteristic pattern of drinking among the Salish as largely indistinguishable from that of their white neighbours: 'This includes drinking to get drunk, drinking until the supply is exhausted, and restless excursions to find more liquor when this happens ... It is also true that many of the Canadian folk who live near these Indians become aggressive and engage in brawling, particularly at dances where drinking is heavy. Sexual indulgence is likewise a part of the white pattern ...'

This 'white pattern' of drinking has most frequently been attributed to specific marginal or undesirable white types, such as traders and construction workers, yet it is assumed to be typical of Aboriginal peoples. Contradictions abound. Hamer and Steinbring (1980: 19) cited an 1811 passage from the journal of a trader among the Carrier to the effect that it was the traders who would get uncontrollably drunk and frighten the Indians with their crazy behaviour. They also argued that the Indians learned from these traders not only how to drink but how to behave when drunk, and hence the responsibility for drunken aggression and violence lay not with Indian inexperience or repressed anxieties and hostilities, but rather with their good teachers. Kuttner and Lorincz (1967) took issue with the view that the Indian harboured 'a sizable reservoir of latent animosities' that were released with alcohol consumption, arguing that this image could not be reconciled with the stereotype of the sober, docile, and placid Indian (Kuttner & Lorincz 1967: 539). Latent animosities were more hypothetical than real, they suggested, adding that white men were known to be aggressive and violent when both sober and drunk, and yet 'reservoirs of hostility are not included in anthropological description of the white man' (539). This led them to the logical conclusion that, 'if aggression is revealed by the Indian only when he is intoxicated, then his control over his emotions is superior to that of the white man when he is sober' (539). It could be argued that the idea of 'frontier' drinking, that Indians learned this pathological style of drinking from unruly Europeans, ironically suggests that the first stereotypically 'Indian' drinkers were actually whites!

The distinguishing of 'white' drinking and 'Indian' drinking is intriguing. As May (1982) has suggested, the pattern of binge drinking, and its consequences, was sufficiently different for ethnographers to appear exotic, and therefore attracted a great deal of scholarly attention; the 'firewater' myth of the earlier historic period was thus perpetuated by scholars whose sensationalist accounts echoed those of earlier traders and missionaries. The belief in a uniform, distinguishable pattern of Aboriginal alcohol consumption has had remarkable resilience, despite obvious conceptual problems. Close attention to the research underscores these. For instance, Westermeyer (1972a) defined not one but three distinct patterns of drinking, each stereotypically faulty: the abstainer, the 'white,' and the 'Indian.' 'White' drinking was described as 'broadly analogous to drinking in the majority society,' which meant 'an occasional beer' or 'daily cocktails before dinner,' restrained behaviour, and bed at an appropriate hour. Acculturated Chippewa often drank this way, he suggested. In contrast, 'Indian' drinking was characterized by loud conviviality and drunken behaviour, followed by depression, anger, sometimes violence, and consumption which often lasted more than a day and involved more than one location. Similarly, Weisner et al. (1984) described 'white man's drinking' as drinking in moderation, often on special occasions only, and with relatively few problems. 'Serious drinking,' presumably analogous to 'Indian' drinking, involved the consumption of large quantities on a regular basis, passing out, binging for several days, violence, and so forth. French and Hornbuckle (1980: 279) more or less equated 'middle-class' Indian drinking patterns with white patterns. Topper (1974) flagged 'traditional' Navajo drinking patterns, by which he meant essentially what has been defined here as 'Indian' drinking, and contrasted these with more recent patterns, learned from white people, such as drinking at dances and sporting events. Topper did not explain why one specific pattern was 'traditional,' however, given that they were all introduced by whites and then rendered compatible with Navajo culture. And just as the 'firewater myth' appears to have been accepted by some Aboriginal people, so too were the ideas of 'Indian drinking' and 'white Man drinking.' Adrian, Layne and Williams (1991) cited a pamphlet produced by Alberta Indian bands which outlined ten 'Indian drinking styles,' including 'drinking for drinking's sake,' 'occasion drinking,' 'drinking to get drunk,' and 'drinking up all there is,' but which failed to offer an explanation as to how these were exclusively *Indian* styles. In fact, this broad range of styles appears to encompass most of those common to non-Aboriginal peoples as well, although this is not mentioned.

May (1982) was one of the few scholars to suggest that there were different styles of white drinking, just as there were differences in Indian consumption, and that a successfully acculturated Indian was likely to drink following the pattern acceptable to a particular reference sub-group of whites, such as lawyers or construction workers. Both Westermeyer (1972a) and Weisner et al. (1984) recognized the existence of abstainers and suggested that an individual's drinking pattern changed over a lifetime. The idea that 'Indian' drinking represents a single, disruptive, and pathological type has been accepted without critical analysis and fails to account for variability. Given relatively high rates of teetotalling, why is it that the Indian style is characterized by boisterous, often violent group drinking and not abstention? Why is it that 'he drinks like an Indian' does not mean very little alcohol, or none at all? Anyone who has lived on or near a university campus is well-acquainted with the alcohol consumption patterns of many fraternities and yet, with the exception of occasional reports of alcohol-related sexual assault or death, this largely escapes our gaze. 'It is accepted that some American Indians engage in abrupt and intense bouts of episodic drinking, or binges, during which large quantities of alcohol are consumed almost nonstop over a period of several days,' trumpet Robin, Long, Rasmussen, Albaugh, and Goldman (1998: 518) in the opening sentence of a recent article. If we substituted 'male college students' for 'American Indians' in this passage, would anyone take issue? While frat boys will be boys, and that is considered an acceptable part of their college experience, Indians cannot be Indians because the exact same behaviour is not acceptable to whites when Indians are doing the drinking. I am reminded of Savishinsky's (1991: 93) description of northern Hare Indians' views of a 'good brew party' which 'echoes some of the requirements for a traditional Irish wake: lots of people, lots of alcohol and at least one good fight!' Tellingly, the English have characteristically looked down upon both Aboriginal peoples and the Irish (see also Scheper-Hughes 1987).

The relative amount of attention paid to sobriety pales in comparison to that pertaining to alcoholism and social pathology. Most studies that have considered the issue of sobriety have done so only as a sidebar to their study of alcohol use (e.g. Westermeyer 1972a, 1974b; Hoffman & Noem 1975; Beltrame & McQueen 1979; Weisner et al. 1984; Moss, Edwards, Edwards, Janzen, & Howell 1985). The absence of drinking, it would seem, is a considerably less glamourous subject than 'warriors without weapons' drunkenly counting coup from the back of a pick-up truck careening down the dusty roads of some off-reservation town after a night at the tavern. Medicine (1982) argued two decades ago that the slight consideration paid to abstinence and sobriety in Aboriginal societies was due to the overwhelming attention devoted to theories of anomie and disorganization. Even today, there are virtually no ethnographic studies that focus on non-drinking individuals specifically. Pessimistic views of the genuiness of abstinence are noteworthy and often betray biases in favour of the 'drunken Indian' myth. Boyer (1964b: 218), for example, noted that 'Although there are a few Apaches who have been teetotallers throughout their lifetimes, the great majority of Indians have been at some period drunkards and promiscuous and violent while intoxicated.'

Social disorganization theories suffer from an implicit assumption that, with respect to alcohol, Aboriginal peoples were only able to make one cultural adjustment, to drink like the white traders and adventurers they encountered, and that several centuries later they remain locked in this form of binge drinking and disruptive behaviour. French and Hornbuckle (1980: 278), for instance, argued that Indians 'have not been allowed to develop acceptable drinking norms' even after several centuries.[9] What these authors really meant was norms acceptable to the larger society, since as we have seen the Indians were very quick to develop their own norms. Kuttner and Lorincz (1967), in contrast, argued that for a population of urbanized Sioux, the passage of time and several generations had rendered historical arguments moot, and suggested that viewing Indian drinking in the city as a result of acculturative stress missed the point that acculturation effectively ceased some time ago, at least for these individuals. Drinking in the city was family-oriented, as it was in the past and on the reserve, and was not a reflection of patterns learned from white people. As noted earlier, it has often been suggested that some Aboriginal groups learned to drink in a certain way because of prohibition: if they adapted their behaviour to the outlawing of alcohol, why can they not adapt to its legalization? Many years ago, Heath (1964) described ways in which the Navajo had altered their drinking styles after the prohibition laws were lifted, including changes in the type of beverages consumed and the places, such as bars, in which to drink. Certainly the intergenerational transmission of problematic drinking patterns exists, as Jones-Saumty, Hochhaus, Dru, and Zeiner (1983) and Mail and Johnson (1993) have suggested, but as these are *learned* patterns, why do so many scholars assume that new, more healthy patterns cannot also be learned? The cultural integration theorists were at least able to recognize some cultural, community, and individual agency in the process, even while accepting that patterns of drinking were introduced by unruly Europeans. Topper (1985) is one writer who, refreshingly, demonstrated that Aboriginal drinking patterns had in fact changed very recently, after the Second World War, and described them as *still evolving*. Similarly, Price (1975) and May (1992a) stressed that change is entirely possible with respect to drinking behaviour among Indians. But these voices remain far too quiet, and the stereotype persists.

Emerging Epidemiological Issues

The search for a grand theory of Aboriginal drinking has been curtailed in recent years, and authors now seem more or less content to simply summarize existing theories (e.g., Shore and Von Fumetti 1972; Brod 1975; Heidenreich 1976; R.G. Lewis 1982; Heath 1983; Lamarine 1988; Silk-Walker, Walker, & Kivlahan 1988; T.J. Young 1989, 1993; May, 1977, 1986, 1999; Beauvais 1998; Robin et al. 1998). The approach to the study of alcohol has also changed, moving away from the ethnographic work of anthropologists and towards the use of epidemiological tools.

In the 1970s, there was an increasing interest in clinical studies employing various instruments designed to assess the extent of alcohol consumption, its outcomes, and its co-morbidity with other disorders. While the ethnographic approach provided rich qualitative data which, not surprisingly, seemed to fit all too conveniently with the researchers' theoretical perspective, the clinical studies provided quantitative data that seemed to abandon the cultural context altogether and which appeared to be considerably less theoretically driven. The problems with these epidemiological studies are the same as those discussed in the previous chapter on psychopathology more generally. They include the use of culture areas as sampling frames, small and unrepresentative sample sizes, and ambiguous criteria for inclusion as 'Aboriginal' and 'white' subjects. There is no real need to repeat the same, detailed critique here – the point has been made. Certainly, the issue of culture remains as muddied in alcohol studies as it does in the other areas examined so far. Although considerably dated, work by Joseph Westermeyer (1972b), which is still cited as seminal, demonstrates how deeply the confusion over culture has penetrated. In his studies of alcoholism in Minnesota, Westermeyer described the Chippewa Indians as compromising a 'distinctive cultural group' in Minnesota while accepting into his study any person claiming to have just 'one-quarter Indian ancestry who identified as belonging to the Chippewa ethnic group' (323). Confusing heritage (blood quantum?) and identity with culture remains a pervasive problem.

One fundamental question has been raised time and again in the literature, and is commonly raised in the community as well: do Aboriginal peoples have a drinking problem? This is a much more complex question than it might appear at first glance. As May (1992a) has charged, the common stereotype is that more Indians drink than non-Indians, even though the data are fairly ambiguous on this question. Manson et al. (1992), like Levy and Kunitz (1974) before them, and many others before and after, have striven to impress that alcohol use varied from tribe to tribe, yet, also like many others, they failed to explain why the tribe was a meaningful unit for comparing Indian drinking in the first place. The question of how, why, and to what extent 'Aboriginal' peoples drink thus begs several related questions. Why does so much of the discourse – in fact, almost all of it – defer to the default position that 'Aboriginal' and 'tribe' are meaningful units for comparison? How frequently do we hear that a particular town has a drinking problem, in contrast to a particular reservation? How often do we hear that 'white' people have a certain level of alcohol consumption?

From the research perspective, Aboriginality appears to be framed primarily by notions of the collectivity, reified as a group, a reservation, or a 'people.' In contrast, non-Aboriginal peoples, white people, are framed by notions of individuality. While alcohol consumption by an Aboriginal person is viewed as a product of their Aboriginality – it is what 'Aboriginal' peoples do – white drinking is never seen as a product of European heritage or collective experience. Although based on anthropological understandings of culture and levels of sociocultural integration, the genesis of this collective/individual dichotomy is appropriately located in cross-cultural psychology and the idea that societies can be categorized as either 'individualistic' or 'collectivist' in orientation (Triandis 1996). This concept fails to accommodate cultural change, however, and its application to Aboriginal peoples suggests that they will continue to exhibit a predominantly collectivist social orientation despite colonization, sociocultural change, and the whole array of contemporary, globalizing forces that impinge on the individual (including several centuries as residents of the most avowedly individualistic nation on earth). Even blood quantum as a measure of Aboriginality is employed to categorize the individual into the collectivist Aboriginal category.

The problem, then, with epidemiological studies of alcohol is partly methodological, and partly conceptual. Heath (1983: 365) has argued that 'The methods for estimating prevalence of alcoholism that are most commonly used with reference to nation-states or other political entities are not well suited for use on Indian populations,' with difficulties including the 'relative smallness of populations and the relative lack of detailed data on causes of death.' Further, he has argued that much of the alcohol epidemiological research which used 'minority' classifications, such as 'Hispanic,' 'Asian,' and 'Indian,' rendered data virtually meaningless at the community level and for national level, comparative purposes (106). Since many alcohol studies are comparative, there is also the issue of what constitutes a suitable comparison group; while sometimes one Indian tribe or population has been compared with another, most frequently some comparison has been made with the 'national' or state/provincial population. Only occasionally has it been suggested that this is inappropriate and that the most suitable comparisons are with neighbouring populations. As we have seen in this chapter, there is also considerable ambiguity as to what constitutes alcoholism and alcohol-related problematic behaviour. In 1985 Beauvais and LaBoueff lamented that there were little reliable data on the extent and patterns of alcohol use among American Indians. Kirmayer et al. (1994), almost ten years later, stated bluntly that accurate prevalence data for most Aboriginal communities simply were not available, and that much of what was determined about Aboriginal alcoholism was derived from indirect measures, especially mortality data. Manson et al. (1992) and Abbott (1998) have made essentially the same argument.[10]

If we were to conduct an uncritical meta-summary of alcohol epidemiological studies to date,[11] comparing Aboriginal to non-Aboriginal peoples, as is almost always the case, we would likely conclude that:

- Aboriginal peoples consume more alcohol overall,
- Aboriginal peoples consume more alcohol per sitting,
- more Aboriginal peoples are heavy drinkers, and men drink more than women,
- more Aboriginal peoples are also abstainers,
- Aboriginal peoples are more likely than non-Aboriginal peoples to engage in consumptive behaviour that leads to other negative consequences, such as accidents and violence, and
- alcohol is more likely to be co-morbid with other psychiatric disorders for Aboriginal peoples.

These observations do not hold in every case, of course, and given the methodological limitations they should be viewed with considerable caution. Researchers have often pointed out that there are important similarities between Aboriginal peoples and other groups, in both their patterns of consumption and their reasons for drinking. Westermeyer and Baker (1986: 277) thus cautioned that 'if one corrects for age, education, and social class, the differences between Indians and non-Indians are often less than the similarities.' Nevertheless, alcohol is considered by many Aboriginal health professionals and scholars, as well as community members, to be a major if not the most important health issue. May (1992a) has taken a reasonable approach in arguing that the problem with alcohol must be conceptualized as one involving both alcoholism (i.e., addiction) and alcohol abuse (typified by problematic behaviours), and this allows us to avoid sinking into the conceptual quicksand of how these concepts should be defined. Simple consumption prevalence is hardly a meaningful measure, and drinking styles explain much more of the resultant problematic behaviour (May 1999).

Conclusion

Much of the literature on alcohol and Aboriginal peoples reflects primitivist themes, with models of civilization and savagery playing off each other in all too convenient ways. Alcohol discourse clearly articulates how the demon rum transformed the Arcadian civilized into the Barbarian savage.

Most of pre-contact Aboriginal North America was virgin soil with respect to alcohol. Unlike many other pathological behaviours, alcohol-related problems are much more readily linked to the arrival of Europeans, and both the biological and the historic/cultural debates on alcohol parallel the notion of the 'virgin soil epidemic,' the belief that Europeans introduced new diseases for which Aboriginal peoples lacked immunities, resulting in dramatic population losses (Waldram, Herring, and Young 1995). Alcohol has been seen as a kind of infectious disease, similar to smallpox, which, like the latter, was deliberately introduced to destroy the Aboriginal population. Accordingly, Aboriginal peoples were thought to be biologically susceptible to alcohol in the same way they were to smallpox and other diseases, and their inexperience with both allegedly contributed to the devastation. This argument requires that we ignore several bits of evidence to the contrary, for example, the facts that pre-contact societies were anything but harmonious utopias (e.g., Edgerton 1992), that some already made alcohol with little ill effect, that alcohol was adopted differentially by individuals and groups over a very long period of time, and that consumption patterns often reflected pre-contact elements of social organization. But ignoring contradictory evidence is nothing new in scholarly research, as I think we have begun to see.

There is also a tension in the literature between those who view alcohol as being primarily destructive of Aboriginal peoples and cultures, and those, far fewer, who recognize adaptive, positive, and functional aspects to drinking. Psychological perspectives, such as the emphasis on personality and anxiety, jostle with sociocultural perspectives, as in the integration of alcohol into pre-existing cultural patterns. Strict biomedical definitions of alcoholism abut sociocultural understandings of what constitutes normative versus problem drinking While it is admitted that some Aboriginal peoples drink for the same and varied reasons as non-Aboriginals, overwhelmingly the argument is firmly anchored in discourses of historical oppression, cultural loss, and economic marginality, processes affecting the collective that have produced unique patterns of consumption and related problems. Indeed, much of the work done has simply *assumed* these causal factors, much in the same way it has assumed cultural and biological homogeneity. I am certainly not suggesting that historical and contemporary social and economic factors are not important. These are rather appealing explanations, for a variety of reasons. Rather, my concern, as it has been throughout this volume, is with the fact that these assumptions have gone relatively unchallenged and the way in which they have guided research and thinking, 'truth,' 'conventional wisdom,' or whatever you want to call it, about Aboriginal peoples and alcohol.

Back in 1977, Philip May described the anomie perspective as 'overly simplistic' (229), yet it still persists in a variety of forms. Social disorganization theories paint such a dismal picture of Aboriginal communities that one must wonder how they can function at all, and how they will sustain themselves in the future. Yet they can, and they will, all the while providing meaning for individual lives. There is faulty logic at work here, as many have recognized (e.g., MacAndrew & Edgerton 1969; Levy & Kunitz 1974; Kunitz & Levy 1974). The observation that Aboriginal peoples drink is frequently used as evidence of social disorganization, or that populations are under acculturative stress, or that they are anxious. Seldom is it determined first that these conditions actually exist, and then if alcohol abuse is the cause, the result, or related in any way. Alcohol studies demonstrate the quickness with which we researchers are prepared to assume that Aboriginal peoples are dysfunctional.

CHAPTER SEVEN

The Depressed Aboriginal

The underlying problem appears to be difficulty in adjusting to a hostile environment. Poverty, unemployment, geographic isolation, cultural conflict, and resultant breakdown of old value systems lead to difficulties in adjusting to life ... (Ogden, Spector, Mozart, & Hill 1970)

As broad-based epidemiological investigations have dwindled, there has been an increase in interest in more focused studies of specific disorders or special populations. Forms of depression as a symptom or co-morbid disorder have, like alcohol, frequently been identified in both generalized epidemiological investigations and disorder-specific studies. Suicide, a problem frequently linked to depression, has been a topic of particular interest, given its standing as one of the most significant mental health issues for Aboriginal peoples and, no doubt, because it often serves as a barometer for other social, cultural, and economic conditions.[1] Although the literature on Aboriginal depression is less extensive than that on suicide and many other disorders, a handful of innovative approaches have emerged which serve as excellent examples of the potential for and pitfalls of combining biomedical and Aboriginal approaches in an attempt to achieve a more culturally appropriate understanding of a particular problem. With depression in particular, considerably more attention has been paid to the existence of indigenous understandings of the problem, both in terms of pre-contact carryovers and contemporary cultural or local idioms of distress. The Arcadian and the Barbarian perspectives still struggle to comprehend why Aboriginal people appear to be so depressed and why they often commit suicide, and we frequently see explanations from a variety of theoretical perspectives cavalierly thrown together, as they are in the quotation from Ogden et al. (1970) that opens this chapter.

Conceptualizing Depression and Suicide

A key question for researchers has been how, if at all, a contemporary psychiatric perspective on depression and suicide could be brought to bear on Aboriginal populations which, hypothetically, continue to exist as culturally distinct. Kleinman and Good (1985) have identified an epistemological confusion characteristic of studies of depression, emphasizing the importance of determining if 'depression' should be conceptualized as a disorder, as in psychiatry, or as an emotional state, as in anthropology. These are two very different perspectives: 'For the clinician, depression is a common, often severe, sometimes mortal disease with characteristic affective (sadness, irritability, joylessness), cognitive (difficulty concentrating, memory disturbance), and vegetative (sleep, appetite, energy disturbances) complaints which has a typical course and predictable response rates to treatment ... This is not the "depression" of the ethnographer, for whom the word denotes a feeling state of sadness, hopelessness, and demoralization that may be as fleeting as a momentary nostalgia or as lasting as prolonged grieving' (Kleinman & Good 1985: 9). In practice, then, researchers have often taken either a psychiatric or an anthropological approach to understanding depression among the Aboriginal population, approaches which reflect their view of the existence or contemporary relevance of depression's antiquity. Only a few, notably Manson and Shore (1981) and O'Nell (1996), have attempted to explore depression using a combined approach, with varying degrees of success. Two leading mental health researchers, James Shore and Spero Manson (1981), have argued that American Indians experienced some kind of depression which was indigenous to them, citing the existence in at least some Indian languages of terms which expressed the concept in some manner. Culturally distinct forms of depression require an ethnographic methodology, at least in the first instance, to elucidate local-level cultural understandings of relevance to a scientifically based psychiatry. However, relatively little weight has been given to the idea that contemporary depression among Aboriginal peoples is in any way related to their cultures per se, that their cultures did, and continue to, generate their own stresses and tensions that might contribute to depression.

Similarly, little weight has been given to the idea that depression exists not as a new disorder but as a universal disorder with ever-changing, contemporary triggers.

Fitting nicely within the Arcadian tradition, then, is the notion that depression and suicide (as well as related pathologies, such as homicide and alcoholism) simply did not exist prior to colonization, or even in the decades and centuries after contact, and most discussions of these problems fail even to consider the possibility. Psychopathology, its seems, begins with the arrival of Europeans and, more specifically, the confinement of Aboriginal peoples to reserves (in Canada) and reservations (in the United States), admittedly a drastic and severe alteration in life-way. However, the evidence that depression, and especially suicide, existed in the past among many Aboriginal groups, and certainly prior to the epidemic outbreaks of recent decades, is compelling.

Devereux (1940), for instance, described the existence of 'heartbreak' among the Mohave as a traditional problem, sometimes leading to suicide. T.H. Lewis (1975), in a study of the Oglala Sioux, described 'wacinko syndrome' as essentially a form of depression characterized by anger, pouting, and withdrawal, accompanied by feelings of despondency and occasionally suicidal ideation. Johnson and Johnson (1965) described 'tawatl ye sni' among the Dakota as meaning 'totally discouraged,' a feeling marked by, among other things, thoughts of death, deceased relatives, and ghosts.[2] Timpson, McKay, Kakegamic, Roundhead, Cohen, and Matewapit (1988) noted that there were several different words in the Nishnawbe (Ojibwa) language for depression, and that elders in northern Ontario described depression as a problem that existed in earlier times, often the result of shame. O'Nell (1996) suggested that the Flathead of Montana experienced intense loneliness and feelings of worthlessness as forms of depression. Storck, Csordas, and Strauss (2000: 589), in a study of Navajo healing, could not find a term that fully corresponded to depression but discovered that some used a word to denote an individual who was worried, sad, or distraught. They also noted that a new Navajo dictionary glossed 'depression' in two ways, as meaning 'lonely and sick' as well as 'something is not right that is giving you a problem making a living and taking care of yourself.' As we shall see in chapter 8, depression has also often been thought to be a symptom associated with several culture-bound syndromes which have allegedly persisted since pre-contact or early contact times.

There is also evidence that many Aboriginal groups had experience with suicide. Pine (1981) provided a valuable, if cursory, review of reports of self-inflicted death, their causes, methods, and societal reactions, across five major culture areas for the pre-contact and early post-contact period (see also Balikci 1961; Foulks 1980; Kirmayer 1994; Levy & Kunitz 1971; May & Dizmang 1981; Wyman & Thorne 1945). Devereux (1969) presented perhaps the most detailed examination of suicide among an Aboriginal population, in this case the Mohave, and identified several different types recognized by the people themselves, including that resulting from being 'heartbroken.' Defining what constitutes 'suicide' is, of course, problematic, especially when dealing with different cultures and fragmentary reports of considerable antiquity. Were the 'Crazy-Dogs-Wishing-To-Die,' a society of men among the Crow who vowed to fight until death, suicidal (Lowie 1913)? Is suicide the appropriate term to describe the actions of aged, infirm Inuit who fell behind the others to die of exposure, so as to not burden the group further (Leighton & Hughes 1955; Foulks 1980)? Are heroic measures undertaken with glory or altruism in mind, and which are likely to lead to certain death, really forms of suicide? While the reasons for such actions may differ from modern reasons for committing suicide, it is difficult to support the contention that Aboriginal groups had no history of experience with the phenomenon of taking one's own life. Nevertheless, there seems to be unanimous agreement among researchers that the rates of suicide have increased in recent decades and have, in many areas, reached alarmingly high proportions. The key question, then, is whether contemporary acts of suicide are qualitatively as well as quantitatively different from historical instances of suicide. If Pine's summary is accurate, many of the reasons for committing suicide, including to seek revenge on another, jealousy, love and marital problems, abuse, grief, and shame, have not changed significantly. Generally, the scant literature on pre-existing understandings of suicide among Aboriginal peoples suggests at least a passive condemnation of the act, except in cases of altruistic suicide.

Certainly we must not jump to the conclusion that these various studies and reports are unequivocal evidence of pre-contact depression and suicide. All of them have sought to elucidate 'traditional' understandings, bits of knowledge and experience from the past which seems compatible with age-old traditions. Yet all of the researchers in question were also working with populations which had experienced the very colonization that the Arcadian perspective suggests is the cause of these disorders. The question of whether or not Aboriginal depression and suicide existed prior to the arrival of Europeans will likely never be answered with certainty. I am proposing here, however, that there is sufficient evidence to suggest that there has been at least a long-standing experience with these disorders, such that knowledge of their existence appears in the discourse as ancient and 'traditional.'

Regardless of any pre-existing experiences with depression and suicide, research clearly demonstrates that Aboriginal peoples currently suffer from high rates of both, and that they are increasing in prevalence (Levy 1965; Havighurst 1971; Conrad & Kahn 1974; Kraus 1974; Ward & Fox 1977; McIntosh & Santos 1981; Peters 1981; McIntosh 1983; Berlin 1985; Hochkirchen & Jilek 1985; Van Winkle & May 1986, 1993; May 1987, 1990; Shore et al. 1987; Bechtold 1988; Garro 1988; Ackerson, Dick, Manson & Baron 1990; Baron, Manson, Ackerson, & Brenneman 1990; Manson, Ackerman, Dick, Baron, & Fleming 1990; Cooper, Corrado, Karlberg, & Pellatier Adams 1992; Kettl & Bixler 1993; Kirmayer 1994; Strickland 1997; Kirmayer, Fletcher, & Boothroyd 1998). This is explained by a variety of factors falling into two broad schools of thought which are largely distinguishable from those related to alcohol abuse. The first school posits the acculturation/anomie/social disorganization model, and suggests that depression and suicide are linked to 'rapid cultural change, epidemic patterns of alcohol abuse, increased rates of physical illness, accidents and deaths, and demoralization secondary to enforced dependency' (Shore, Manson, Bloom, Keepers, & Neligh 1987: 4; see also Beiser & Attneave 1982). This view has been strongly influenced by several predominantly sociological paradigms highlighting the inherently functional, integrative, and healthy character of 'primitive' and pre-industrial society, including Durkheim's notion of 'mechanical solidarity' and Ferdinand Tönnies's ideas of *Gemeinschaft*, as well as anthropologist Robert Redfield's conceptualization of 'folk' society, all broadly evolutionist perspectives within the Arcadian tradition (Harris 1968). The gist of these well-known formulations was that such communities were relatively free of social pathology until contaminated by industrialization or contact with industrial nations, and by the concomitant social, economic, and cultural changes. Built in, then, was the idea that change in the direction of the society of the colonizer was a priori a bad thing.

Related to the anomie and social disorganization explanation is the idea that the level of social integration is a contributing factor; in other words, the more socially integrated a society is (meaning that individual and collective needs are fulfilled), the lower the suicide rate, especially when the society is undergoing acculturative changes (Smith & Hackathorn 1982; Van Winkle & May 1986, 1993). An acculturation paradigm was therefore added into the theoretical mix to provide a more concrete explanation of what was actually happening in the transition of these apparently harmonious societies, describing a process of culture change in which traditional norms were replaced by those of the dominant white society. In other instances, the problem seems to be one of inadequate replacement of cultural items, even a lack of replacement, so that not just individuals but entire communities or societies suffer from anomie.

Jilek (1981) (see also Jilek & Todd 1974; Jilek-Aall, Jilek, & Flynn 1978; Hochkirchen & Jilek 1985) argued for the existence of 'anomic depression' among Coast Salish peoples, caused largely by acculturative stress, loss of identity, the absence of an effective normative structure, relative deprivation, and frustration at the lack of ability to succeed in the white world. Topper and Curtis (1987) took this one step further and, building on the idea of 'caught-between-two-worlds' discussed earlier in the book, identified 'synergistic dual anomic depression' among Navajo who lived in agency towns on the reservation, 'a disorder that arises out of the young person's frustration at not being able to achieve economic success either in the westernized wage-work sector or in the native-subsistence sector of the reservation economy' (335). Townsley and Goldstein (1977: 459) described a form of 'dependency depression,' that is, the 'parasitic dependency' fostered in Indians by government which has rendered the Indians incapable of exerting control over their lives. Dependence on the federal government, they argued, had created the 'adult-child' – the child metaphor again – and these individuals developed a 'lifelong negative evaluation of self' as a result, leading to depression. Timpson et al. (1988: 6) described the loss of Ojibwa spirituality as a cause of depression and suggested that this loss was 'remarkably similar to the concepts of normlessness and anomie.' Brant (1990) believed that grief caused by the sudden loss of family members, which had accelerated in recent years, was a major cause of depression. Johnson (1994: 30) agreed, expanding the concept of loss to the 'personal, tribal, and cultural level' to 'combine into unresolved grief and anger and ultimately into a deeply embedded depression.'[3] Fleming (1996), working through the new 'cultural formulation' that appeared in the DSM-IV, presented the case of a Coast Salish woman suffering from depression related to grief and alcoholism. Finally, co-morbidity has frequently been cited as a common occurrence, particularly depression with alcohol and substance abuse and, frequently, suicide (Sack, Beiser, Phillips, & Baker-Brown 1993; Dinges & Duong-Tran 1993; Sack, Beiser, Baker Brown, & Redshirt 1994).

The majority of scholars writing about suicide have partially or wholly embraced the disorganization paradigm, in which the failure to retain traditional ways combined with increasing use of alcohol are often seen as central, precipitating factors (Levy 1965; Devereux 1969; Ogden, Mozart, Spector, & Hill 1970; Havighurst 1971; Resnik & Dizmang 1971; Conrad & Hahn 1974; Parkin 1974; Ward & Fox 1977; McIntosh 1983; McIntosh & Santos 1981; Berlin 1987; Davenport & Davenport 1987; Garro 1988; Kettl, & Bixler 1993; Keane, Dick, Bechtold, & Manson 1996). Exactly *how* acculturative pressures and stress affect the pathogenesis of suicide is somewhat debatable, however. Most suggest that as proximity to non-Aboriginal peoples increases, so too do suicide rates (Conrad & Kahn 1974). However, contradictory reports occasionally emerge that suggest that isolation from the dominant society, combined with the persistence of traditional cultures, is associated with higher suicide rates rather than lower ones (Bachman 1992; Berlin 1987), findings which not only demonstrate the complexity of the issue but which also suggest the importance of cultural continuity as a risk factor, to be elaborated in more detail below. Kirmayer's (1994) 'inverted U' pattern postulate of the relationship between traditionalism and suicide, in which the rates appear lowest for the most traditional and most assimilated, obviously does not hold in every instance. Plaguing all such analyses moreover is the imprecise operationalization of key concepts such as what constitutes a 'traditional' versus 'acculturated' community, but embedded within these constructs can no doubt be found important clues to the relationship between cultural processes and mental health.

We also find suggestions that anomie and related depression and suicide are connected to contemporary socio-economic issues, such as poor housing and lack of employment (Bagley 1991; Bagley, Wood, & Khumar 1990). Indeed, it is in the field of Aboriginal suicidology that we find one of the few attempts to provide a socio-economic explanation within the broader psychopathological research, no doubt the product of the dominance of sociology and Durkheimian theory in this area. While the quotation from Ogden et al. (1970) which opens this chapter would suggest a hypothesized relationship between socio-economic explanations and acculturation/anomie/social disorganization explanations, efforts to connect these two broad frameworks have been rare.

The second school of thought on the development of social and psychological pathologies such as suicide suggests that specific Aboriginal cultures have predisposed individuals to experience certain pathologies and not others, and that contemporary psychopathology must be viewed within the context of continuing cultural traditions, not severed ones, and their adaptation to new circumstances (Levy & Kunitz 1971). This idea was developed in the previous chapter as the 'cultural continuity/integration' paradigm. The idea of levels of social integration, as described above, is also visible. This argument is an important one, since it recognizes that culture for Aboriginal peoples did not cease to be a dominant factor in their lives with the arrival of Europeans or the construction of reserves. Levy and Kunitz (1971), the foremost advocates of this approach, argued that contemporary psychopathology must be interpreted within a framework of continuing cultural adaptation by Aboriginal groups, and the fact of widespread contemporary cultural heterogeneity combined with unique, local historical experience goes a long way in explaining why, for instance, there are such disparities in suicide rates and patterns among Aboriginal groups (Shore 1975; Webb & Willard 1975; McIntosh 1983; McIntosh & Santos 1981).[4] In the case of the Navajo, Levy (1965) suggested that the traditional lack of social integration of males within the matrilineages, a cause of suicide in the past, was exacerbated in recent years by cultural changes causing the disintegration of the matrilineages themselves. T.J. Young (1991) has likewise accepted that both contemporary poverty and anomie, on the one hand, and social learning in the form of traditional cultural elements, on the other, combine to offer the best explanation of suicide and homicide among Native Americans. But without an explicit acceptance by scholars that Aboriginal societies harboured their own forms of deviance and pathology which continue to be reflected in their patterns of suicide, as Levy and Kunitz maintain, this argument has largely failed to attract followers.

Cultural continuity has, occasionally, emerged in other arenas as an explanation, but frequently these formulations have suffered from conceptual difficulties. In a recent study of 'cultural continuity as a hedge against suicide in Canada's First Nations,' psychologists Michael Chandler and Christopher Lalonde (1998) attempted to understand how the persistence of cultural traditions might explain the lower rates of suicide in some British Columbia Indian reserves relative to others. Their measures of cultural continuity, however, were anything but, and included such items as involvement in land claims, self-government, and control over education, police, fire, and health services. While none of these demonstrates continuity with a cultural past in which such institutions were non-existent, they do demonstrate, contrary to the authors' assertions, that positive cultural *change*, especially one that addresses issues of economic and social deprivation, can have a profound effect on suicide rates. Their focus on what makes a community *healthy*, as opposed to sick, should also be applauded.

Overall, then, a disorganization hypothesis dominates explanations of Aboriginal depression and suicide. Little effort has been expended to explore a biological explanation, despite the significant attention paid to individual biological factors in research with non-Aboriginal populations (Shore & Manson 1981). While Armstrong (1993) has suggested that the relative lack of exposure to sunlight in the winter for Canadian Indians was possibly a contributing factor, even he gave paramountcy to social and cultural factors in the search for a causative explanation. The fact that studies of Aboriginal depression have generally not looked at biological explanations is telling, given the importance of biological factors in contemporary psychiatric explanations of the problem and prevailing attempts to define depression as a 'disease' (Kleinman & Good 1985). This discordance is particularly striking when one compares the preponderance of interest in biology as an explanation for Aboriginal alcoholism and various other measures of psychopathology with the relative lack of interest in biological explanations of depression. Perhaps depression has simply not attracted researchers schooled in the belief of Aboriginal inferiority; the intense focus on alcohol may also have prevented researchers from recognizing a co-morbid depression even where alcohol and suicide have been linked. Indigenous forms of depression and suicide, while acknowledged by some to have existed, have garnered little attention relative to a more contemporary interpretation which places blame almost entirely not just on the consequences of colonization, but on relatively *recent* causes. The connection between past cultural history and traditions and contemporary psychopathology is simply not made (see, e.g., for instance, Dizmang 1967).

The extent to which the concept of depression has any cross-cultural validity has been questioned, of course (e.g., Kleinman & Good 1985), and some mental health research among Aboriginal peoples has focused on determining both local, culture-specific understandings of the concept and idioms of distress and the utility of existing diagnostic instruments developed for non-Aboriginal populations. These two approaches have occasionally been at odds and both contain some conceptual problems. Let me turn first to the use of psychometric instruments.

Measuring and Treating Aboriginal Depression and Suicide

There has been a flurry of activity on the issue of Indian depression and suicide in the last few decades, centred on the important work of Spero Manson, James Shore, and their colleagues affiliated with the National Center for American Indian and Alaska Native Mental Health at the University of Colorado. Much of this work has focused on testing the utility of existing diagnostic instruments, modifying them where appropriate to better fit local contexts, and even developing a new, Indian-oriented scale.

The validation of existing instruments to diagnose disorders in Aboriginal communities has garnered a great deal of attention. Shore et al. (1987), for instance, undertook a study of the usefulness of the Schedule for Affective Disorders and Schizophrenia-Lifetime Version (SADS-L) in identifying index cases of depression as a precursor to the development of a more culturally sensitive instrument. They were primarily concerned with allowing for 'intertribal comparisons,' and to this end three American Indian reservation communities were selected, using the culture area concept as a guideline for demonstrating their distinctiveness. Specific details of the three communities were withheld to ensure anonymity, and they were designated simply as the Plains, Plateau, and Pueblo tribes. Local medical officials in each community identified individuals suspected of suffering from depressive disorders, and these individuals were invited to participate. Out of a total of 104 SADS-L interviews across the three communities, 86 cases of major depression were identified through the instrument. The researchers concluded that there were few differences between tribes or by sex and suggested the existence of 'a core depressive syndrome' (11) among these patients, which is compatible with more general views of similarly depressive symptomology across cultures. Sociodemographic and cultural differences might modify the content of major depressive disorder, but not the form. However, like other studies which have showed higher levels of psychopathology among Plains Indians, Shore et al. noted that the Plains group appeared to have a higher rate of 'complicated depression ... a major depressive disorder superimposed upon an underlying chronic depression,' possibly explainable by 'unique cultural and genetic factors' (13). The fact that some groups lacked a semantic equivalent for 'depression' was not seen by the researchers to necessarily indicate the lack of the disorder.

Shore et al. (1987) stressed several important limitations in their study, including that the interviews were undertaken in English and that a 'high level of transcultural experience among the four research psychiatrists was essential to judge accurately patients' responses' (11). They also noted that 'patients generally had difficulty in distinguishing between subtle differences in SADS-L probe questions, especially for affective symptoms associated with the personality disorders,' and that they were 'uncertain about the reliability of Indian patients' recall of symptom duration since time perception may be significantly affected by cultural experience' (11). Thus, while arguing that there appeared to be a common depressive symptomology across American Indian cultures, they also presented tantalizing evidence that cultural or linguistic differences, either individual or across all three communities, affected the performance of patients on the SADS-L instrument. In fact, since virtually no data were presented on the cultural orientations of any of the patients involved, it is impossible for the reader to glean any useful insight regarding the potential role of culture in the formation or expression of depression. Their argument that these American Indian patients demonstrated similar depressive symptomology could well be simply an artifact of the instrument's homogenizing of cultural and linguistic differences. Equally problematic is the decision to withhold important information about the specific communities to protect their identities and prevent the potential harm that could be caused if knowledge of psychiatric issues was to become widespread. This decision cannot easily be criticized, and it is a common, though not unanimous, practice in community-based studies of psychopathology, but it does have the effect of rendering impotent any allusion to the importance of culture. Studies in which specific communities have been identified, such as the case of suicide in the Cree and Métis community of Norway House, Manitoba, allow us to think more concretely about both cultural issues and historical processes (Ross & Davis 1986).

In contrast to the SADS-L, the Center for Epidemiologic Studies Depression Scale (CES-D) is a self-report screening instrument. Manson et al. (1990) employed it in a study of 188 American Indian boarding school students. The springboard for this study was their concern that instruments such as the CES-D were being transferred to American Indian populations without modification or 'with little thought devoted to the difference that culture may make in the performance of such instruments' (232). Five unspecified tribal groups were represented in their southeastern United States sample, consisting of students in the high school years. While the instrument demonstrated good internal consistency, differences between the research population and data from adult populations, as well as major gender differences, led the researchers to advise caution in the use of the CES-D with American Indian adolescents. But there was little in the research to suggest that these issues were related to the fact that the subjects were, indeed, American Indians, and, as in the Shore et al. (1987) study, the lack of specific cultural detail for each of the groups once again renders it impossible to judge the validity of their caution. In what appears to be a related study, Keane, Dick, Bechtold, and Manson (1996: 739) undertook to test the predictive validity of the Suicide Ideational Questionnaire, noting that some 52% of their high school respondents were from 'one of the five culturally similar tribes living in the area,' and that a further 33% 'were distributed between two other tribes from this group.' The assumption of a significant cultural similarity among these tribes, and hence a further but unstated assumption of cultural similarity among the *individuals* from these tribes, guided their decision that a tribal-specific analysis was unnecessary. Such assumptions, I would suggest, require considerably more empirical support than was provided here, as they speak to the centrality of the issue of testing for the cross-cultural validity of standardized instruments.

The assumption of cultural homogeneity is also evident in a parallel study with the same subjects by many of the same members of the research team on the use of the Inventory to Diagnose Depression (IDD), a self-report instrument based on DSM-III-R (Ackerson, Dick, Manson, & Baron 1990). Arguing that the paper 'offers additional insight into the performance of instruments like the IDD when employed across disparate cultural populations' (601), they apparently believed that the five tribes involved were not themselves 'disparate' but rather reflected a single cultural group. Once again, no concrete rationale was provided. More cultural data were provided in a subsequent publication on the use of the CES-D for older American Indians (Baron, Manson, Ackerson, & Brenneman 1990). This study involved four Pacific Northwest reservation populations, the Confederated

Tribes of the Warm Springs Indian Reservation, the Yakima Indian Nation, the Lummi Nation, and the Nooksack Tribe. However, both the Confederated Tribes and the Yakima Nation were actually comprised of several different tribes, making the use of these entities as proxies for culture particularly problematic. Further, as is common in many studies, all the subjects were aggregated into one category and there was no indication the researchers explored the cultural differences between the various groups or the existence of intracultural variability. Subjects were treated as if they were all culturally 'Indian' in exactly the same way. In concluding that the CES-D demonstrated some internal validity problems and that the data yielded different factor analytic results than those obtained in other studies of non-American Indians, the researchers hinted that Indianness was in some way the relevant explanatory factor. But the vagueness of the discussion calls into question the extent to which they achieved their stated goal of providing some insight into the issue of the generalizability or external validity of the CES-D. This is a ubiquitous problem: in another study of the CES-D and 605 American Indian college students, the cultural or tribal backgrounds of the subjects were not even mentioned (Beals, Manson, Keane, & Dick 1991), demonstrating clearly a view that American Indians represent, in their words, a unique, bounded 'special population' (623).

Similar problems are evident in a study of the CES-D related to earlier work described above among an anonymous Northwest Coast cultural group (Somervell, Beals, Kinzie, Boehnlein, Leung, & Manson 1993b; see also Somervell, Beals, Kinzie, Boehnlein, Leung, & Manson 1993a). In this study the SADS-L was used as the criterion for evaluating the CES-D among a sample drawn from a single village. The instruments were deployed using English since the community was almost entirely monolingual in this language. While the performance of the CES-D was considered to be 'encouraging,' the researchers cautioned that it could not be assumed that these results were replicable for other Indian communities because of the 'great diversity' that existed. This study is one of the few to raise the issue of acculturation as a confounding factor, although it was not explored further. However, in describing the community as essentially monolingual in English with a very long history of contact with non-Indian people, the authors noted that 'it is at least plausible that instruments of white/Anglo origin such as the CES-D may perform better in such a community than in one where the Native language is still dominant or where intense non-Native influence has been more recent' (264). This issue, which in my view is one of prime concern in the debate over the 'cultural' appropriateness of instruments such as the CES-D, remains largely undeveloped in the literature. It is conceivable that these instruments work in appropriate fashion as their developers intended when the target population is culturally closest to that of the population for whom the instrument was normed, and that therefore the extent to which populations perform within normative boundaries highlights these instruments as measures of acculturation. What is particularly frustrating is how little 'culture' is discussed and analysed in studies which avow to shed light on the appropriateness of these techniques cross-culturally.

A further example of this contradictory process can be found in the work of Wilson, Civic, and Glass (1995). These authors employed the Inventory to Diagnose Depression in a study of an anonymous primary outpatient clinic at an Indian Health Services facility in an unnamed southwestern United States reservation; all we are told about the population that is vaguely cultural is that it was 'of a southern Athabascan people' (2), and that the traditional culture remained strong. However, they noted that there had also been significant Caucasian influences on that culture and that the majority spoke English as the primary language in the home, two factors that confound our understanding of just how traditional or Athabascan they really were. Nevertheless, the authors expressed concern that their finding that the epidemiology of depression among patients in this clinic was similar to that found in other studies of clinic populations could be limited by the 'potential for cultural differences in the expression of depressive syndromes between American Indian and Alaska Native people and the majority population' (8). 'If significant differences exist,' they continued, 'the IDD might not be a valid instrument for defining depressive syndromes despite the fact that it is based on DSM III-R criteria' (8). They concluded by advocating that the 'wide variety of cultures and situations in the American Indian primary care populations [necessitates] replication studies ... to determine the epidemiology and characteristics of depression in other IHS primary care settings' and to determine the validity of self-report questionnaires 'among people with varying cultures' (10). But they actually disclosed virtually nothing about culture in their study.

Despite the ongoing attempts to utilize, sometimes in modified form, existing instruments, concerns about their validity lead Manson and Shore to develop a new instrument which they called the 'American

Indian Depression Scale,' and later the 'Indian Depression Scale' (Manson & Shore 1981; Manson, Shore, & Bloom 1985). Utilizing the explanatory model framework developed by Kleinman (1980) which at the time was increasing in popularity in medical anthropology, the researchers were guided by the view that the development of 'reliable, culturally valid diagnostic instrumentation has to take into account the explanatory models to which American Indian people themselves subscribe in making sense of their illness' (Manson et al. 1985: 332). This was a somewhat radical departure in the development of psychometric instruments, assuming as it did that there was more to generating a culturally appropriate instrument than simply translating an existing one into a local language. The work began in 1980 among the Hopi, utilizing a form of ethnosemantic interviewing to elicit illness categories and understandings. Five categories were determined which, expressed in English, were 'worry sickness,' 'unhappiness,' 'heartbroken,' 'drunkenlike craziness with or without alcohol,' and 'disappointment or pouting' (336–7). Worry sickness most closely approximated the English equivalent of mental illness, but the researchers stressed that the terms were only glosses for a variety of states which were often situation specific. Similar symptoms existed across these categories, but since no single set of symptoms was common to all, the researchers concluded that the categories represented distinct entities. These cultural data were then combined with elements of an existing instrument, the Diagnostic Interview Schedule (DIS), designed to generate diagnoses of disorder over specific periods of time (such as at present, the last two weeks, the last month, etc.). Those items of the DIS to be used were translated not into Hopi but into a form of English deemed comprehensible by the Hopi, even though for most English was their second language. Modifications were required, of course. For instance, some questions on sexual behaviour were deleted because they were inappropriate in a Hopi context, and one item which combined the concepts of guilt, shame, and sinfulness had to be broken down into separate items to reflect Hopi affective nosology.

The Indian Depression Scale that emerged from this exercise consisted of five sections and included understandings of indigenous psychopathology as well as the selected items from the DIS. This is without question an innovative approach. Concern for validity (in terms of both indigenous categories and those emanating from Western nosology) and reliability were central to the exercise, and another existing instrument, the Schedule for Affective Disorders and Schizophrenia – Lifetime Version (SADS-L) was used to establish criterion validity.[5] Among the final conclusions of the study were that while many Hopi recognized the indigenous categories only some of the defined illnesses were related to depression, and no conceptual equivalent to 'depression' seemed to exist. One form of illness, 'heartbroken,' was most strongly associated with symptoms of depression and occurred with the greatest frequency among those diagnosed with major depressive disorder according to DSM-III.

The important work of these researchers illustrates the potential in combining indigenous and Western understandings in a diagnostic instrument. Of course, by definition the instrument was really a *Hopi* Depression Scale rather than an *Indian* Depression Scale. The fact that the instrument was by necessity anchored in a singular cultural context defines how such work should be done and perhaps explains why the approach has not been used in other studies. Ethnography and psychiatric epidemiology have been shown to be compatible, yet the difficulties encountered in the multiple methods approach to developing such an instrument might frighten off many who are supportive of the general idea and who might wish to adapt it to a different cultural context. Manson et al. (1985: 361) concluded their interesting paper with the following criticism: 'in its rush to generate highly specified criteria by which to reliably diagnose disorder, psychiatry has failed to consider the cultural dimension of illness: how it is conceptualized, experienced, manifested, explained, and treated.' While their work has demonstrated how some aspects of indigenous understanding can be captured in an instrument, does this really represent the 'cultural dimension' in any meaningful way? Even the authors admit that there is considerably more to Hopi understandings of illness than their research uncovered or that could be included in their instrument. Broader, and I think more insightful, questions remain unaddressed. Why try to force indigenous understandings into Western frameworks? While the validity and reliability of a specific instrument can be proven using standard methodologies, what about the validity of the general technique itself? Why use an instrument at all? In so far as these fundamental questions remain unaddressed they testify to the inherently scientific and Western bias that the researchers seem to want to eschew. Nevertheless, the impact of their work has been profound: being 'heartbroken' among the Hopi was introduced into DSM-IV in the mid-1990s as an example of the way culture can influence the experience of depression and the communication of its symptoms (American Psychiatric Association 1994: 324).

In a study of depression among American Indian elderly utilizing the CES-D, Chapleski, Lamphere, Kaczynski, Lichtenberg, and Dwyer (1997) (see also Curyto, Chapleski, Lichtenberg, Hodges, Kaczynski, & Sobeck 1998) explicitly acknowledged the difficulties in generalizing a unidimensional view of the disorder across Indian cultural boundaries and especially within the context of acculturation. They utilized a multi-group comparative strategy which identified three categories of individuals – urban residents, rural off-reservation residents, and those living on reservation – each of which was viewed as a separate 'cultural context.' In so doing they explicitly rejected as too simple the rural-urban or on-reservation–off-reservation dichotomies that guide much comparative work. Overall, 125 urban, 83 rural, and 101 reservation elderly in Michigan were interviewed. The specific tribal backgrounds of participants were not provided, unfortunately, and although the authors suggested that the target population lived in areas 'which are representative of the major tribal groups in the state, Potawatomi, Ojibwa, and Odawa,' no analysis by tribe was presented (Curyto et al. 1998: 27). Instead, the researchers argued that since the vast majority of the participants came from tribes to be found in the woodlands culture area, 'the sample offers a group of American Indians with similar biological and cultural roots' (Chapleski et al. 1997: 471). This is a perplexing and disappointing assertion, given the relatively progressive approach to the issue of cultural change adopted by the researchers. While arguing that there is great cultural variability and that intermarriage with non-Indians had resulted in a 'polycultural' rather than a mono-cultural or even bicultural reality, they nevertheless reverted to the culture area concept, even implying that these areas represent not just cultural continuity but *biological* continuity. The issue of culture was muddled even further when they suggested that the same CES-D measurement model found to be superior with a Mexican American sample was also superior for this sample of American Indians, which they believed might 'reflect cross-cultural similarities shared between minority groups living among a dominant culture' (Chapleski et al. 1997: 482). Finally, they argued that some items in the CES-D 'may not be conceptually congruent with the group-centered worldview of American Indian culture' (481). Retreating to the commonly held view that there are core, essential cultural traits characteristic of *all* American Indians, they suggested that Indian cultures were 'cooperative and group-oriented,' in contrast to 'highly individualistic cultures,' and that this affected Indian performance on several interpersonal items. The inclination to talk through issues, they added, 'is similarly of questionable validity for a culture known to be more reflective and nonconfrontational' (481). While none of these concerns affected their conclusion that the CES-D can discern differences across the three residential groups, and that urban residence was a significant predictor of depression, in point of fact the research does not allow us to say anything about culture at all.

Language translation is always an issue in the utilization of instruments in cross-cultural settings. In a study of depression, anxiety, and alcohol abuse among residents of a Canadian Inuit community, Haggarty, Cernovsky, Kermeen, and Merskey (2000) employed a multilevel technique to ensure that the depression instrument they were testing, the Hospital Anxiety and Depression Scale (HADS), was as linguistically and culturally appropriate as possible. The Structured Clinical Interview (SCID) for DSM-III-R was also utilized to assess criterion validity. A trained government translator was first employed to transform the HADS into Inuktitut, and then a local interpreter worked to render it compatible with the community's dialect. Back translation into English was also used to help ensure content validity. The HADS, a fourteen-item self-report survey designed to differentiate between anxiety and depression, was then administered by local, trained interviewers in either English or Inuktitut. The instrument was highly regarded for this use because of its simplicity and the ease with which it could be translated. Perhaps surprisingly, most of the 163 respondents (64 per cent) chose to use English in the interview (a reflection of the bilingual nature of the community), a potentially confounding factor which the authors failed to address adequately. The choice of language was not related to the prevalence of depression, however. Fully a quarter of those interviewed were diagnosed with depression, and the authors recognized that Inuit cultural factors represented an 'unmeasured effect which may have influenced symptom reporting' (Haggarty et al. 2000: 361). Recognizing the limitations of the community-based epidemiological approach, they advocated the use of local ethnographic research to assess the limitations of instruments like the HADS and the SCID in cross-cultural settings.

In contrast to research on diagnosis, there is relatively little literature on approaches to treating Aboriginal peoples with depression. Manson (1992) described a cognitive-behavioural strategy for chronically physically ill older American Indians suffering from depression, the 'Coping with Stress Course,' which was modelled on a similar project for non-Indian people. There was no pretense that this represented a 'traditional' approach to treatment: the course involved lectures, class activities, a textbook, and even homework, all of which would have been familiar to most participants from their school days. Coping skills that were taught included social skills, assertiveness, increasing pleasant and decreasing negative activities, anxiety reduction, and time management. According to Manson (1992: 87), 'past claims that such skills are alien to most American Indians and cannot be learned by them have crumbled in the face of mounting evidence to the contrary.' Whether this is due to misconceptions of 'traditional' Aboriginal cultural abilities or to more recent processes of cultural change was not made clear. Manson did note that 'indigenous forms of healing and various religious traditions' often included such skills (87), nevertheless, the delivery mode of the course was clearly based on a non-Indian model.

Although Manson (1992) described several 'traditional' methods for treating depression and related mental illnesses, his description of these was brief and non-specific to particular disorders. Storck et al. (2000) looked more specifically at the experiences of Navajo patients, depressed according to DSM criteria, with traditional or 'religious' healing activities. These activities, while ensconced within a Navajo cultural framework, offered therapeutic strategies which were similar in many ways to those of Western psychotherapy, including psychodynamic and cognitive-behavioural modalities. But in the Navajo understanding of depression, symptoms included not just individualized pain or depressed affect, but also a negative event or setback, and these were rendered interpretable and treatable within the traditional context. While the idea that the genesis of a mental disorder can exist outside the physical body is not unusual, the belief that symptoms can poses a challenge to a DSM-governed view of psychopathology. Extending our view of depression beyond the DSM represents both a methodological and a conceptual challenge.

An Ethnographic Approach to the Study of Aboriginal Depression

The ethnographic approach to understanding depression has provided a qualitatively different view of this disorder among Aboriginal peoples and demonstrated how cultural continuity, in some instances at least, remains integral to our understanding of contemporary distress. Theresa O'Nell (1993; 1996), an anthropologist grounded in the work of Arthur Kleinman and an associate of Manson and Shore, adopted such an approach in research among the Flathead of Montana. The springboard for her research was the view held both within and outside the Flathead community that the majority of Flathead people were 'depressed.' In attempting to understand how this could be, O'Nell admittedly approached the issue from a DSM framework, but came to realize the shortcomings of the biomedical approach to depression within this other-cultural context. Some eighteen months of fieldwork on the Flathead reservation led O'Nell to conclude that there were some problems in the rote administration of DSM criteria for depressive disorder.[6]

O'Nell (1996) cautioned that the fact that the Flathead spoke English and used English-language terminology to describe their pathology was misleading and disguised a very different, indigenous understanding of the problem.[7] For the Flathead, a feeling of loneliness was the central affective symptom in depression. Loneliness was conceived of as a broad concept that included not only feelings of loss or bereavement, occasioned for instance by the loss of a loved one, but also feelings of aggrievement related to past injustices, rejection, and neglect. 'Feeling worthless,' in the sense of feeling abandoned by family, friends, and even the Creator because of an inherent 'unworthyness,' was the most serious form of loneliness. A particular strength of O'Nell's work was the situating of Flathead depression in both an historical and a cultural context. The history of loss related to colonization was integral to their current world-view; this included fundamental changes in what it meant to be 'Indian,' and even who qualified as an 'Indian' at all. This is one of the few examples of research that clearly articulates the need to understand *contemporary* Aboriginality and which does not gloss over intracultural difference or assume the existence of a single, bounded Indian culture even at the community level.

Not all loneliness was seen as pathological by these Flathead; indeed, according to O'Nell (1996: 205), 'Flathead narratives of depression seem to resonate as much with positive moral meanings as with ego-centered pain.' The sense of loss was not to be worked through or forgotten, but rather 'should remain in their hearts as reminders to have pity on others' (177). 'Thus Flathead people discipline their hearts to remember their pain and yet to transcend it,' O'Nell argued (177). Even loneliness accompanied by such DSM markers as sleeplessness, tearfulness, and loss of appetite was often seen as a sign of maturity as a human being and demonstrative of one's Indianness; in other words, these symptoms were positive, normative, and psychically sound. To the Flathead, a disturbance in social relations, for instance in a lack of compassionate feelings for another person, was seen as a more significant marker of pathological depression, yet DSM is silent on the issue of disturbed or disordered social relations. In a powerful critique of the perspectives on emotions which dominate the DSM and the biopsychosocial perspective, O'Nell (1996: 180) argued that Euro-Americans are largely blind to the way cultural others experience emotional states, and tend to view only the differences between themselves and these others as 'cultural.' In this process of exoticizing, while 'the emotions of others' are seen as 'cultural,' the emotions of Euro-Americans are considered 'natural.' Further, she noted that this perspective defines emotions as inherently internal to the individual, as 'precultural,' which was incompatible with the social orientation of Flathead epistemology. Loneliness for the Flathead must be seen within its broad social, cultural, and historic contexts to be understood, but such an understanding is beyond the framework of a DSM approach. In fact, she argued persuasively that 'the unexamined use of DSM criteria for research purposes can lead to the medicalization or pathologizing of alternate visions of normality, or to the trivialization of profound human misery' (O'Nell 1996: 207).[8] O'Nell's attempt to generate DSM-like Flathead diagnostic criteria for 'pathological mood disturbance' stressed the limits of the DSM in such a cross-cultural setting: the rich cultural context in which the Flathead conceptualization was anchored did not translate well into signs and symptoms, and the complete absence of a reference to Flathead history, considered by O'Nell as central to their understanding, further underscored the narrowness of the DSM approach (203). In the end, comprehending how the Flathead people view something which DSM calls depression does not necessarily mean the constructs are equivalent, no matter how noble the inquiry.

In an attempt to compare Flathead and DSM criteria for depression, O'Nell (1996) employed a small experiment involving twenty individuals who had identified themselves as suffering from depression. She determined whether or not the person was experiencing 'pathological loneliness,' in other words, 'depression' as the Flathead would understand it. This was done, in her words, 'on several bases that include subjective accounts of distress, the atypical usage of Flathead idioms, subjective accounts or evidence of disordered social relationships (whether in terms of affection or material reciprocity), the extent of help-seeking for reported distress, and family or community judgements about the individual.' These results were then compared with a strict application of DSM-III criteria. Her conclusion: 'Among the cases

I reviewed, there were respondents who met criteria for a depressive disorder but who evidenced little or no pathology according to the cultural criteria noted above. There were also respondents who met criteria but whose narratives of loneliness included locally significant signs of distress that the DSM criteria failed to capture. Finally, there were respondents who at some level of accuracy could be diagnosed with a depressive disorder with DSM criteria but for whom an assessment of the severity or pathology of individual symptoms or symptom patterns could easily be misjudged' (O'Nell 1996: 196). Granted, this was hardly a gold standard kind of experiment, but it dramatically underscored the importance of grounding any determination about the cultural appropriateness of the DSM or other instruments in actual, not hypothetical or stereotypical, cultures. By incorporating culture more centrally into her analysis, O'Nell avoided the pitfalls that haunt research which purports to talk about cultural appropriateness without ever discussing culture in any meaningful way. Back in 1981, Shore and Manson (1981: 11) argued that there was 'substantial evidence that the differences in American Indian subcultures significantly affect behavior,' and that 'the spectrum of depressive behaviors represents a variety of responses with multiple etiologies.' 'Future research,' they suggested, 'should focus on methodological developments that emphasize both subcultural specificity and multiple etiologies of depressive reactions' (Shore & Manson (1981: 11). Apart from the work of O'Nell, little progress seems to have been made in this important direction.

If the Flathead were truly depressed according to DSM criteria, and to the extent that those criteria suggested they were, theirs would have been a profoundly dysfunctional community. Yet O'Nell's analysis did not succumb to such a pessimistic view: the Flathead people were portrayed as leading functional and fulfilling lives even while dealing with difficult circumstances. That their conceptualization of depression could include a very positive, affirming element partly explains this reality. We must look critically at local contexts before rushing to the judgment that an Aboriginal community is caught in a spiral of psychopathology.

Conclusion

The study of depression and suicide provides one of the best examples of the very different approaches to mental health topics taken by psychiatry and anthropology. These differences are both conceptual (depression as universal versus depression as particularistic) and methodological (the use of diagnostic instruments versus ethnography). Kleinman and Good (1985: 8), in their review of the issue of culture and depression, argued that 'the single most troublesome problem plaguing the cross-cultural study of affect and affective disorder is the failure to take an anthropologically sophisticated view of culture.' Such a view would start from a realistic understanding of human culture and behaviour, recognizing that culture creates stresses and life circumstances which, for some individuals, prove problematic. It would also recognize that cultures do not cease to exist or to adapt with the arrival of new cultural stimuli.

Unfortunately, the overall conclusion seems to be that while we understand that depression and suicide have become significant mental health problems for the Aboriginal population, especially in recent decades, we still know very little about the intersection of culture, history, depression, and suicide. We have yet to develop an integrated explanation for why some communities have much lower suicide rates than others, why suicide patterns vary so widely, or why some individuals, but not others, suffer so much distress. Instead, there is a tendency to embrace panoptic explanations which uncritically attribute psychopathology to broad historical and cultural phenomena while ignoring local cultural heterogeneity, continuity, and adaptation. The use of existing diagnostic instruments, or variants thereof, betray an underlining assumption of at least a sufficient degree of Aboriginal homogeneity of culture and experience. While they provide us with quantitative data for those self-declaring to be Aboriginal, or who are so designated by researchers, we must reject the kinds of manipulations that lead us to believe that these studies necessarily deal with *cultural* groups or cultural explanatory factors. The promise of elucidating the role of culture in Aboriginal depression and suicide studies has yet to be fulfilled, although a start has been made by researchers such as O'Nell and Manson and Shore. A cultural epidemiological approach that combines ethnography with psychiatric epidemiology is at the heart of this initiative.

CHAPTER EIGHT

The Culture-Bound Aboriginal

The Indian is a big child, credulous, impressionable, sensitive, imaginative. (Saindon 1933: 2)

Are some mental disorders restricted to specific cultures? Do cultures produce unique forms of disorder? These are the key questions behind the concept of culture-bound syndromes. As we have seen in previous chapters, Aboriginal North Americans have served as important sources of data that have helped frame both theory and method in anthropology, psychology, and psychiatry, and this trend continues with the culture-bound syndromes. Three Aboriginal syndromes in particular have demonstrated a tenacious resilience: windigo psychosis, *pibloktok*, and ghost sickness. On the surface, these three seem to be examples of culture-bound syndromes par excellence. Upon closer inspection, however, it appears as though these constructions have their origins in the imaginations of scholars rather than the cultures of the original inhabitants of North America. Saindon, this would suggest, had it backwards.

The Culture-Bound Syndromes

Culture-bound syndromes have been the subject of anthropological and psychiatric attention for many decades, with the earliest formulations dating back to the early 1800s (Prince 2000). Discussions of 'ethnic psychoses' and other labels exhibiting exoticism (Devereux 1971; Prince & Tcheng-Laroche 1987; Prince 2000), primarily anthropological in orientation, have given way in more recent years to a resoundingly psychiatric delineation. Psychiatrist Pow Meng Yap (1967) is usually credited with coining the expression 'culture-bound reactive syndrome,' from which the current concept is derived. The most recent version of the DSM (DSM-IV-TR; American Psychiatric Association 2000) defined culture-bound syndromes as 'recurrent, locality-specific patterns of aberrant behavior and troubling experience that may or may not be linked to a particular DSM-IV diagnostic category ... culture-bound syndromes are generally limited to specific societies or culture areas and are localized, folk, diagnostic categories that frame coherent meanings for certain repetitive, patterned, and troubling sets of experiences and observations' (898). While they may or may not be 'indigenously considered to be "illnesses," or at least afflictions' with local names, there is obviously a strong bias in favour of the view that they are in some way recognized within local, folk taxonomies. There is little consensus as to their genesis. The DSM seems to imply that they represent naturally occurring, ontological phenomena that spring from cultural processes intrinsic to bounded, somewhat isolated cultures and demonstrates an ahistorical view of their development. Some scholars have posited a more dynamic explanation, however, arguing that culture-bound syndromes are 'reactive to sociocultural circumstances' (Fabrega 1982; Jilek & Jilek-Aall 1985). The extent to which these conditions are truly culture *bound* has also been questioned (much more than the extent to which cultures themselves can be bound), as evidence has mounted that many so-called culture-bound syndromes are in fact disorders with local names but a more commonly shared, cross-cultural distribution (Hughes 1996). Perhaps more importantly, it has been argued that 'any efforts to represent psychiatric disorders as unique to particular "cultures" leads rapidly to cultural essentialism, stereotyping, and increased possibilities of stigmatization' (Good 1996: 129). Whatever the explanation, in general these disorders have been treated as real, if mysterious and exotic phenomena. It seems as though much of the debate regarding culture-bound syndromes has focused on the issue of their *uniqueness* and not their *existence*. As I shall demonstrate, this has led to the reification in scholarly publications, public culture, and even on the Internet, of several Aboriginal North American syndromes as genuine psychiatric phenomena characteristic not only of ancient or historic but also of contemporary Aboriginal peoples. Just how 'real' are they? Let me turn first to windigo psychosis.

Windigo Psychosis

The story of the windigo,[1] a cannibal monster with a heart of ice inhabiting the northern woodlands of Canada, has fascinated Algonquian specialists for a century or more. From the early works of famed ethnologists such as A.I. Hallowell (1934, 1936, 1955) and Ruth Landes (1937, 1938) through work by James G.E. Smith (1976) and Richard Preston (1980), there has been a singular fascination with this aspect of northern Cree and Ojibwa folklore. The notion of windigo *psychosis* has also entered into the medical history of northern Canada (Margetts 1975). This transformation of windigo from fable to psychiatric disorder is quite contentious.

The genesis of the idea that windigo represented something more than folklore can be found in the work of Landes and especially in that of J.E. Saindon (1933), a Catholic priest. Saindon published a highly influential paper in the Catholic anthropological journal *Primitive Man* in 1933, in which he described his observations of 'abnormal psychic phenomena' among the Cree on the west coast of James Bay. Saindon was one of the first to associate windigo mythology with psychiatric disorder and, perhaps more surprisingly, apparently to present an eyewitness description of an individual allegedly affected by windigo psychosis, the only such account in print even to this day. Saindon's (1933: 1) observation that there was 'a good deal of hysteria, particularly among women' of the northern Cree was explained, in part, as the product of their cognitive limitations as 'big children.' 'While he is intelligent and is gifted with a marvellous memory,' Saindon (1933: 2) suggested, 'on the other hand his powers of judgement are in many respects little exercised and little developed' (2). As a result, 'his undisciplined imagination delivers itself up to the worst excesses, to the most foolish and most fantastic vagaries' which 'envelop and permeate the whole field of consciousness and block rational thought and judgment' (2). Windigo-based insanity, according to Landes (1937), was rife among the northern Ojibwa population.

Windigo psychosis was characterized by an individual's belief that he or she was turning into the cannibal monster, as evidenced by a compulsive desire to eat human flesh. Interestingly, Saindon's lone sufferer did not exhibit a desire to eat humans per se, but rather wild animals into which, the individual believed, humans had transformed. Nevertheless, by the time Seymour Parker penned his article on 'wiitiko' psychosis almost thirty years later, it had evolved, in Parker's

words, into 'a bizarre form of mental disorder involving obsessive cannibalism,' the initial symptoms of which were 'feelings of morbid
depression, nausea, and distaste for most ordinary foods, and sometimes periods of semi-stupor' (Parker 1960: 603). Parker continued:

> Gradually, the victim becomes obsessed with paranoid ideas of being
> bewitched and is subject to homicidal (and occasionally suicidal)
> thoughts. He feels that he is possessed by the wiitiko monster, a fierce
> cannibalistic being, to whose will he has become subjected. The convic-
> tion of the existence of a wiitiko monster itself is not evidence of pathol-
> ogy, since this is a socially shared belief among the Ojibwa. If the illness
> progresses beyond this stage, the individual begins to see those around
> him (often close family members) as fat, luscious animals which he
> desires to devour. Finally, the wiitiko sufferer enters a stage of violent
> homicidal cannibalism. It is commonly thought that once this stage is
> reached and the person has tasted human flesh, the craving will not leave
> him and he must be killed. (Parker 1960: 603)

Parker (1960) suggested that the disorder was most likely to affect
males because of the stresses of their solitary existence hunting in the
bush; authors such as Hallowell and Landes, as expected, argued that
the phenomenon was a logical extension of the suspicious individuality
characteristic of the northern Algonquian personality, as detailed in
chapter 3.[2] Parker (1960: 603; emphasis added) then added that wiitiko
psychosis had 'been reported by *many* investigators' in the north, citing
both Hallowell and Landes, who had not actually witnessed a case of
the disorder and were themselves reporting from distant, vague
accounts offered by informants. Parker also utilized the work of
another Catholic priest, John M. Cooper (1933), whose discussion of
'wiitiko' was published in the same journal issue of *Primitive Man* in
1933 as Saindon's piece. Cooper described the disorder as a 'common
psychosis' among the eastern Cree, one related to periods of intense
starvation during which individuals resorted to eating their dead associates as a means to stay alive, despite strong social sanctions against
such an act. This view was based on his discussions with the Cree
themselves, combined with occasional reports in documents of the
resort to cannibalism. Saindon's discussion contains the only reported
case interview of the disorder; as Lou Marano (1985) demonstrated in a
scathing critique of the construction of the 'emic-etic' confusion over
the notion of windigo psychosis, there appear to be no other reports

and certainly no documentation of actual cannibalism. Even Parker lamented that none of the previous commentators had ever been able to interview an actual windigo patient. What did exist, simply put, was a wealth of stories. Little did the Cree and Ojibwa know that their stories would cause such a tidal wave in the waters of transcultural psychiatry!

An alternative interpretation of windigo psychosis was presented by Kiev (1972) and subsequently accepted by leading scholars Shore and Manson (1981: 7). Emphasizing the existence of melancholia, Kiev (1972: 84–5) determined that windigo psychosis represented 'the classical depressive disorder, showing a specifically prominent secondary symptom of self-deprecation and need for punishment with a culturally available explanation.' However, Kiev then added that 'while cultural influences determine the nature of the symptoms, there is no evidence available that the form of the illness is caused by cultural factors, nor any evidence that the Windigo belief itself has an etiological role.' In other words, this was *not* a culture-bound syndrome but rather a culturally localized expression of a universal condition, depression. Shore and Manson (1981: 6) nevertheless still referred to it as a 'culture-bound disorder.'

Marano's (1985) deconstruction of windigo psychosis remains one of the best reminders of the importance of critically reconsidering accepted constructs in the field of Aboriginal mental health. Marano carefully examined all materials written about the disorder, tracing connections between articles, only to discover the windigo house of cards. His conclusion: windigo psychosis was based on nothing more than 'hearsay reports and folktales' and likely never occurred! 'It could even be argued that the windigo phenomenon is more of an example of mass suggestibility among anthropologists than among Northern Algonkians,' he argued insightfully (418). On this point he quoted Richard Preston (1980; as cited in Marano 1985: 436), who wrote: 'We have made the diagnosis without seeing the patient ... Some kind of compulsion and transformation is believed in by the Northern Algonkians, but their words are too often taken as literal (rather than magic or symbolic) representations of events, which we then use to construct our definition of a Witiko psychopathology ... It seems that we have taken an exotic notion out of its native context of the images of terror, and with much seriousness we have overinterpreted the meagre data.' Marano accepted that elements of windigo folklore might have emerged in accounts of mental instability as a means of emically explaining aberrant behaviour, but he rejected the idea of a psychosis connected to the windigo theme. Marano did concede that, in addition to the existence of windigo in folklore, *accusations* of windigo were made, a kind of serious name-calling which served to isolate and ostracize undesirable individuals, be they sick, weak, or disruptive. Occasionally, such accusations may have led to the execution of the accused during difficult times, on the grounds that they were turning into windigos and hence were a threat to the security of the group. Marano employed the concept of 'triage homicide' to explain this, suggesting it was similar to the European witch trials of several centuries ago. He suggested that windigo accusations reached a peak *after* several hundred years of contact with Europeans, especially through the fur trade, and were concomitant with an increase in mortality and morbidity from European-introduced disease. The Ojibwa were 'traumatized,' in Marano's words, and 'the windigo belief complex was the Northern Algonkian manifestation of the collective witch fear that is predictable in traumatized societies' (440). This alternative hypothesis required more investigation than Marano was able to provide, but as conjecture it did not detract from the strength of Marano's critique of the concept of windigo psychosis. The critique should have had a profound influence on understandings of this so-called disorder, but as I shall demonstrate shortly, there is life-after-death for psychotic cannibal monsters.

Pibloktoq

Pibloktoq, sometimes referred to as 'Arctic hysteria,' was originally ascribed to the Greenlandic Eskimos but, through time, came to be thought characteristic of most Eskimo and Inuit populations and, within medical anthropology and related fields, was seen as a prime example of a culture-bound syndrome (e.g., Foster & Anderson 1978). One of the most influential presentations of this disorder is found in a 1913 article by noted American psychoanalyst A.A. Brill, who had been heavily influenced by Freud and who had translated the latter's works on hysteria into English (Shorter 1997). Brill (1913) utilized the text of Admiral Robert Peary's Arctic expeditions between 1891 and 1909, along with interviews with a member of Peary's crew, to construct this new disorder. *Pibloktoq* was taken to refer to hysteric acts, usually perpetrated by women, in which the individual tore off or destroyed clothing and ran off with abandon despite the harsh cold of the Arctic winter. Attacks could last up to one and a half hours, eventually concluding with the victim calm and quiet, or trembling and weeping. The sufferer then fell asleep. A prodromal period was typical, in which the individual could be seen softly singing, rocking, and rhythmically pounding the fist. The cause, according to Brill's informant, could be found in the characteristic abuse of women by men. Brill's informant offered that 'it reminded me of a little child discouraged and unhappy because it imagines that no one loves it or cares for it and therefore runs away' (517). The Aboriginal-as-child metaphor struck a chord with Brill, as it did with so many other commentators. His Freudian training led him to conclude that the nature of Eskimo society deprived females of strong, loving relationships (including sex) with their partners. They were denied 'the elements of love so essential to feminine nature' (518), and hysteria was the consequence.[3]

Several important works were published on *pibloktoq* subsequent to Brill's pioneering efforts. Psychiatrist Zachary Gussow, in 1960, added information with regard to the prodromal period (e.g., tiredness, depressive silence, weeping) and the symptomology (e.g., glossolalia, rolling in the snow, eating faeces), and noted that while men sometimes suffered from the disorder the women's experience was more 'florid' (279). Gussow (1960) described the disorder as a culturally patterned response to culturally defined stressors and anxiety ('Eskimo culture institutionalizes "hysteroid" behavior,' he wrote (280)), such as fears of winter starvation or being lost. 'The pibloktoq performance,' he explained, 'represents a culturally patterned panic reaction to such trauma' (283). Following Brill's lead, and consistant with Freudian theories, Gussow summarized that, 'in pibloqtoq the traumatized ego reacts in a psychologically primitive and infantile, but characteristically Eskimo, manner. In other words, though the psychological mode is ontogenetically primitive, much of the behaviour is congruent with adult ethnic personality' (284). Freeman, Foulks, and Freeman (1978) and Foulks, Freeman, and Freeman (1979), while accepting Gussow's interpretation of Eskimo childhood, argued that the children grew into over-dependent adults who experienced great anxiety when separated from others; hysteria, then, was a form of regression to an infantile state of comfortable dependence.

Seymour Parker (1962), whose influential views on windigo psychosis were discussed above, described the Eskimo culture as characterized by a reliance on mutual aid and nurturance; the individual had reason to believe he or she would always receive the necessary support to survive. Eskimo society was also characterized by the lack of severe early socialization practices, an emphasis on communalistic values, and a religious system in which hysteria-like behaviour among shamans was accepted. Foulks (1972, 1985) likewise saw shamanic performances during times of stress as accepted behaviours that inspired others to behave in a similar fashion; in his attempt to update the situation of North Alaskan Eskimos, he suggested that alcohol was replacing the traditional shamanic behaviours and, by extension, the role model function which defined Arctic hysteria. Since females, it was believed, experienced lower self-esteem and were disadvantaged, they were more prone to hysteria. In a psychiatric study of southern Baffin Island Eskimos (Sampath 1974: 365–6), an astounding 70 per cent of the females were determined to have an 'hysterical type of personality disorder, particularly with histories of dissociative reactions,' which was presented as evidence that *pibloktoq* was still extensive in the area. *Pibloktoq*, then, as a form of hysteria, was seen as a culturally sanctioned means of calling attention to oneself, a cry for help that the individual knew would be answered. The individual running off into the tundra both hoped and expected to be retrieved. This acting-out was contrasted by Parker (1962) to the more sullen, depressive experience of northern Indians.

According to Abel, Metraux, and Roll (1987: 56), 'in contrast to the existing data on windigo psychosis, data on Eskimo arctic hysterias are grounded in actual observation and informed discussion ...' This assertion cannot be sustained, however. On the contrary, like windigo psychosis, *pibloktoq* also seems to have a dubious empirical background. Vallee (1966) noted that he could find only one Eskimo in his research on the east side of Hudson Bay who had ever heard of this Inuktitut word, and perhaps tellingly this individual had heard it from a white nurse. Dick (1995: 11) also found a general lack of Inuit knowledge of the word, although he did discover evidence of '*pivdlerortoq*,' and variations thereof, which he glossed as 'madness.' Boag (1970) chastised authors who had created inaccurate stereotypes of Eskimo peoples and overgeneralized from one group to another in describing them as essentially wracked with psychopathology and, especially, hysteria. '*Pibloktoq*' was one such hysteria, created from anecdotal reports of anthropologists, traders, and explorers; it was 'primarily of historical and technical interest *and not currently significant*' (116; emphasis added). 'One may question the extent to which they ever were a significant part of the total load of psychopathology in the population,' Boag ascertained (116). Hippler (1975) lamented the unreliable data, problems of under-reporting, and the problem of alcohol use masking psychotic symptoms. Kirmayer, Fletcher, Corin, & Boothroyd (1997: 18), in a study of three Inuit communities in northern Quebec, failed to discover a single case of *pibloktoq*. Their informants found the whole idea of such behaviour odd, although conceivable in the case of someone who was intoxicated. These authors made the important point that whatever *pibloktoq's* prevalence in the past, 'the classic accounts of exotic culture-bound syndromes bear little resemblance to the current psychiatric problems of the Inuit.'

Dick (1995) took this argument further in his Marano-like critique of *pibloktoq*, the kind of analysis which I believe is too infrequent. In a review of twenty-two scientific articles on the topic, encompassing forty reported cases, Dick (1995) argued that '*pibloktoq*' was in fact a term used for a broad variety of disorders, some real and others clearly imagined by the European commentators. Among many penetrating conclusions he determined that a semantic analysis pointed to the misinterpretation of a variety of Inuit utterances, such as hunger, as *pibloktoq*; there were cases in the historic record of staged observations and photographs; in some cases the afflicted individual was experiencing a recurring episode, reducing the overall number of unique reported cases; what was actually observed in several instances was shamanic trance and not hysteria; the stresses of contact with Europeans were responsible for many of the reported episodes, including those of women faking hysteria to avoid engaging in sexual relations with Europeans. Referring specifically to Foulks's (1972) clinical description of ten cases, Dick (1995) argued that both Foulks's data and his clinical observations suggested a variety of alternative explanations for hysteric-like behaviour, including epilepsy in at least three cases. My own examination of Foulks's cases found such a wide variety of symptomatic behaviours as to raise doubts about the utility of grouping them together into a single syndrome, regardless of the underlying cause. Dick's cases, eighteen men and twenty-eight women, contradicted the prevailing notion within the historic record as well as the psychiatric literature (e.g., Alarcon, Foulks, and Vakkur 1998) that this form of hysteria was common and that it primarily afflicted women, a view informed by a long-standing, male, European conviction that hysteria in general was a female affliction (as Brill and others argued) (Nuckolls 1998). 'Euro-American semantic associations surrounding the term "hysteria",' Dick (1995: 12) wrote, 'formed an important part of the perceptual repertoire which American observers carried with them when they first witnessed episodes of "pibloktoq".' Dick's (1995: 1–2) analysis was incisive:

The proliferation of commentaries [on *pibloktoq*] is itself one of the most interesting aspects of 'arctic hysteria.' As with the voluminous psychoanalytical literature deriving from Freud's famous case report on Dora, the small number of reported 'pibloktoq' episodes enabled the construction of an entire discourse on arctic hysteria on the base of a few fragmentary textual narratives. Yet, these original reports of 'pibloktoq' were filtered through the specific cultural perspectives of their Euro-American writers and shaped by the history of their own experiences of early contact with arctic peoples ... Whatever its specific character, 'pibloktoq' would not have achieved such prominence in the literature if social scientists and physicians had not viewed it as both widespread and integral to the personality of the Inuit.

Pibloktoq, in Dick's eyes, explained more about European-Inuit relations than it did about Inuit psychopathology.

Ghost Sickness

Ghost sickness has not been subject to the same intensive critical treatment by scholars as have windigo psychosis and *pibloqtoq*. Unlike the latter two disorders, ghost sickness has been considerably less pathologized in the Western sense. Indeed, there is little evidence that it has been investigated to determine how it fits with Western nosologies, and it has frequently been explicated in terms compatible with what Westerners believe to be the traditional indigenous context.

Ghost sickness was primarily considered to be a Navajo disorder, although there have been suggestions that variants of it existed among the Mohave and the Chiricahua, Mescalero, Jicarilla, Lipan, and Kiowa Apache, all in the American southwest. Trimble, Manson, Dinges, and Medicine (1984), in a paper that is frequently cited as authoritative, cited the work of Morgan (1936), Opler (1936, 1938, 1945, 1946), Fathauer (1951), Opler and Bittle (1961), Boyer (1964a, 1964b), and Kaplan and Johnson (1964) in their description of ghost sickness, establishing it as a bona fide mental disorder. But a closer look at these sources reveals a number of problems.

William Morgan (1936: 7), for instance, is quoted by both Trimble et al. (1984) and Kaplan and Johnson (1964) as describing a 'typical' case of ghost sickness: '[T]he individual enters a period of anxiety and generalized fear. This fear seems to emanate from a feeling of helplessness, and in some cases terror, which precedes and accompanies the involuntary eruption of unconscious impulses where the individual has little or no control over his mind and body. He may have delusions about sights and sounds in the dark. He may have repetitive nightmares. He may have hallucinations' (Morgan 1936: 6–7; quoted in Kaplan & Johnson 1964: 212; Trimble et al. 1984: 209–10). Several important problems emerge immediately with this 'typical' description. First, as Morgan (1936) himself noted, the data were derived from just a dozen personality studies in a single extended Navajo family in 1933, and he was at pains to emphasize that it was not possible to generalize beyond this small group. Second, and more importantly, a careful reading of his text suggests that Morgan may not have been talking about 'ghost sickness' at all. Rather, he was discussing a phenomenon which he related to the existence of generalized anxiety and the repression of emotions and interpersonal aggression among the Navajo, in which the belief in witchcraft was central. As we have seen, this was a very common theme in psychoanalytical personality studies of Aboriginal North Americans. Indeed, the text immediately preceding and following the strategic quotation tells a different story. At the risk of repetitiveness, here is the full passage, with the additional text in italics:

> *There is a common phenomenon evincing itself sporadically among Navaho. This phenomenon consists of an interval when repression weakens and unconscious impulses appear on the threshold of consciousness.* The individual enters a period of anxiety and generalized fear. This fear seems to emanate from a feeling of helplessness, and in some cases terror, which precedes and accompanies the involuntary eruption of unconscious impulses where the individual has little or no control over his mind and body. He may have delusions about sights and sounds in the dark. He may have repetitive nightmares. He may have hallucinations. *In any case, it is imperative that the culture recognizes his fears as valid; that it identifies and names the sources of them, and provides the means of alleviating them. The quicker the culture intervenes, the less likelihood there will be that an individual's condition will progress into phobias, compulsions and psychogenic symptoms of sickness, all of which, however, can be found in the Talking Rock area.* (Morgan 1936: 6–7)

Not only is there no reference to ghosts in the complete passage, it is not clear that Morgan is even talking about a specific, let alone single, idiom or disorder.

There are problems in the other literature used to construct ghost sickness as well. Fathauer (1951) talked very generally of 'ghost sickness' among the Mohave, suggesting that the illness could result from 'violating the funeral taboos or dreaming of dead relatives or friends' (605). 'People afflicted with the ghost sickness were afraid of darkness, experienced nightmares, were unable to sleep at night, and cried for long periods of time,' he wrote (605). Individuals dreaming of their dead relatives could also become insane. But he added that the shaman could *produce* these same symptoms by witchcraft. He further suggested that symptoms of ghost sickness and another disorder, 'enemy sickness,' were essentially the same, leading him to speculate that these two might be different aspects of the same problem. No case material was presented.

Morris Opler provided some of the best detail on ghost sickness, but even this was scant. He described the Apache peoples as having 'a terror of ghosts and, indeed, of anything associated with death' (1945: 123) and, like Fathauer, argued that shamans could cause the disorder as well as treat it (Opler & Bittle 1961). However, he also noted a 'tendency to explain *anything* frightening or obscure in terms of ghosts' (Opler 1945: 133–4; emphasis added), including 'anything eerie or inexplicable, or hysterical seizures and evidences of extreme terror' (133), thereby casting considerable doubt on the specificity of ghost sickness as a singular syndrome. Opler frequently noted that ghosts, often of deceased relatives, sometimes came back and caused illness or otherwise bothered the living, but he offered little detail with respect to what this illness was or looked like. The idea that spirits can cause illness is explained to all first-year anthropology students as a belief common to peoples the world over. That the Mohave, Navajo, or anyone else would have a name for the problems caused by ghosts should not be particularly noteworthy. Opler also noted that the onset of the disorder characteristically followed the death of a friend, leading to depression in a surviver who then dreamed of the deceased or of his or her own death. If the symptoms remained depression and bad dreams, common remedies for dealing with ghosts were employed. But more serious cases might involve 'hysteria, insanity, or paralysis, particularly facial paralysis' (Opler & Bittle 1961: 392). Paralysis and a racing heart caused by fright when encountering a ghost could also be a symptom (Opler 1946). Opler (1936: 94; 1946: 464) even suggested that the Mecalero Apache preferred to call the disorder 'darkness sickness,' or 'owl sickness,' in part because they simply did not like to talk about ghosts, even in the abstract. The three terms, taken together, explained 'illness attributable to persecution by the ghosts of the dead' (1936: 94). No real case examples were presented, and Opler offered only anecdotal comments of group members recalling incidents. This is compatible with research on White Mountain Apache healing rituals published several decades later by Everett (1970), who uncovered only one ritual of fifty-one that even pertained to ghosts.

Trimble et al. (1984: 210) cited several sources in suggesting that ghost sickness was characteristic of several other groups. They noted that Fathauer (1951) described ghost sickness among the Mohave as a 'slight variant' of the Mohave notion of soul loss, adding that in ghost sickness the individual found him- or herself in close proximity to the deceased, who take the form of owls. They also cited Bryce Boyer (1964a, 1964b) to corroborate the earlier work by Opler. Boyer under-took research with the Mescalero Apache in the late 1950s, and he described their belief in witches and malevolent ghosts that could 'frighten or inconvenience the living, ultimately to drive them crazy,' possibly leading to suicide or a foolish death (Boyer 1964a: 401). 'Ghosts affect people with great fear and create psychic disturbances,' he noted (401). Is this reported belief indicative of a mental disorder? Boyer seemed to think so. Applying a psychoanalytic framework, he offered: 'It is my opinion that belief in a religion which involves the concept of diffuse supernatural power and the retention of infantile notions of animation of the inanimate, requires relatively indiscriminate projection of infantile omnipotence onto surroundings, conditions which are consistent with confusion of ego boundaries. People who retain such defects of ego growth are subject to the development of character disorders and psychoses' (Boyer 1964b: 247). But he was speaking very generally here about beliefs in the spiritual, a weak basis upon which to construct a culture-bound syndrome.

Perhaps the most influential article published on this disorder was by Bert Kaplan and Dale Johnson (1964), based on three years of research among the Navajo. According to these authors, this 'mental illness' was 'closely associated with the influence of evil power and witches.' Further, 'what is apparently supposed to happen to the victim of witching or a ghost is that the witch's power or the ghost itself comes into the victim and takes over, either causing him to behave in strange ways or to weaken, sicken, or have troubling thoughts' (214). 'It is a clear case of possession,' they added, 'although this term is not used directly.' In addition to symptoms that included 'a great many of the physical illnesses known to Western medicine,' which they did not define, the following symptoms were noted: 'weakness, bad dreams, feelings of danger, confusion, feelings of futility, loss of appetite, feelings of suffocation, fainting, dizziness, fear' (212). This is a very broad range of symptoms, perhaps because ghost sickness is in fact neither a single disorder, as Everett's (1970) research suggests, if it is one at all in the Western sense, nor bound to any specific culture. Kaplan and Johnson (1964) presented three cases in their discussion, two of which involved individuals preoccupied with thoughts of deceased family members, but only one of which included the idea of being harassed in some way by a relative's ghost. The third case involved the use of 'love-magic.' So only one of the three cases involved a ghost, only one involved witches, and one seemed to have nothing to do with either. We are limited, of course, by the data provided by Kaplan and Johnson, but these are the cases presented by them to support the idea that the malady 'ghost sickness' existed.

Does 'ghost sickness' really exist as a culture-bound syndrome? The evidence is certaintly not compelling. To begin with, there is little case material, normally expected by psychiatrists when considering the potential of a new disorder. It is quite possible that some authors confused witchcraft and ghost sickness, two somewhat different problems. And clearly ghost sickness, or something that looks very much like it, is reported in the literature for many other Aboriginal groups and, as we shall see in a later chapter, around the world. The ambiguities surrounding this so-called culture-bound syndrome are best exemplified in Putsch's (1988) assertion that what he calls 'ghost illness' was a culture-bound syndrome characteristic of the Navajo, the Coast Salish and, perhaps even more surprisingly, the Hmong![4]

Why the Culture-Bound Syndromes Persist

The European construction of culture-bound syndromes such as windigo psychosis, *pibloktoq*, and ghost sickness is beyond dispute. Boag (1970) showed great insight when he questioned the contemporary usefulness of the idea of *pibloktoq*, and we should extend this concern to the other two 'syndromes' well. These culture-bound syndromes have existed in an ahistorical, synchronic, and exoticized past (H.B.M. Murphy 1973; Littlewood & Lipsedge 1985; Littlewood 2000). Saindon's (1933) informants in the early part of the twentieth century suggested that windigo 'sickness' was already rare. However, separate from the question of whether or not they existed in the past, the psychiatric literature continues to foment the idea that these are current and significant psychopathologies affecting Aboriginal peoples. In a recent review article on American Indian and Alaska Native mental health care, for instance, Manson (2000: 618) deferred uncritically to DSM-IV's listing of American Indian culture-bound syndromes, describing them as *'frequently* encountered idioms of distress' (emphasis added). Both remarkable and exotic, the culture-bound syndromes described here were magnets for Europeans of all backgrounds. As Marano (1985) so eloquently demonstrated in his deconstruction of windigo psychosis, the lack of real evidence of actual psychoses, as opposed to folklore, the genesis of emic/etic confusion, did not stand in the way of the development of some truly alien, even gruesome, psychiatric syndromes. What is remarkable is how these syndromes have persisted through time as medical 'facts,' despite the comprehensive work of scholars like Marano (1985) and Dick (1995).

The psychiatric community's acceptance of culture-bound syndromes is clearly acknowledged by their inclusion in DSM. While windigo psychosis never made it into the manual, *pibloktoq* and ghost sickness appeared as culture-bound syndromes in the 1987 third revision (DSM-III-R), when culture was first addressed (American Psychiatric Association 1987). *Pibloktoq* and ghost sickness can still be found in the most recent edition, DSM-IV-TR (American Psychiatric Association 2000); their descriptions demonstrate very little change since, and not even a shadow of a doubt is cast concerning their validity.[5] Further, their inclusion in DSM suggests that the psychiatrist in the new millenium could conceivably encounter a patient suffering from such a disorder! Both *pibloktoq* and ghost sickness are presented in the same psychiatric language used to describe other disorders in the manual, bestowing contemporary legitimacy on their existence. *Pibloktoq* is defined as follows: 'An abrupt dissociative episode accompanied by extreme excitement of up to 30 minutes' duration and frequently followed by convulsive seizures and coma lasting up to 12 hours. This is observed primarily in arctic and subarctic Eskimo communities, although regional variations in name exist. The individual may be withdrawn or mildly irritable for a period of hours or days before the attack and will typically report complete amnesia for the attack. During the attack, the individual may tear off his or her clothing, break furniture, shout obscenities, eat feces, flee from protective shelters, or perform other irrational or dangerous acts' (American Psychiatric Association 2000: 901). Ghost sickness is defined as: 'A preoccupation with death and the deceased (sometimes associated with witchcraft) frequently observed among members of many American Indian tribes. Various symptoms can be attributed to ghost sickness, including bad dreams, weakness, feelings of danger, loss of appetite, fainting, dizziness, fear, anxiety, hallucinations, loss of consciousness, confusion, feelings of futility, and a sense of suffocation' (American Psychiatric Association 2000: 900).[6] These entries, in an appendix that Kirmayer and Minas (2000: 439) justifiably referred to as a colonialists 'museum of exotica,' were included despite the fact that many leading scientists have openly questioned not only their existence as specific syndromes or disorders, but also the whole notion of culture-bound syndromes (Hughes 1985; Hahn 1995).

Although windigo psychosis is not in DSM-IV-TR, it has not disappeared altogether, and frequently resurfaces along with other contemporary discussions of the culture-bound syndromes. Prince (1993), for instance, while admitting to having never encountered a case of a culture-bound syndrome in ten years of psychiatric work among the James Bay Cree, surprisingly cited Marano (1982) as an authority on the existence of windigo psychosis to *support* his clinical interpretation of a Cree psychiatric case. J.W. Thompson, Walker, and Silk-Walker (1993), in a volume aimed at training clinicians about the role of culture in mental illness and treatment, described both *pibloktoq* and windigo psychosis, citing Marano's work but deferring to earlier work by Shore and Manson (1981) and Trimble et al. (1984), which suggested the existence of these disorders. Konner (1995), in a chapter on 'Anthropology and Psychiatry,' presented a description of windigo psychosis, along with *pibloktoq*, in a popular psychiatry textbook, even though he noted that the existence of windigo (but not *pibloktoq*) was in dispute. In the same edited volume, Mezzich and Lin (1995), the former a leading scholar in cultural psychiatry who helped shape the DSM IV's cultural formulation, mentioned both ghost sickness and *pibloktoq*. The editors of the volume in question, Kaplan and Sadock, have also authored several other recent psychiatry textbooks which included descriptions of both *pibloktoq* and 'wihtigo' (Kaplan & Sadock 1996, 1997, 2000). 'The growing sophistication and cultural sensitivity of modern psychiatry has led to renewed interest' in culture-bound syndromes, suggested Levine and Gaw (1995: 523), who cited both *pibloktoq* and ghost sickness, the former as a culture-bound syndrome, the latter as an 'illness of attribution' and both as 'neither rare nor unusual ... in their respective cultures' (534). Other recent psychiatry texts likewise contain uncritical references to *pibloktoq* and windigo (Sutker & Adams 1993; Tasman, Kay, & Lieberman 1997; Puri, Laking, & Treasaden 2002). Psychiatrists are not alone in perpetuating the concept of culture-based syndromes, however. In a recent volume linking 'psychiatric observation' and 'anthropological understanding,' Martínez-Hernáez (2000), who was trained in both anthropology and psychiatry, listed *pibloktoq* and 'wiitiko' as culture-bound syndromes without further comment. Helman (2000: 186), in the fourth edition of a very popular medical anthropology textbook, also listed windigo, 'a compulsive desire to eat human flesh among the Algonkian-speaking Indians of central and north-eastern Canada,' as a culture-bound syndrome. Likewise, Spector (2000), in the fifth edition of her popular cross-cultural health text, presented *pibloktoq* and ghost sickness.

Assertions by influential scholars inevitably fuel subsequent discussions and constitute the scientific expertise to which others unquestioningly appeal for authority. For instance, Alarcón et al. (1998), in a volume entitled *Personality Disorders and Culture*, cited Kaplan and Sadock in their uncritical discussion of windigo psychosis and *pibloktoq*. Windigo psychosis, they suggested, 'is *particularly common* among North American Native Americans' (Alarcón et al. 1998: 198; emphasis added). In a volume emanating from a conference designed to provide expert advice to the editors of a revised DSM-III-R (i.e., DSM-IV), and published by the American Psychiatric Press (a company connected to the American Psychiatric Association, who also publish the DSM), *pibloktoq* was referred to in current psychiatric parlance as a 'dissociative syndrome'with a '*documented* prodromal period that may last several days and that is characterized by feelings of lethargy, depression, and anxiety' (Gonzalez & Griffith 1996: 140; emphasis added) (see also Hughes, Simons, & Wintrob 1997). *Pibloktoq* also appeared in a recent psychiatric textbook published by the American Psychiatric Press (Hales, Yudofsky, & Talbott 1999).

Other, more broadly based medical reference sources have similarly included largely uncritical discussions of culture-bound syndromes. The sixteenth edition of the venerable *Merck Manual of Diagnosis and Therapy* (Berkow & Fletcher 1992: 2595), in a section on 'Cross-Cultural Issues in Medicine,' contained a generalized discussion of 'spirit disease' as a 'disorder of the soul or spirit' which was believed to be quite common among several groups, including 'native North Americans'; this could be caused by the intrusion of a ghost into the body, the loss of the soul, or retribution for broken taboos.[7] The tenth edition of the International Classification of Mental and Behavioural Disorders, published by the World Health Organization, provided descriptions of both *pibloktoq* and windigo, including suggested International Classification of Diseases codes for categorizing the disorders. While the manual noted that the existence of windigo was contentious, it nevertheless suggested, 'if a code is needed, use ... Other specified disorders of adult personality and behaviour' (WHO 1993: 186).

Information on disorders such as windigo psychosis and *pibloktoq* can also be found on the Internet. Entering any of these terms into an Internet search engine results in dozens of 'hits.' Mosaic Minds, for instance, an organization formed by 'dissociative survivors of childhood trauma,' maintains a website in which *pibloktoq* is listed as a 'dissociative trance disorder' (citing DSM-IV as the source) (*www.mosaicminds.org/rroom/diag_crit.html*; accessed 9 April 2003). Another site (*www.parkpub. com*; accessed 9 April 2003),[8] designed as a 'search engine for medical professionals of over 500 *current* medical questions and answers in 20 different categories,' in a section called 'Clinical Q and A: Answers to clinical questions that come up in *day-to-day* medical practice' (emphases added), provided the following answer by a psychiatrist to a question about the existence of Arctic hysteria: 'Culture-bound syndromes really do exist. Not only do they have explanations and labels which are culturally unique, they are so bound up with their cultural meaning that they can not exist outside of their particular cultural framework. Windigo is found in Algonkian Indians and involves a fear of becoming a cannibal by being possessed by the mythic Windigo. Arctic hysteria or Pibloktoq, found in the Inuit of northern Greenland, involves wild excitement ending in seizures, stuporous sleep and amnesia.' A website linked to the University of California at San Diego also identified windigo psychosis, *pibloktoq*, and ghost sickness as culture-bound syndromes without commenting on their controversial nature. The site's discussion of Marano's work on windigo, for example, failed to note that Marano questioned the very existence of a psychosis (*www.weber. ucsd.edu/~thall/cbs_glos.html*; accessed 9 April 2003).

Lucas and Barrett (1995) have described how the culture-bound syndrome known as 'amok,' the murderous rampage first described in the Malay archipelago, has been absorbed by the West such that the term is now commonly used here with essentially the same meaning. The notion of windigo psychosis has also recently entered Western popular culture, in part as a metaphor for Western consumption, an idea put forward by American Indian scholar Jack Forbes, among others (Forbes 1992; see also Root 1996). Windigo, in the persona of 'Wendigo,' has even been transformed into a misunderstood superhero of sorts in the Spider-Man comic book series.[9]

It should not come as a surprise that the three culture-bound syndromes most commonly said to afflict Aboriginal North Americans are characterized by forms of fear, anxiety, and hysteria. Anthropologist Lewis Langness (1976: 56), for instance, referred to both windigo psychosis and *pibloktoq* as 'hysterical psychoses,' and grouped them with a variety of other culture-bound syndromes from around the world, such as *latah*, *amok*, and *koro*. In the influential compendium by Simons and Hughes (1985), windigo psychosis was exoticized as a member of the 'cannibal compulsion taxon,' while *pibloqtoq* represented the 'running' taxon. Windigo in particular fits well with earlier historic images of North American Indians as wildmen and 'monstrous races' (Jahoda 1999: 24), an Enlightenment-inspired idea that half-human, half-animal beings inhabited the far reaches of the globe (Barnard 2000). What could be more monstrous than a cannibal giant with a heart of ice, except perhaps a family member turning into one! The link between contemporary psychiatric and older anthropological views of the nature of these cultures is clear: early anthropologists and psychoanalysts viewed Aboriginal peoples as inherently superstitious, irrational, childlike, and anxious; psychologists and psychiatrists, it seems, accepted these essentialisms when it came time to pathologize indigenous knowledge and beliefs.

It should also come as no surprise to the reader at this stage in the volume to learn that the culture-bound syndromes outlined in DSM IV-TR do not generally encompass afflictions of white, middle-class northerners in the United States. Therefore, Rogler's (1996: 148) assertion that the DSM presents culture-bound disorders 'not as alien exotic disorders but as part of the cultural landscape, including modern industrial societies'[10] is difficult to support. Indeed, the references to groups within the United States refer specifically to Latinos, groups in the 'southern' United States, and recent immigrants such as Greeks. How exotic! It is as if culture shapes affliction only in other cultures. While it is true that DSM is primarily a North American product, and we might graciously accept that the 'average' American is the normative standard to which all others are compared, the fact remains that DSM has been presented as a globally appropriate system of classification of mental disorders.[11] The colonial roots of both North American society and the DSM persist in the guise of the culture-bound syndromes, a form of primitivist medicalization. And, assuming for arguments sake that windigo psychosis, *pibloktoq*, and ghost sickness were real mental disorders, even the most generous literature suggests that they were extremely rare in the past, and are likely more so today. Why, then, do DSM and psychiatry textbooks bother to discuss them at all? Is there really much of a likelihood that a North American psychiatrist will encounter an Inuk with *pibloktoq*, or a Cree with windigo psychosis? The fact that, separate from the question of their existence, these pathologies exist as *syndromes* within DSM, rather than as concrete *disorders*, affirms their status as exotic cultural legacies which continue to confound as they titillate psychiatry.[12]

Some researchers have apparently grown quite uncomfortable with the notion of culture-bound syndromes, and have begun using the term 'idioms of distress' in its place, at least for certain syndromes (e.g., Levine & Gaw 1995; Manson 1997). DSM-IV speaks of both culture-bound syndromes and idioms of distress without explaining how, if at all, these are different. Idioms of distress, according to Nichter (1981), represent localized expressions of distress, be they psychiatric or somatic. He posits the existence of multiple idioms within given societies, and the existence of cultural change in their expression, rather than the single, culturally bounded, spatially and temporally fixed syndromes that the DSM-IV glossary presents. Thus, when Jilek and Jilek-Aall (1985) defined contemporary Coast Salish spirit dancing as a culture-bound syndrome that was in fact a reaction to fairly recent socio-political problems, including alcoholism and the effects of the historic suppression of the ceremony, they were allowing for a more dynamic understanding. Spirit dancing in the 1980s was not what it was in the past, it had changed and adapted. Tellingly, spirit dancing never seemed to make it into discussion of culture-bound syndromes in Aboriginal North America.

I am not arguing here against the proposition that cultures shape forms of mental illness. My concern lies in part with the problem of defining certain syndromes as *bounded* in any meaningful way, both spatially and temporally. While DSM-IV-TR (American Psychiatric Association 2000: xxxi) in general emphasized that any given category of mental disorder should not be seen as 'a completely discrete entity with absolute boundaries dividing it from other mental disorders,' the manual lapsed when considering the consequences of suggesting the existence of indigenous syndromes that can be culturally bounded. For two of the culture-bound syndromes discussed here, windigo psychosis and *pibloktoq*, there is compelling evidence of their construction by

Europeans, that the behaviour they purport to describe was, to be generous, quite rare, and that they may never have existed within the cultures themselves either as indigenously recognized mental disorders or as any other realistic phenomenon. Ghost sickness was ascribed to many different Aboriginal societies without attention to the question of cultural boundedness. While DSM has argued that culture-bound syndromes can be attributed to both singular and grouped cultures (employing the 'culture area' concept), no attention was paid to the need to identify these entities as meaningful cultures in the first place. The notion of ghost sickness as a culture-bound syndrome, then, is predicated on the shaky foundation that the many Aboriginal cultures in which a variant of it is found represent a singular cultural formation, or at least are closely related in the cultural sense to allow for boundedness. Several decades ago, Arctic researcher and anthropologist Frank Vallee (1968) warned against the temptation to 'overdescribe' a single form of illness such that it becomes the 'classical' form for that cultural group. Apparently no one was listening.

Why have these culture-bound syndromes persisted in light of the fundamental problems addressed in this chapter? Why do they still appear, uncritically, in standard works of psychiatry, psychology, and medical anthropology, even in the new millennium? I believe that there are two explanations. The first, regrettably, relates to shoddy research on the part of those who have written these texts and created the websites. This is not finger-pointing, for the problem lies not so much with individuals as with the exigencies of scholarly publishing. While within the scientific intellectual tradition it is expected that new knowledge will be built upon the foundation of the old, critical assessments of older knowledge are relatively rare, particularly in the social sciences. Reports of explorers and traders, and published research findings, are rarely scrutinized for methodological or conceptual problems. These culture-bound syndromes continue to exist because scholars continue to write that they do, building successively on earlier works making the same assertions. Critical studies, such as those by Marano and Dick, are not noticed by those who frame the DSM and write the textbooks. Perhaps it is unfair to expect authors to undertake extensive research into concepts which, frequently, simply appear in other published lists of culture-bound syndromes. But the consequence of this is that primitivist ideas continue to be nourished.

The second reason for the persistence of windigo, *pibloktoq*, and ghost sickness pertains to the broader theme of this book. These syndromes are intensely, voyeuristically exotic. An ongoing fascination with things 'primitive' insidiously permeates the culture-bound syndrome discourse, culminating in a belief that these disorders must, by definition, be characteristic of these cultural others. Exotic conditions are what 'primitives' have, and for many there is no reason to think otherwise. Despite the warning offered by Trimble et al. (1984: 210) that these disorders did not necessarily pertain to contemporary Aboriginal societies, an alarming lack of attention has been paid to contemporary cultural contexts. Apparently the 'primitive's' past is also his or her present. These syndromes thus appear in the literature to be pertinent to Aboriginal peoples today in a way as equally meaningful as depression, alcoholism, or schizophrenia. The literature seriously suggests that a mental health practitioner has a reasonable likelihood of encountering the hoary face and icy heart of a Cree windigo, in his or her very office, next week!

Conclusion

The three culture-bound syndromes I have examined, windigo psychosis, *pibloktoq*, and ghost sickness, stand as unparalleled examples of wayward psychiatric mythologizing, the construction of new disorders on the tangled ruins of folklore, errant historical documents, and naive scholarship. While there might well be something real buried underneath, the story told here is not so much of the existence or nonexistence of these disorders, but rather the tenacity with which their supposed existence and persistence, and even widespread applicability, has been embraced by scholars. Like Frankenstein's monster, having been given life by the good doctors, they are proving difficult to dispatch.

CHAPTER NINE

The Traumatized Aboriginal

The world has not acknowledged the Holocaust of native people in this hemisphere. (Duran & Duran 1995: 30)

This chapter examines one of the most significant disorders du jour, post-traumatic stress disorder (PTSD). In recent years the notions of trauma and PTSD have entered the Aboriginal mental health discourse, and as these concepts have been applied, appeals to culture, and to history in particular, have given them a somewhat unique Aboriginal flavour. The existence of two differing understandings of trauma is evident. One focuses on the individual and is diagnosable as a disorder within the criteria set out in the DSM; the other exists metaphorically within the popular realm and conceives of whole communities and even cultures as being affected. There has also been a tendency to assume that Aboriginal peoples have been and continue to be severely traumatized even when available data suggests the contrary, and, not surprisingly, given my discussion up to this point, little attention has been paid to existing social and cultural mechanisms for coping with difficult circumstances. After briefly describing PTSD and some of the pertinent issues surrounding its construction and implementation as a psychiatric diagnosis, I will turn to how it has been employed in the attempt to understand current psychopathology among Aboriginal peoples, ultimately arriving at a newly emerging construct known as 'Residential School Syndrome.'

Conceptualizing Trauma and PTSD

The history of the development of PTSD has been well-documented and I will not recount it in any real detail here (see Young 1995; Kutchins & Kirk 1997; Leys 2000). While the precursors to PTSD, such as 'shell shock,' have existed for some time, as anthropologist Alan Young (1995) has demonstrated, the disorder now known as PTSD is a relatively recent construct. Developing out of the Vietnam war experience of soldiers exposed to a variety of battle-related traumas, it has subsequently been extended by others (e.g., Herman 1992) to encompass a wide variety of stressful human experiences. PTSD was first recognized in 1980 and entered the DSM in the third revision. DSM-IV-TR (American Psychiatric Association 2000: 463) described PTSD as follows:

> The essential feature of Posttraumatic Stress Disorder is the development of characteristic symptoms following exposure to an extreme traumatic stressor involving direct personal experience of an event that involves actual or threatened death or serious injury, or other threat to one's physical integrity; or witnessing an event that involves death, injury, or a threat to the physical integrity of another person; or learning about unexpected or violent death, serious harm, or threat of death or injury experienced by a family member or other close associate ... The person's response to the event must involve intense fear, helplessness, or horror (or in children, the response must involve disorganized or agitated behavior) ... The characteristic symptoms resulting from the exposure to the extreme trauma include persistent reexperiencing of the traumatic event ... persistent avoidance of stimuli associated with the trauma and numbing of general responsiveness ... and persistent symptoms of increased arousal ... The full symptom picture must be present for more than 1 month ... and the disturbance must cause clinically significant distress or impairment in social, occupational, or other important areas of functioning ...

Examples of traumatic events that can precipitate PTSD include combat, violent personal assault (including sexual assault), kidnapping, terrorist attack, torture, natural disasters, accidents, and even life-threatening illness. The trauma need not be experienced directly: the witnessing of traumatic events or being given news of traumatic events, such as the death of a family member, can also precipitate PTSD. Kirmayer (1996a) has suggested that the trauma may consist not of a single, terrorizing incident but rather a series of lesser stresses or incidents. Precisely what constitutes a traumatic event varies from individual to individual and community to community. In previous editions, the DSM stated that the traumatic event had to be outside 'normal' experience, but the ambiguity and bias inherent in this criteria was soundly criticized, leading to its omission in DSM-IV. The lifetime prevalence for PTSD was estimated to be 8 per cent of the adult population in the United States (American Psychiatric Association 2000: 466).

It is clear that DSM focuses in one way or another on *individual* experience, with the individual body as the locus of distress; the 'social body' and the 'body politic' play no meaningful role within the psychiatric conceptualization of the disorder (cf. Lock & Scheper-Hughes 1996). There has been no attempt to comprehend the historical dimensions of trauma or the existence of community trauma, other than as directly experienced by the individual. The one possible exception would be the formulation of the concept of intergenerational or multigenerational trauma (Danieli 1998), which posits the possibility of generating a family legacy in which the experiences and reactions of one individual are transmitted to his or her children or significant others, with the potential for emotional and behavioural consequences to reshape individuals in subsequent generations. Although history must enter into the formulation, at least for purposes of diagnosis, the unit of treatment invariably remains at the level of the individual. However, DSM-IV-TR (American Psychiatric Association 2000: 466–7) acknowledged for the first time the existence of 'a heritable component to the transmission of Posttraumatic Stress Disorder,' adding that 'a history of depression in first-degree relatives has been related to an increased vulnerability to developing Posttraumatic Stress Disorder.' This idea was not developed further, however.

Arthur Kleinman (1995: 179–80), a psychiatrist/anthropologist, has argued that the DSM individualizes what is essentially a social matter, that is, the experience of collective violence, and medicalizes the commonplace human experience of suffering. In his words, PTSD represents 'a colonization of the lifeworld by professional discourse' (1995: 181). Suffering, as a normal reaction to trauma, has been 'refigured, for policy and intervention programs, as psychological and medical pathologies' (177). The entire responsibility for this medicalization cannot be laid at the feet of the DSM and those who have framed it, however, for the manual has been constructed and revised in response to social and political movements and even outright lobbying by special interest groups.[1] Furthermore, individuals who have experienced trauma have sometimes campaigned to have their experience formally recognized as a medical condition; this is precisely what happened in the original formulation, as Vietnam war veterans advocated to have their suffering acknowledged, in part, so they could receive treatment.

PTSD thus exists as an important marker of mental illness which allows the individual to attain treatment (Kleinman 1995; Kutchins & Kirk 1997). But central to this process is the concept of memory: the trauma allegedly exists in the past (and there is concern that some memories of trauma are false), but is interpreted in the present. Antze and Lambek (1996: vii) have argued that 'memories are never simply records of the past, but are interpretive reconstructions that bear the imprint of local narrative conventions, cultural assumptions, discursive formations and practices, and social contexts of recall and commemoration.' Kirmayer (1996b: 189) has written that 'There is a crucial distinction between the social space in which the trauma occurred and the contemporary space in which it is (or is not) recalled.' And the individual also has some agency here, at least in laying claim to the traumatic event and even the diagnosis. As Young (1996: 97–8) has suggested, 'individuals rediscover and rework their memories of past events as a means of accounting for their present distress ... Individuals "choose" PTSD for this purpose, to reorganize their life-worlds, because it is a widely known and ready-made construct, it is sanctioned by the highest medical authority, it is said to originate in external circumstances rather than personal flaws or weakness, and (in some situations) it earns compensation.' In this sense, acts of remembering are political – 'indictments or confessions, or ... emblems of a victimized identity,' according to Antze and Lambek (1996: vii) – perhaps even economic. There is a performative aspect as well, in which the individual or group demonstrate both the pathology and victimized outrage at the experience, all for the consuming audience. As such, memory is also inherently contestable: not all individuals 'at risk' will confirm the trauma, admit to having experienced it, or admit to suffering because of it, and because much of the trauma discourse is about laying blame, the alleged perpetrators frequently act to silence the victims, to deny the event, or to recast the trauma in terms that deflect attention, blame, and liability from themselves. At the very least, individualizing trauma reduces the potential for legal liability, since collective trauma is frequently seen as the consequence of organized, conspiratorial action, whereas individual trauma is more readily personalized as individual weakness.

Trauma and Aboriginal Peoples

The introduction of the concepts of trauma and PTSD into the Aboriginal mental health discourse is at once exciting, innovative, and troubling. All of the issues and tensions discussed above emerge when we look at the discourse of trauma and PTSD among the North American Aboriginal population. As Manson et al. (1996) have suggested, PTSD has clearly been conceptualized differently for American Indians and Alaska Natives. It has become ubiquitous and pervasive: 'Trauma and its consequence for individuals, families, and communities,' they have stated, 'shadows the daily lives of American Indians and Alaska Natives' (1996: 255). Trauma, then, is quotidian, lived experience and not simply the intrusion of traumatic memory representative of past events. They offered evidence which encompasses both individual experience and historic memory: high suicide rates, sexual abuse by teachers, the disruption caused by the Exxon Valdez oil spill, widespread alcohol abuse and violence, life-threatening illness, and the unrecognized experiences of Indian Vietnam veterans. Indian people also harbour 'a deeply ingrained sense of oppression spanning several centuries and the repeated violation of presumably ironclad agreements [i.e., treaties] that displaced this special population from ancestral lands' (256). As the concept of PTSD emerged, Indian peoples latched on to it 'as an idiom or metaphor for the consequences of the enormous social and psychological burdens under which they labor' (256). However, while this is an important point, vernacular expressions of trauma are not the same thing as empirically based psychiatric diagnoses of PTSD.

Overall, while trauma discourse has become increasingly popular, there has been little research on the prevalence of Aboriginal trauma and PTSD, and the findings so far have not been at all consistent. While some have discovered relatively high rates of PTSD, many others have been troubled by apparently low rates. High rates were found in a prevalence study of 247 adults from an unnamed southwestern tribe by Robin, Chester, Rasmussen, Jaranson, and Goldman (1997a), who utilized a psychiatric interview and the Traumatic Events Booklet (derived from DSM-III-R) to investigate the relationship between both the frequency and type of traumatic events experienced and the prevalence of PTSD. The booklet details a variety of specific events, such as combat, accidents, fire, natural disaster, assault, witnessing death, and so on, and the subject is asked to respond with a simple yes or no to the question of whether they have experienced these events. The results indicated a lifetime PTSD prevalence of 21.9 per cent and a point prevalence of 5.7 per cent; the median number of traumatic events for those with lifetime prevalence was twenty-three, and only two for those without lifetime prevalence. The most frequently reported traumatic events were automobile accidents and receiving news of trauma afflicting a loved one (such as their violent death), but physical assault also proved common for women. Military combat clearly represents a qualitatively different trauma experience, and virtually all of the men who had experienced combat had developed PTSD. The authors concluded that the prevalence rates of PTSD were considerably higher among this population than for non-Indian populations generally, and were on par with rates found in populations which had undergone extreme stress, such as survivors of mass shootings or combat. Furthermore, they determined that the risk of developing PTSD was greater for individuals with a history of multiple traumatic events.

In a related study of 'intimate violence,' Robin, Chester, and Rasmussen (1998) (see also Robin, Chester, Rasmussen, Jaranson, & Goldman 1997b) determined that both men and women reported high rates of lifetime intimate violence (91 per cent) and recent (within twelve months) violence (31 per cent), yet their data demonstrated no statistical relationship between intimate violence and PTSD or other psychiatric disorders. We also find in this work a reluctance to accept the low rates of PTSD, especially in the face of reports of high exposure to traumatic events. This is perhaps due in part to a conceptual flaw, that is, the confusion of reports of events that researchers or even community members would say are 'traumatic' and the notion of 'trauma' as a psychiatric disorder. Indeed, Robin et al. (1998) admitted that intimate violence could be common enough to make it inconsequential, or at least not unusual, from the perspective of reporting it as trauma. But they also suggested that other forms of interpersonal violence, such as child sexual abuse, rape, homicide, and suicide, could also be so common as to obscure the relationship between intimate violence and psychiatric disorder.

The apparent existence of low rates of PTSD has without question perplexed many researchers. Manson et al. (1996) detailed several research projects that looked at trauma and PTSD, and in which this issue clearly emerged: a health survey of Indian boarding school students; the Flower of Two Soils Reinterview project; a project with Indian teens; and work with American Indian Vietnam veterans. The 1988 boarding school survey, employing the Diagnostic Interview Schedule for Children (DISC-02.1C) and its PTSD module, was designed to determine the prevalence and incidence of several disorders, including depression, anxiety, and suicidal behaviour (see King, Beals, Manson, &

Trimble 1992; Dick, Manson, & Beals 1993). The majority of the sixty-one students interviewed about their mental health status were from 'five local, culturally similar tribes' in the southeastern United States; once again, specific tribal identities were not disclosed. Conduct disorder (18 per cent), alcohol dependence (18 per cent), and major depression (15 per cent) were the most common diagnoses, and some 25 per cent had made a suicide attempt in the past. No data on the prevalence of PTSD was offered, however. The Flower of Two Soils restudy project (in 1991) was designed to examine the relationship between school dropout and risk of emotional disorder in four 'culturally distinct reservation communities in the United States and Canada' (Manson et al. 1996: 258). This study included 109 children from a Northern Plains reservation who were interviewed with the DISC-2.1C and PTSD module (see Sack, Beiser, Clarke, & Redshirt 1987; Sack, Beiser, Baker-Brown, & Redshirt 1994). Overall, 43 per cent were given a DISC diagnosis of at least one major disorder, with disruptive behaviour disorders (22 per cent), sub-stance abuse disorders (18.4 per cent), and anxiety disorder (17.4 per cent) leading the way. Yet only 5 per cent were diagnosed with post-traumatic stress disorders. The Foundations of Indian Teens project focused more on trauma than had the previous two (see Manson, Shore, & Bloom 1985; Ackerson, Dick, Manson, & Baron 1990; Manson, Acker-son, Dick, Baron, & Fleming 1990). Utilizing a version of the PTSD inter-view from DSM-III-R, 297 adolescents in an unnamed southwestern Indian community were interviewed. The students were prompted to disclose traumatic events with the following query: 'Have you ever experienced something that is so horrible that it would be very upset-ting to almost anyone?' (259). Examples of such incidents were offered to the subjects, and included feeling threatened, feeling that one might die, and witnessing someone's injury or death. Some 51 per cent of the students reported having experienced at least one such traumatic inci-dent, and of these half endorsed eight or more of a possible seventeen PTSD symptoms. However, only one student fulfilled the necessary cri-teria to be diagnosed with PTSD. In contrast to these relatively low rates of PTSD, while only preliminary data could be offered in the Vietnam veterans project, the authors noted that some 70 per cent of the 600 vet-erans in two communities, one from the southwest and the other from the northern plains, exhibited PTSD.[2]

The pattern of high report of exposure to traumatic events combined with low diagnosis of PTSD was also found in a study of 109 adoles-cents from an unnamed Northern Plains reservation by Jones, Dauphinais, Sack, and Somervell (1997). The method of reporting traumatic events was essentially the same as that employed in the studies above. Overall, 61 per cent reported having witnessed or experienced a traumatic event, and of these some 62 per cent reported more than one event, yet only 3 per cent met the DSM-III-R criteria for a diagnosis of PTSD. Furthermore, the researchers determined that having witnessed or experienced at least one traumatic event bore no relationship to school performance or attendance, both measures of social functioning. Interestingly, in comparing these data with that derived from a Detroit study, an environment the authors characterized as being known for high levels of stress, it was found that only 39 per cent of the Detroit sample reported a lifetime traumatic event, and yet the prevalence rate for PTSD was three times higher in Detroit. The authors offered three possible explanations for the discrepancy between reports of traumatic events and diagnoses of PTSD: in addition to possible problems with the methodology, including the instrument, which 'may have over included stressors not belonging to the DSM definition of the stressor criterion, thus inflating this discrepancy,' they also posited that 'cultural factors may have influenced the way this sample of Indian youth reported symptoms' (170). To wit: 'The cultural environment of this reservation, along with elements of poverty, unpredictability and disruption may, paradoxically, have made the reported stressors less "outside the range of usual human experience" than would be the case in other settings, and therefore less liable to generate symptoms' (171). They also suggested that, because the research subjects were adolescents, they may have been reluctant to report symptoms in a first interview. These are all plausible explanations. The first one comes closest to stating that, perhaps, there was simply less PTSD in this population. But as in many studies, evidence of low rates of PTSD was accompanied by an emphasis on high rates of social pathology which make otherwise traumatic events seem experientially unremarkable. Manson et al. (1996: 262) have suggested that, perhaps, the 'degree of trauma itself is sufficiently greater in many Native communities so that the individual threshold for clinical response has been reset at higher levels as trauma has become more the norm than the exception' (262). Does this mean, then, that they truly exhibit less trauma, or does it mean they are numbed by the ongoing experience? If trauma represents the quotidian existence of these people, it is possible that any single event, or even the cumulative consequences of many events, fails to elicit a psychiatric response. If there is no such response, is there still a problem?

It is hard to escape the feeling that many researchers harbour a firm conviction that there must be extensive PTSD among the Aboriginal population, and that the explanation for under-reporting lies primarily with inappropriate conceptualizations and methods. In the boarding school study, for instance, Manson et al. (1996) suggested that there could be a problem with the types of stressors deemed likely to precipitate PTSD, as comprehended in the DSM-III-R that they were using. 'There are no specific criteria as to what constitutes a sufficient stressor,' they wrote, adding that 'Clinical experience, in fact, demonstrates considerable individual variability in response to a comparable stressor' (261). But, having questioned the appropriateness of the stressors, they also questioned whether there might be a cultural bias in the operationalization of PTSD criteria which explained under-diagnosis despite reports of a high exposure to traumatic events. Reaching for an explanation seemingly based on the old culture and personality studies, they asked, for instance, if the Indian tendency towards 'limited disclosure and stoicism' might mask the presence of psychic numbing, a characteristic symptom of PTSD (262). They also posited that the high rates of various other psychiatric disorders documented for the Indian population might obscure a co-morbid PTSD. And they raised the possibility that use of standardized instruments for American Indians is unreliable.

An adequate explanation for the apparent discrepancy between exposure to traumatic events and prevalence rates of PTSD still eludes us. This discrepancy suggests several possibilities: that these individuals are dealing with the trauma without evidence of psychiatric dysfunction; that they are experiencing and then recovering from PTSD without psychiatric intervention; that they are expressing the consequences of trauma in ways that existing diagnostic procedures miss; or that they are simply not measurably traumatized by the kinds of events DSM anticipates. Speaking of an elevated threshold for trauma-related PTSD clearly suggests the existence of a comparative standard of normative experience against which the Aboriginal population is being measured, an approach which fails to comprehend the inherently cultural nature of life experiences such as personal misfortune and disaster. Only a few studies have considered the possibility that cultural factors, and perhaps cultural history, may explain a different type of reaction to such events, that some Aboriginal individuals may think of apparently traumatic events in entirely different terms, or that these cultures may contain healthy, positive mechanisms for dealing with trauma. Manson (1997), for instance, has pointed out that, among the Navajo, the traditional anxiety caused by being near dead bodies could conceivably lead to heightened trauma resulting from the relatively rare experience of combat or traffic accident. Long (1983), in contrast, in a study of traumatic loss among Crow children which seems, by today's standards, rather insightful, described the importance of the extended family network among the Crow. Due to the deaths of their parents, these children were required to move to the care of non-parents, but these were invariably adults who had in the past assumed parental roles (and who, within Crow kinship terminology, may have been referred to as 'mother' or 'father'). Parental continuity was maintained, mitigating the trauma experienced by the children. Suggestions that culture is indeed important, such as those offered by Manson and Long, underscore the apparent problem of cultural obliteration that appears to result from the use of psychometric measures of trauma.

The assumed relationship between the self-reporting of exposure to allegedly traumatic events, the subjective experience of being traumatized, and the clinical diagnosis of PTSD requires re-examination. Clearly, what constitutes a traumatic event for an individual or community cannot be defined a priori, and the confusion of trauma as an event with trauma as a reaction to an event seems pervasive. Reactions to potentially traumatizing events are shaped by culture, yet cultural analyses of the phenomenon are sorely lacking. It is also crucial to consider that Aboriginal peoples may exhibit low rates of diagnosed PTSD *because* they have low rates of PTSD.

Historic, Cultural, and Collective Trauma

There is another way of looking at trauma, one that seems at odds with the empirical, DSM-based approach discussed earlier. This alternative pays greater attention to history and the expression of different forms of experiencing trauma. Trauma is removed from the level of the individual and becomes embedded in community, in culture, and in history. It becomes something that is shared, taught, and embraced as well as experienced. Continuity with the past is expressed primarily in terms of the intergenerational nature of the trauma, the manner in which it can be passed down through the generations to be successively re-experienced. It is also at this juncture that the issue of memory becomes pertinent, as history becomes contested ground for differing versions of truth.

As noted earlier, in its current form, DSM remains committed to the idea of a single, traumatic event as the catalyst, with an emotional or somatic response commencing soon after. Not all would agree, however. According to Robin, Chester, and Goldman (1996: 246), 'as a diagnostic category, PTSD fails to describe the nature and impact of severe, multiple, repeated, and cumulative aspects of trauma common to many [American Indian] communities.' One of the first to articulate the general notion of cumulative trauma, Judith Lewis Herman (1992) argued that long-term, sustained exposure to terrifying stressors was just as damaging as exposure to single incidents, especially if the stressors involved individuals known to the victim and in a relationship of trust. She proposed the idea of 'complex post-traumatic stress disorder' to describe the effects of this sustained trauma, an idea that has yet to be picked up by the framers of DSM. In my study of Aboriginal men in prison (Waldram 1997), I documented the life histories of many men who experienced this form of trauma and argued that PTSD needed to be reconceptualized in terms of lived experience and not just traumatic memory. Trauma may indeed be the result of a ton of stressful feathers, and it follows that a disabling response to these events may likewise take some time to emerge. In other words, as the traumatic events unfold, so too do the reactions. And because we are talking about a timeline, often years, over which this happens, some individual agency is implied. The individual in combat has few options open to him to alter or reduce the stress, as does the observer of a violent death or the survivor of a plane crash. But an individual who repeatedly experiences traumatic events over longer periods of time is afforded the opportunity to act, to react, to interpret, and to reinterpret.

Emerging parallel to the idea of cumulative and intergenerational PTSD has been the idea of trauma experienced not simply at the individual level but also at the community, and even a cultural, level. One of the first to identify this phenomenon was Kai Erikson (1976), a sociologist who studied the aftermath of a catastrophic flash flood in an Appalachian valley that wiped out several close knit communities and irreparably altered their way of life. He described a 'collective' trauma resulting from the loss of 'communality;' while individual losses were substantial (most saw their homes obliterated), and many experienced symptoms of PTSD after the event, it was the sense of loss with respect to the community and way of life that seemed most traumatizing. The loss of meaningful cultural symbols can also lead to grief and depression. Robin et al. (1996) described the case of an elderly Navajo woman who lapsed into depression when forcibly moved from her home, which had a view of a sacred mountain. The relocation of Aboriginal individuals and communities, a pervasive process on both sides of the border, has often been portrayed as intensely traumatic for those involved (e.g., Loney 1995).

Into this mix we now add history, perhaps the most problematic form of memory. The colonization of North America by Europe remains the most powerful symbolic trigger for the collapse of Aboriginal societies. In a contentious and clearly debatable move, some scholars have likened the violence, disease, and subsequent demographic changes to the Jewish Holocaust of the Second World War (e.g., Thornton 1987; Legters 1988; Braveheart-Jordon & DeBruyn 1995; Duran & Duran 1995; Brave Heart 1998; Brave Heart & DeBruyn 1998; Gray 1998), employing emotionally laden terms like' 'genocide' and 'mass slaughter,' which some might argue do a disservice to the differing histories of Aboriginal peoples, not to mention the Jews. Yet arguments for a North American holocaust continue to be made, clearly a nod to the broadly based view that what the Jewish people experienced set the standard against which all other collective trauma should be measured. Colonialism also provides Aboriginal peoples with a symbolic benchmark (albeit an ambiguous one throughout the continent) to demarcate an Arcadian era of trauma-less harmony from an era characterized by disharmony, terror, and trauma. I have yet to uncover a single discussion of trauma among Aboriginal peoples that suggests the possibility that interpersonal and intergroup conflict, harsh living conditions, and natural disasters *prior* to contact with Europeans could also have been traumatizing, that trauma was not a new phenomenon. Interestingly, some discussions of traditional approaches to healing do imply a continuity with the past, as in Manson's (1996) description of the 'gourd society,' a men's support group for warriors, or the Navajo Enemy Way ceremony, which, Manson, Beals, O'Nell, Piasecki, Bechtold, Keane, and Jones (1996: 275) noted has 'explicitly evolved in response to the trauma experienced by warriors' (see also Silver & Wilson 1988). The existence of ages-old methods for dealing with trauma disproves the idea that Aboriginal trauma is associated only with colonization; that Aboriginals have been dealing with trauma for a very long time is self-evident and provides a possible explanation for the relative lack of current PTSD.

The interplay of history and trauma has been most stridently advanced by Pueblo/Apache psychologist Eduardo Duran and his associates. Duran and Duran (1995), in an influential book provocatively titled, *Native American Postcolonial Psychology*, adopted a framework in which the past was firmly embedded in interpretations of the present and projections for the future. The discourse eschewed the relatively passionless accounting of methods and results characteristic of the prevalence studies described earlier and employed impassioned rhetoric. The book stands, in part, as an indictment of the field of psychology and its role in the promotion of intergenerational trauma: 'The past five hundred years have been devastating to our communities; the effects of this systematic genocide are quickly personalized and pathologized by our profession via the diagnosing and labelling tools designed for this purpose. If the labeling and diagnosing process is to have any historical truth, it should incorporate a diagnostic category that reflects the effects of genocide. Such a diagnosis would be 'acute and/or chronic reaction to colonialism' (Duran & Duran 1995: 6). This work underscores some of the profound contradictions inherent in the reification (fetishization?) of history and memory:[3] it is interesting to see these scholars speak of the existence of an absolute 'truth' on a page opposite one extolling the ideas of Michel Foucault, for instance, and to see the authors condemn DSM while advocating yet another new disorder![4] While Duran and Duran (1995) argued that American Indians continued to be mis-diagnosed in part because of a lack of historical perspective, they also presented us with a singular, reductionist historical perspective which they saw as the 'truth' to be applied to this diagnosis in all circumstances.

Duran and Duran (1995) adopted a 'post-colonial' theoretical framework, according to which the colonizer had come to dominate knowledge about the colonized, including their history. To correct this problem the knowledge of the colonized should be accepted as valid in its own right, and not only in reference to that of the colonizer. Hence, these authors sought to introduce an indigenous understanding of the history of colonization to explain both the degree and extent of trauma within the Aboriginal population and the appropriate methods of treatment. But this proved difficult to do, it seems, without appealing to a European standard, the Jewish Holocaust: 'Many of the Native American people who survived the onslaught were not only physically abused but also psychologically tormented. The level of abuse could have easily provided a workshop on technique even for the most sophisticated diabolical minds in Hitler's regime' (Duran & Duran 1995: 31). In addition to suggesting that American Indians experienced genocide and suffered even worse abuse than the Jews, Duran and

Duran hastened to add that there were two key differences in the experience of Aboriginals and Jews: 'the world has not acknowledged the Holocaust of native people in this hemisphere' (30), and the Indian experience predated the Holocaust by several generations. Severity, primacy, and recognition were the platforms upon which these authors constructed the Indian 'Holocaust' experience.

At the centre of the historical trauma is the concept of a 'soul wound.' Ambiguously synonymous with terms like 'historical trauma,' 'historical legacy,' 'American Indian holocaust,' and 'intergenerational posttraumatic stress disorder,' the soul wound, as described by Duran, Duran, Brave Heart, and Horse-Davis (1998: 341) had existed since Columbus. American Indians had experienced generations of unresolved trauma and grief, including 'disenfranchised grief' that cannot openly be acknowledged or mourned (Brave Heart 1998), and had internalized dysfunctional emotions and behaviour to the point where they had become normative. Intergenerational trauma was the logical consequence of the genocidal policies of the colonists, and the damage was cumulative. Not only do individuals suffer the consequences of trauma inflicted on their parents and grandparents, who may be alcoholics and dysfunctional parents, but they also must deal with trauma being inflicted upon themselves and perhaps even their children. Their soul, their very essence, becomes wounded. Individual symptoms included depression and suicidal ideation, but also included phenomena not immediately recognizable within the DSM formulation: 'guilt and concern about betraying the ancestors for being excluded from the suffering, as well as obligation to share ancestral pain, a sense of being obliged to take care of and being responsible for survivor parents, identification with parental suffering and a compulsion to compensate for the genocidal legacy, persecutory and intrusive Holocaust as well as grandiose fantasies, dreams, images, and a perception of the world as dangerous' (Duran et al. 1998: 342). Borrowing from the work of psychologist John Berry, these authors argued that acculturative stress also contributed to the historical trauma, often leading to symptoms such as 'anxiety, depression, feelings of marginality and alienation, heightened psychosomatic symptoms, and identity confusion' (343). Finally, they added that 'the aftereffects of racism, oppression and genocide' were also pertinent. Ironically, they ultimately transformed this indigenous conception of 'soul wound,' a constellation of history and symptoms, into something looking suspiciously like a DSM category, that is, 'chronic and acute reactions to colonialism' (346).

Duran et al. (1998) outlined a schema for the history of colonization as a means of explaining the development of this historical trauma.[5] They suggested that at 'first contact' there was 'a total environmental and lifeworld shock' as the 'lifeworld of Native people was systematically destroyed through genocidal military actions' (343). Several subsequent historical processes, such as subjugation and confinement to reservations, forced relocation, and termination, then served to exacerbate the situation. It is essential, they argued, that therapists address, rather than deny, this history, which has the effect of removing individual blame for problems. The therapist should work at 'exorcizing ... the internalized oppressor' (350). My own work with Aboriginal offenders in prison certainly suggested that acknowledgment of colonial history for Aboriginal men was an essential stepping-stone towards the establishment of trust between therapist and patient (Waldram 1997). In the prisons, Aboriginal Elders frequently used history to help the individual contextualize his problems so that he would feel less 'bad.' But Duran et al. (1998) appeared to be advocating for a highly essentialized historical 'truth' that is not compatible with local histories and experiences. These histories and cultural traditions, especially as remembered and reified in the present, exist as disputed terrain. Scurfield (1995) documented traditional treatments among American Indian war veterans and the development of a schism between traditionalists and assimilated veterans in their approach to sweatlodge ceremonies and other healing and spiritual activities. I discovered that there was frequently wide divergence in colonial experiences as understood by men from very different regions of Canada, and that several foundational 'truths' were openly debated among men from different tribal backgrounds. Historical treatments on both sides of the border demonstrate vast differences in the colonial experiences of Aboriginal peoples (see, e.g., Trigger & Washburn 1996). If the therapist becomes charged with educating Aboriginal individuals about history, whose version represents the 'historical truth'?

Duran et al. (1998) also argued that the Vietnam war added additional trauma to the lives of American Indians, and that treatment of these combat veterans also required a historical perspective. However, the American Indian soldier was not only sent to fight the colonizer's war, he was also sent to fight other Indigenous peoples, 'close cultural relatives who were fighting the onslaught of colonialism' (Duran & Duran 1995: 173). The suggestion that there was any cultural connection between Indigenous peopless in Vietnam and American Indians implies acceptance of the Bering Strait theory of the populating of

North America (and a very liberal interpretation of the theory at that), a model developed by the colonizer! By extension, implicit also is a confusion between biological and cultural populations.

'Historical unresolved grief' is a key component of the soul wound. Brave Heart (1998) (see also Braveheart-Jordon & DeBruyn 1995; Brave Heart & DeBruyn 1998) argued that, for the Lakota peoples, the suppression of traditional spiritual and healing ceremonies in the past prevented the resolution of 'traumatic grief resulting from cataclysmic events,' including the assassination of one of their leaders, Sitting Bull, and the Wounded Knee massacre, both in the late nineteenth century. As a result, the Lakota 'collective ego identity as bereaved, victimized, and traumatized ... anchored in the historical and cultural past' had been 'transmitted through the intergenerational experience of unresolved grief and trauma' (291) in a process referred to as 'transposition' (Brave Heart & DeBruyn 1998). In effect, Brave Heart and her collaborators argued that not only was the memory of certain historic events transmitted from generation to generation, a very normal cultural process, but so too was the affective and somatic reaction to those events. 'Like children of Jewish Holocaust survivors,' Brave Heart and DeBruyn (198: 68) argued, 'subsequent generations of American Indians also have a pervasive sense of pain from what happened to their ancestors and incomplete mourning of those losses.' This is a complex idea. In her treatment program, Brave Heart utilized videotapes about Lakota history which 'stimulated ... traumatic memories' among her patients. Some of these memories, such as boarding school experiences, may well have represented the lived experience of some of those present, but others, such as the Wounded Knee massacre, would exist only in historical memory. Could Brave Heart actually be educating individuals to develop grief reactions to events that occurred outside their lifetime or which were otherwise of little concern to them, similar to those therapists who 'recover' trauma memories within their patients? Precisely how unresolved grief, as opposed to historical knowledge, transmits from generation to generation is not made clear. This is unfortunate, as it seems central to an acceptance of the broader conceptualization.

'Trauma is an integral part of American Indian life,' Norma Gray (1998: 396) has written. But are North American Aboriginal peoples simply victims, passively accepting their fate as colonized beings, internalizing pathology to the point where it becomes the norm in families and communities? Much of the literature discussed above certainly suggests this. I think in the attempt to establish the history of oppression and the damage done, and to have this legitimated in the eyes of the larger society, a victim persona has emerged. But post-colonial theory calls for decentring historical analysis which, following along the lines of Foucault and others, means that there must be individual agency and resistance. Very few have acknowledged this fact. One who has, Allan Wade (1995), argued that in attempting to understand historical trauma and effectively heal individuals, it was essential that resistance to oppression be conceptualized. Duran and Duran (1995) would certainly agree with his assertion that conventional psychotherapy 'can consolidate a victim status ... by displacing recognition of his/her resistance to the oppression she/he experienced' (Wade 1995: 168). Trauma narratives, then, in so far as they can be informative and therapeutic, must detail not simply the trauma but the ways in which the individual dealt with and also opposed it. Otherwise, the individual remains a 'passive recipient and damaged product of oppression, thus entrapping her in a narrative of decline and terminal change' (Wade 1995: 175). Trauma victims become reconceptualized as trauma 'survivors.' Earlier it was noted that few researchers seemed interested in exploring the possibility that low rates of PTSD in their studies might be indicative of coping or adaptation to stress and trauma, possibly even the invocation of cultural mechanisms to protect or rehabilitate individuals. Wade's analysis suggests that embedded in the discourse of resistance might be found the key to understanding the relatively low rates of PTSD despite difficult living circumstances.

Trauma and the Construction of 'Residential School Syndrome'

Kirmayer (1996b: 175) has defined the 'culturally constructed landscape of memory' to mean 'the metaphoric terrain that shapes the distance and effort required to remember affectively charged and socially defined events that initially may be vague, impressionistic, or simply absent from memory.' 'Landscapes of memory,' he continued, 'are given shape by the personal and social significance of specific memories but also draw from meta-memory – implicit models of memory which influence what can be recalled and cited as veridical.' At a recent conference on the consequences of residential schools that I attended, one individual stood to address the group after several others had given very emotional testimonials of the abuse they had suffered. 'I used to think my residential school experience was positive,' she related sombrely, 'but now I realize I'm in denial.' For this individual, and many like her, meta-memory had just shifted, and a new 'truth' was revealed. In many ways the stories of the trauma and abuse suffered by individuals at Indian residential schools in Canada and the United States represents just such a shift in the use, shape, and politicization of memory as the archetypal trauma narrative has unfolded. In this section I wish to look a little more closely at a disorder under construction, a form of trauma colloquially known as 'residential school syndrome.'

In both Canada and the United States, education was seen by government authorities as the key to Aboriginal assimilation. In recent years, various aspects of that educational process have been criticized by scholars and Aboriginal peoples as a form of genocide. One type of educational institution in particular, the residential school, has come under fire because of apparent widespread physical, sexual, and emotional abuse perpetrated on students while in care. In recent years, several individuals have been charged and convicted of abusing Indian children in these institutions.

According to a study of residential schools in Canada by the Assembly of First Nations (AFN 1994), the number of such institutions increased from eleven in 1880 to seventy-seven in 1909, with sixty in operation in the 1960s before the movement to close them was initiated. The last residential school was only closed in the 1970s. It has been estimated that by the early 1900s over 3000 children were attending residential schools, out of a population of 20,000; by the 1940s, roughly half of all eligible children were in residence (AFN 1994: 1). In the 1960s, some 10,000 children were still enrolled. The evidence suggests that at no point during their history were a majority of Indian students attending these schools, and further there were some regions in Canada in which students did not attend at all. Nevertheless, the numbers were substantial and, it is argued, the legacy profound. The residential school experience has come to characterize the experience of all Indian peoples in Canada, to be a claimed status of survival even among those who did not attend. The experience has become something of a marker of Indianness.

Residential schools have been described as 'total institutions' in the language of Goffman (1961), 'not unlike penitentiaries' (AFN 1994: 4; see also Chrisjohn and Young 1997), facilities in which every aspect of the child's life was regulated. Students lived at the facilities, often at some distance from their homes; but visiting with parents was tightly controlled and, therefore, physical distance largely irrelevant. Sleeping, eating, playing, working, and learning were all regulated as well, often supported by strict codes of conduct and corporal punishment. As these schools formed part of an assimilationist agenda, children were forced to wear European-style clothing (sometimes military-style uniforms) with European-style haircuts and were typically prohibited from speaking their own languages, on penalty of strict punishment. Many of the schools were operated by various churches, especially the Anglican, Catholic, and United churches, as well as the federal government, and schools sometimes changed hands over the course of their history. Not surprisingly, Christian education was a cornerstone in the programming. Several excellent studies on the history of the residential school system in Canada and the experiences of children are now available, and much of my discussion here is based on them (e.g., Haig-Brown 1988; Furniss 1995; Miller 1996; Nuu-Chah-Nulth Tribal Council 1996; Fournier & Crey 1997; Milloy 1999).

The story of the residential schools is a tangled web of accusations and counter-accusations, testimonials and denials, contested truths and agreed upon facts. Nevertheless, emerging from this web has been a story of widespread abuse that is no longer seriously questioned. These abuses included:

- physical punishment, involving caning, whipping and the use of various other objects, and burning
- sexual abuse, including forced sodomy, intercourse, fondling, and masturbation
- inadequate food and nutrition
- forced labour
- physical confinement
- emotional abuse, such as public humiliation, and denial of emotional support.[6]

Abuses of these types were both experienced and witnessed. Most frequently, the perpetrators were the care-givers: school superintendents, teachers, priests, nuns, brothers, and lay staff hired to maintain the facilities. But students themselves also became abusers, and engaged in the physical and sexual abuse of other students (Miller 1996; Nuu-Chah-Nulth Tribal Council 1996). The result was a daily life of fear and terror for many. Of course, there were also everyday acts of resistance at the schools, from stealing food to running away. Some authors, such as Haig-Brown (1988), have preferred to focus as much on resistance as on victimization, which in itself has created some controversy, as 'victim' and 'resistance' discourses carry somewhat different political currencies.

How widespread was the abuse? That is a difficult question to answer. For many years little was said about these experiences: some were fearful they would not be believed (after all, in some instances the abusers were priests and nuns), others were embarrassed or believed they were somehow to blame, others still were in denial or simply unable to discuss the abuse. The 'landscape of memory' has not proven to be readily open to the kinds of social challenges that these experiences would entail, and individuals have dealt with their personal histories in different ways. These differential reactions were underscored in a 1991 study of Williams Lake, British Columbia, in which, of 187 adults interviewed, many of whom had been students in residential schools, 89 admitted to being abused as children, 38 denied being abused, and 60 refused to answer the question (Miller 1996). It is also apparent that many individuals had positive experiences in the schools, or at least now have mixed feelings about their experience. The AFN's (1994) report even admitted that, in some instances where children were being neglected or abused at home, residential schools may have been a benefit to them. Miller (1996) has suggested that there is some conflict between those with negative and those with positive experiences, revealing the inherently contestable nature of the experience itself. Others reject the idea that a positive exerience was possible. Wade (1995: 173), for instance, argued that 'the fact that some survivors of residential school clearly state that they benefited from attending residential school is less a reflection of the value of these institutions than it is a testament to the remarkable ability of human beings to create something positive even in the most oppressive conditions.'

For its part, the AFN seemed less concerned with actual numbers, or determining the damage caused by residential schools in comparison to other causes, accepting that the residential schools were without question an important element in the overall health and psychological profile of Aboriginal peoples. They suggested in their report that 'the application of objective measure – numerical quantification – does not address a significant dimension of residential school impact ... In fact, objectifying the outcome of an experience such as residential school in this way reduces the meaning of it to numbers, and consequently, trivializes both the experience and its significance in the lives of those who

have lived and continue to live through it' (AFN 1994: 5). Chrisjohn
and Young (1997: 245) have argued the same point, but they have gone
further in disputing the need for, or appropriateness of, research. They
challenged the idea that 'the long-term consequences of what First
Nations peoples endured in residential school can be reduced to a
handful of Western-derived, culturally-myopic variables,' adding, 'As
such, the experience is accessible to anyone who can read' and 'this is a
dangerous delusion' because it allows 'bureaucrats' to equate 'their
days at strict, upper class private boarding schools with residential
school practices.' But authors such as Chrisjohn and Young (1997) have
been prepared to equate residential schools with non-Aboriginal parallels, such as the Jewish Holocaust and other horrible acts, that make
their case more forcefully. And many Aboriginal individuals have
launched lawsuits against the federal government and the churches,
either individually or as part of class action suits, which require them
to very specifically attribute certain personal difficulties to their experience in the residential schools. These stories will likely become as
much a part of the public record as the financial compensation the
individuals receive.

The door to disclosure was opened considerably in 1990, when Phil
Fontaine, Grand Chief of the AFN, publicly admitted that he had been
abused in residential school (Miller 1996: 328). Then, in 1992, a royal
commission was established to investigate a variety of Aboriginal
issues in Canada, and one of its priorities was to learn the truth about
residential schools. According to the co-chair of the Royal Commission
on Aboriginal Peoples (RCAP), Georges Erasmus, 'Everywhere we
have gone, we have been told about the impact of residential schools ...
Most of the stories we are hearing are negative; 99% of them ...' (AFN
1994: 3). Yet the AFN also disclosed a view of memory as constructed,
challenging their own assertion that the 'truth' of the residential school
experience required acknowledgment: 'Truth is built and rebuilt over
time through the stories we tell, individually and together in community, about our experience of a particular event such as residential
school. As individuals, families and communities, it is the meaning, the
interpretations or understandings found in our stories which determines, at least to a certain point, the impact of that experience on our
lives' (AFN 1994: 5). As Kirmayer (1996b: 189–90) has suggested,
'trauma shared by a whole community creates a potential public space
for retelling ... A public space of trauma provides a consensual reality
and collective memory through which the fragments of personal mem-

ory can be assembled, reconstructed, and displayed with a tacit assumption of validity.' It is apparent that while the public hearings of RCAP were created as a 'public space of trauma,' relatively few embraced the opportunity. An examination of the transcripts of the public hearings reveals that residential schools and their impact was indeed an important theme, but many still had difficulty talking openly in any great detail about their painful experiences. Some, too uncomfortable to speak on their own, had others speak for them. Quite likely, the very formal process of a royal commission hearing was far beyond what many considered to be an acceptable public space in which to tell these stories.

Nevertheless, many individuals placed responsibility for problems on the schools, and the notion of 'residential school syndrome' surfaced at many points. At one of the RCAP public hearings, Erasmus was brought to wonder aloud where the expression 'residential school syndrome' had come from, and how best to interpret its meaning. RCAP, in its final report, refrained from the use of this expression entirely, preferring to speak of the various traumas that the residential schools had inflicted upon Indian children, and how the effects of these traumas had permeated through subsequent generations. However, the expression 'residential school syndrome' itself has endured. Subsequent to the release of the RCAP report, a federally funded initiative, the Aboriginal Healing Foundation (AHF), was established to support projects designed to assist individuals in recovering from the trauma and related effects of the residential schools.[7] Utilizing primarily a survivor discourse, the AHF understood the notion of intergenerational trauma to encompass not only descending trauma, those generations following the experience of an individual confined to a residential school, but also ascending trauma, the parents of that individual, who may have suffered from the effects of having a child forcibly removed. While the AHF does not use the expression 'residential school syndrome' in its official documents, many of the projects it has funded use the expression liberally.[8] It has clearly become a part of the public lexicon in Canada.

Does 'residential school syndrome' exist, and if so, what does it look like? As its history continues to unfold, it resembles the history of other controversial trauma-related syndromes, and the syndrome remains contentious and recognized only by some. The public has, in recent years, been bombarded with media stories of the schools and their impacts, with litigation and the trials of abusers. The legacy of residential schools has been firmly established by media fiat. Yet the mental health professions have remained sceptical. Some have actively acknowledged residential school syndrome to be a serious psychological disorder: a psychologist in western Canada, for instance, advertised that he had developed an instrument to assess it, and invited those who felt they might have the syndrome to contact him.[9] Chrisjohn and Young (1997), in contrast, suggested it does not exist at all, that the experiences of students ranged so widely as to fail to meet the required uniformity of reaction required in the concept of a 'syndrome.' Just as the metaphor of trauma has developed to describe a whole litany of historical events and their consequences for Aboriginal peoples, so too has the metaphor of residential school syndrome. Where individuals suffer from alcoholism or substance abuse, depression, or hysteria, or engage in criminal activities, are violent, or neglect their family responsibilities, these behaviours are frequently articulated in accordance with a belief that residential schools constituted a pivotal moment in the transformation of Aboriginal societies from relatively trauma-free and functional to traumatized and dysfunctional. That dysfunctional behaviour can be passed on through the generations is well-accepted, and hence the notion of intergenerational trauma related to the residential schools has some currency, but to date there have been no empirical studies focused on its intergenerational nature among Aboriginal peoples. The existence of lawsuits has muddled the picture even more: beyond the apologies of churches and government lies possible compensation, and it is widely believed that some individuals have fabricated trauma, and argued for its intergenerational nature, in order to join class action suits.[10] Like PTSD before it, and like many other disorders which at various times have been included in and/or removed from DSM, residential school syndrome is, in part, a political idiom, a post-colonial tool employed by the oppressed to exact contrite and compensatory responses from the oppressor. It serves to keep colonialism and its consequences alive in the public consciousness while providing a more concrete explanation for contemporary troubles than allusions to a murky, distant past of unscrupulous settlers and Indian wars. Residential school syndrome, in effect, overlays an authoritative psychiatric-sounding diagnosis on the historic processes of colonization and assimilation.

Conclusion

There are certainly problems in the formulation of trauma as it has been applied to North American Aboriginal peoples, least of which is an obvious lack of consensus on what constitutes an acute traumatic event or, alternatively, a chronic state of trauma. There have been relatively few studies of trauma in general, or PTSD in particular, and these have been fraught with methodological difficulties. The idea of trauma as both experienced and witnessed, combined with the idea of cumulative and collective trauma, points persuasively to the existence of trauma-related disorders among some Aboriginal peoples living in troubled communities. One must question, however, the strong tendency to define Aboriginal populations as wracked with trauma and, by extension, PTSD, since the evidence suggests that the picture is considerably more complex. We must distinguish more clearly between trauma as a common, known element of human experience and PTSD as a psychiatric disorder. We need to work harder to understand how individuals continue to find meaning in life despite having apparently dealt with experiences which to many of us would seem unimaginable. The image of the traumatized Aboriginal, experiencing not the turmoil of millennia-old human existence on this continent but rather the ills that have accompanied colonization, haunts the trauma discourse. The traumatized Aboriginal has truly fallen from the Eden of Arcadia, as conceptualized and measured within the construct known as PTSD. But the Barbarian Aboriginal still looms at the fringe of the discourse, for while the Arcadian cannot visualize a pre-contact, traumatized Aboriginal individual, the Barbarian has trouble acknowledging that Aboriginal peoples were sophisticated enough to have effective systems for dealing with traumatizing experiences.

Approaching trauma through DSM by and large precludes a meaningful discussion of culture, and virtually excludes notions of history and collective, community, or cultural trauma. Post-colonial approaches, while bringing history into play, do so in a reductionist way that implies not only a uniform history of colonial experience but also a uniform reaction to that experience, and which fails, like DSM, to consider culture in any meaningful way. Just as disputes over the appropriateness of the psychiatric diagnosis of PTSD in specific circumstances exist, so too do disputes over the nature of the historical trauma that, it is argued for Aboriginal peoples, lead to it. Within the public realm, however, history, culture, and trauma are all brought together, not seamlessly by any means, but certainly with enough integrity to attract attention as a comprehensive explanation for all the ills affecting Aboriginal peoples today. In public trauma discourse, history and culture are central.

Clearly there are two traumas in evidence in this discussion. The first is the clinical one, PTSD, based on the conceptualization of the DSM and applied exclusively to individuals. Residential school syndrome may yet emerge as an important, recognized variant of PTSD. Related to this is an emerging lay understanding of trauma, not just as experience but as a condition, one that individuals can lay claim to even in the absence of a psychiatric diagnosis.

The second trauma is metaphorical and has come to mean a broader understanding of historical and collective trauma imbedded in colonialism. The discourse of residential school syndrome harbours elements of this metaphorical trauma, and challenges our understanding of what constitutes a psychiatric disorder. Can cultural bereavement, grief over the loss of the culture of one's people, be seriously thought of as 'traumatic' as psychiatry would understand it, or is this something altogether new and outside psychiatric parameters? Can individuals learn, or be taught, to be traumatized after the fact, because of historic injustices? Just as DSM's PTSD became a mechanism legitimizing the suffering of Vietnam veterans, so too has it become a means of legitimizing Aboriginal experiences, history, and suffering.

Not surprisingly, the application of PTSD frameworks to Aboriginal peoples has been open to manipulation and evolution in meaning. The emergence of 'residential school syndrome' represents just this type of development. Conceptual and methodological problems abound in the trauma research and discourse, but the lessons are clear: history is memory, and people take their history seriously. Many Aboriginal peoples have embraced this particular disorder, not always as a pathological condition, but as a metaphor for their historical relationship with the European settler society. To ignore that history, or to discount or challenge it, while purporting to treat a disorder of memory would be folly.

PART C

Treating the
Aboriginal

CHAPTER TEN

The Clinician's Aboriginal

People can tell just by looking at us what we want, what should be done to help us, how we feel, and what a 'real' Indian is like. (Deloria 1969: 9)

As we have seen throughout this book, anthropologists, psychologists, and psychiatrists alike have been fascinated by the personality of *the* Aboriginal for a century or more. Much of the emphasis has been placed on the generation of group profiles and generalized statements of personality and psychopathology, as well as the development and application of instruments designed to capture these effectively. An extension of this interest can be found in the generation of blueprints for understanding Aboriginal peoples as individuals, particularly those who are troubled and in need of treatment. This chapter turns, then, towards the more grounded concerns of mental health practitioners confronted by the cultural other, an 'Aboriginal,' in their clinics and offices. Who is this individual, and how should he or she be treated? What does the clinician's Aboriginal 'look' like? My focus in this chapter is on the problematic generation of ethics, values, and behavioural profiles of Aboriginal individuals and groups as alleged tools for effective therapeutic intervention. What emerges is a disturbing portrait of *the* singular Aboriginal client, a ubiquitous 'other' who is both everywhere, and nowhere.

The Anthropological Roots of Aboriginal Values Research

The study of Aboriginal ethics, values, and behaviours was originally the domain of anthropologists, heavily influenced by sociologists such as Talcott Parsons and his view that values in particular were at the core of the culture concept (Kuper 1999). Boasian anthropologists like Alfred Kroeber and Clyde Kluckhohn agreed, and values research became central to much anthropological inquiry. There was some debate on the flexibility of values, however, especially in reaction to culture contact. In the first half of the twentieth century it was commonly believed that value systems were heavily resistant to change, that values were the last traits to be altered, and the influential 1954 Memorandum on acculturation placed considerable emphasis on understanding this apparent intransigence in researching culture change situations (Summer Seminar on Acculturation 1954; Bee 1974). Values, being inherently psychological phenomena, were also central to emerging research in psychological anthropology. The basic or modal personalities of cultures were logically seen to reinforce, and to be reinforced by, modal or core values, and rote descriptions of the values of particular tribes, often presented as lists, became common.[1] Hallowell (1955: 360), for instance, described the 'central value' of northern Saulteux society as 'life in the fullest sense, life in the sense of health, longevity, and well-being, not only for oneself but for one's family.' Similarly, Aberle (1951), whose work was often cited by later psychologists, described Hopi values as including strength, self-control, poise, tranquillity, cooperation, unselfishness, kindness, and non-aggression. However, while Hallowell's and Aberle's work was focused on tribal-specific traits, and based on extensive periods of fieldwork, eventually the idea that the sum of these tribal specific studies was something more general, more universal, began to emerge.

Not surprisingly, the idea that there were common Aboriginal values and related behaviours across tribal groups had its origin in the work of anthropologists. Such assertions were typically accompanied by references, however oblique, to intercultural variability. When Honigmann (1961b: 124) argued that 'a high degree of psychological homogeneity characterizes the American Indian,' he also conceded that this was especially so within specific regions, such as the northern Algonkians and Athapaskans. Honigmann cited the work of Spindler and Spindler (1957), who 'hypothesized' the existence of a 'pan-Indian psychological core,' particularly for the 'least acculturated segments of contemporary tribes.' Their work focused on certain specific ethics, values, and behaviours, such as 'nondemonstrative emotionality and reserve accompanied by a high degree of control over interpersonal aggression within the in-group;' 'ability to endure pain, hardship, hunger, and frustration without external evidence of discomfort;' 'a generalized fear of the world as a dangerous place, and particularly a fear of witchcraft;' and 'attention to the concrete realities of the present' (503). Yet Spindler and Spindler stressed that these ethics, values, and behaviours were not 'fixed psychological constants' and that they varied 'by context and serve[d] somewhat different purposes in somewhat different ways in each culture' (504). The willingness of anthropologists to ignore variability was often quite striking. Wilcomb Washburn (1975: xv–xvi), in the preface to his book, *The Indian in America*, advised, 'there was and is no single Indian culture.' 'The languages, customs, personalities, and beliefs of Indians varied (and vary) widely, and have been subject to numerous modifications over time. Anthropologists are also discovering an increasingly wide range of individual behaviour within the context of supposedly monolithic tribal culture.' Surprisingly, Washburn added, 'Nevertheless, it is possible to isolate unifying and consistent patterns of behavior among Indian individuals as well as among Indian tribes ...'

In a paper that had considerable influence on the field of psychology, Rosalie Wax and Robert Thomas (1961) sought to establish the ways in which American Indians were different from 'white people,' especially in the area of communication.[2] Appealing to classic, almost Hollywood stereotypes, they described how the Indian, when confronted with a strange or dangerous situation, had been 'brought up to remain motionless and watch.' A kind of paralysis set in. 'Outwardly he appears to freeze,' they added, while 'inwardly, he is using all of his senses to discover what is expected of him' (1961: 306). The 'white man,' in contrast, reacts to such a situation by springing into action, to alter the situation or to escape from it. The white man acts, presumably to think later; the Indian freezes and thinks before acting. Similarly, in describing the ethic of 'non-interference,' they outlined an amusingly bizarre scenario in which an Indian passenger in a car would refrain from alerting the driver to a dangerous obstacle on the road ahead, allowing an accident to happen. Social paralysis and refusal to comment prevailed, according to these authors, and 'as the car rolls merrily into the ditch all that may be heard is a quiet exhalation of breath' (311).

Even more influential was Florence Kluckhohn and Fred L. Strodtbeck's 1961 anthropological study. Guided by earlier work by anthropologists including Hallowell, Clyde Kluckhohn, and Benjamin Whorf, these authors defined value orientations as 'complex but definitely patterned (rank-ordered) principles, resulting from the transactional

interplay of three analytically distinguishable elements of the evalua-
tive process – the cognitive, the affective, and the directive elements –
which give order and direction to the ever-flowing stream of human
acts and thoughts as these relate to the solution of "common human"
problems' (1961: 4). These principles were seen as cultural universals,
differing only in their ranking patterns within specific cultures. Furthermore, the authors made several key assumptions in their work, for
instance, that all societies experienced a limited number of common
human problems and harboured a limited number of universal solutions. Differences in value orientations between cultures, therefore,
represented different preferences drawn from among these universals.
Kluckhohn and Strodtbeck (1961: 11–20) outlined five universal
human problems for purposes of their research:

1. 'What is the character of innate human nature? (human nature orientation)' [options were 'evil,' 'neutral' or a 'mixture of good-and-
   evil,' and 'good']
2. 'What is the relation of man to nature (and supernature)? (man-
   nature orientation)' [options were 'subjugation-to-nature,' 'har-
   mony-with-nature,' and 'mastery-over-nature']
3. 'What is the temporal focus of human life? (time orientation)'
   [options were 'past,' 'present,' and 'future']
4. 'What is the modality of human activity? (activity orientation)'
   [options were 'being,' 'being-in-becoming,' and 'doing']
5. 'What is the modality of man's relationship to other men? (relational
   orientation)' [options were 'lineal,' 'collateral,' and 'individualistic']

Every culture member was assumed to harbour a rank order of value
orientations which were influenced by his or her culture. Logically,
then, one could learn something about a culture as a whole by examining individual value orientation rankings, and this is what Kluckhohn
and Strodtbeck did. Utilizing a twenty-two-item questionnaire, they
undertook research in the American southwest among five different
communities: Spanish-Americans, Texans, Mormons, Navajo, and
Zuni.[3] The assumption that value orientations were essentially universals that differed only in rank in specific cultures allowed the researchers to justify working with only a handful of subjects: between twenty
and twenty-five adults in each community, split more or less equally
between men and women.[4] While Kluckhohn and Strodtbeck admitted
that the sample sizes prevented an analysis of intracultural variation,

Table 10.1
Selected Comparison of Value Orientations – Kluckhohn & Strodtbeck 1961

Universal Human Problems	Value Orientations		
	TEXAS	ZUNI	NAVAJO
RELATIONAL	Individualistic	Collateral	Collateral
TIME	Future/Present	Present/Past	Present
MAN-NATURE	Over Nature	With/Subjected to/Over	With/Over/Subjected to
ACTIVITY	Doing	Doing/Being	Doing

they seemed somewhat oblivious to other problems inherent in drawing a random sample of only twenty-two Navajo, given the immense size of that population and the extensive regional and local cultural variations.[5] An assumption of discreet and bounded cultures also characterized the study, as if there had been no meaningful contact between the various groups despite several centuries of co-habitation within the region.

Table 10.1 contains partial value interpretations for the Texans, Zuni, and Navajo, and gives us a good idea of the take-off point for much of the psychologically based literature that follows (the slashes indicate ranked but essentially equal preferences).

This type of schematic comparison of value orientations subsequently became extremely popular among psychologists who accessed studies such as this, and often glossed over the very detailed methodological and statistical discussions, ignored the small sample size and the exploratory nature of the work, and drew broad conclusions regarding Aboriginal values.

The Psychologist's Approach to Aboriginal Values

The waning of Aboriginal culture and personality studies in anthropology opened the door for the psychologists, who were concerned with both comprehending the universals of human behaviour, and, by the 1980s, with developing 'culturally competent' modes of therapy (e.g., Sue et al. 1982; Sue & Sue 1990, 2003; Sue, Arrendondo, & McDavis 1992; Pedersen 1994, 1997; Helms & Richardson 1997; S. Sue 1998; Marín & Gamba 2003).[6] Psychologists were intellectually predisposed to accept without question the anthropological assertion that groups of humans could be defined by core value orientations and behavioural rules, and that these could be determined in large part from the existing anthropological database. Unlike the fieldwork-based in situ observations of the anthropologists, psychological observations were more likely to be based on clinical or laboratory research experiences. Sometimes their treatises on the topic of values seemed to be little more than the blind reproduction of common stereotypes about Aboriginal ethics, values, and behaviours derived from the literature. While cross-cultural surveys of value orientations also became popular in psychology, with a few exceptions (such as Kluckhohn & Strodtbeck 1961), there was, and remains, surprisingly little connection between the work of the anthropologists and that of the psychologists in this regard (Krause 1998: 173). Values became far more central to psychological inquiry than to anthropology in the latter decades of the twentieth century.

The way in which Aboriginal ethics, values, and behaviours would be handled was set by the beginning of the 1970s. One of the first major treatments was offered by John F. Bryde, an educational psychologist working in South Dakota. His main work, *Modern Indian Psychology* (1971), was based on twenty-three years of clinical work among the Indian population, listening to and writing down 'everything the old time Indians told him' (i). Unabashedly, then, the work was based on recollections of elderly individuals, presumably reflecting on the past. Bryde was a universalist, and stressed that 'the great Indian value system runs through most of the Indian tribes from Canada to the tip of South America' (65); his major theme seemed to be the need for Indians to revisit these lost values and adapt them to the 'modern' world of employment and education. Old values were therefore revamped by him to provide lessons for modern living: 'bravery,' for instance, a value anchored in a past of horse stealing and 'counting coup' (these people were presumably Sioux), was redefined as 'doing a hard thing without showing fear or running from it' (31). Many Indian fathers had lost sight of this value, he noted, as evidenced in their propensity to abandon employment, to run from the 'hard thing' of keeping a steady job. Another old value identified by Bryde was 'individual freedom,' which he redefined as the individual making the right decision (not just any decision) in order to survive in the best way possible (1971: 42). Education represented one of these right decisions.

Edwin H. Richardson (1977, 1981), a psychologist of 'Abnaki/Ute extraction' whose work we have already discussed, also published influential work on Indian values in this early period. Richardson, like Bryde, argued that despite some tribal differences, there were strong

Table 10.2
Selected Comparison of Indian and White Values – E.H. Richardson, 1977
(quotation marks original)

Indians	Whites
Happiness – paramount	Success – generally involving security, wealth, obtainment
Sharing	Ownership – would rather own an outhouse than share
Tribe and family first	'Think of number one' syndrome
Humble – causing them to be passive-aggressive	Competitive and believers in – 'if you don't toot your own horn who will'
Discrete – dating, for example is restrictive	Flouting and an Openness – 'What you see is what you get'
Look backwards to traditional ways	Look to the future – tie your wagon to a star and keep climbing
Work for a purpose – once you have enough then quit	Work, earn money, save; make routine and habits a part of your life
Be as free as the wind	Don't be a 'boat rocker'
Intuitiveness	Empiricism
Mystical	Scientific
Live natural, eat things raw, remember your brother the fox	Be sophisticated, eat your foods well prepared

similarities in values among American Indian peoples. Richardson also imported the issue of values more directly into the realm of counselling, and his work represented one of the first treatments of this issue. Many of his studies exist in the form of unpublished conference papers, or indirectly credited book chapters, but his work was considered seminal by those who subsequently wrote on the topic. While Bryde (1971) provided a short, detailed list of American Indian ethics, values, and behaviours, often comparing them to their non-Indian American counterparts, Richardson took this idea to a new level. And, though his work appeared to be based on Sioux peoples, Richardson also asserted the commonality of basic values in all American Indian groups. Without citing a single source or indicating how he determined them, Richardson (1977: 6–9) presented a list of thirty-seven Indian values and corresponding 'white' values. Table 10.2 reproduces several of these comparisons to provide the reader with a feel for how this was done.

This is obviously a somewhat amateurish list, making actual comparison difficult. Directly comparable contrasts do not always appear (e.g., 'Don't be a boat rocker' versus 'be as free as the wind'), and similarities in values are also not mentioned; that Richardson believed there were no similarities is suggested in his comment, 'No two races could so grossly differ in value systems than the Indian and the white' (1977: 6). The sum of the American Indian values was a primitivistic portrait of a people who were seen as egalitarian, free from interpersonal constraints, mystical and intuitive, and who were 'natural' people, preferring to eat their food raw.

The construction of values lists was not simply a scholarly exercise. Rather, the point was to provide guidance for culturally competent treatment, although in retrospect the guidance frequently appears absurd. In a book chapter more widely available and targeted towards counsellors, Richardson (1981; in Sue 1981)[7] indicated why these values were important for counselling Native Americans. How the office was configured was considered important; Richardson (1981: 235) advised that 'Since the Native American is humble and unpretentious, we suggest you have a small, homey, and lived in office,' with pictures of Indians on the walls. When greeting a Native American, a soft handshake was preferable because 'it is typical of humble people to shake hands in such a manner' (236). In a reference to nonverbal behaviours, he emphasized the need to listen to and carefully observe Native American clients. 'Native Americans will give you clues with their bodies, eyes, and tone of voice; but do not expect them to be as ostentatious, flamboyant, and dramatic as white clients. Rather, the clues they give are on a subliminal basis that many people miss' (1981: 233). But, he cautioned, 'American Indians can almost feel a phony person. It is almost as if they had antennae that pick up signals, or as if the insincere person gave off a chemical that betrayed her or his insincerity, or maybe it is something like infrared or electrical vibrations' (248).

Joseph Trimble, a psychologist and one of the most prominent researchers on American Indian mental health, was critical of the work of the culture and personality anthropologists, especially Clyde Kluckhohn, A.F.C. Wallace, George Spindler, and Louise Spindler, which he argued served to homogenize American Indians rather than to elucidate their heterogeneity (Trimble & Medicine 1993). In an early paper, he also criticized the kinds of comparative presentations offered by the likes of Bryde and Richardson (although he did not specifically refer to these authors), insightfully arguing that cross-cultural research operated with the 'tacit belief that the host people are in fact culturally different,' in the absence of empirical proof (Trimble 1975: 304). He continued by arguing that 'the search for differences [has] been the main thrust of research on the American Indian.' 'Most of the studies,' he added, 'attempt to isolate sets of discriminating variables that serve to differentiate one cultural group from another' (304). A 1981 paper, coauthored with several other leading mental health researchers, reinforced this point: 'there are, already, too many stereotypes in the cross-cultural counseling literature (e.g., Navajo won't look you in the eye; Sioux aren't competitive) to mislead the non-Indian mental health practitioner. Minimal experience with either tribe would demonstrate the situational effects on eye contact or competitiveness and belie the collective personality absurdities' (Dinges, Trimble, Manson, & Pasquale 1981: 244). In a chapter published in 1976 and reprinted in 1981, Trimble argued that because of the extensive cultural variability there was no sense in trying to list American Indian values (Trimble 1981), and he subsequently lamented the consequences of 'collective grouping' (Trimble & Fleming 1989: 178). Presenting the Sioux as a case in point, Trimble indicated that there were dialect differences, differences between urban and rural individuals, and differences in clan identification. 'Each reservation has its idiosyncrasies, gestural references, and norms that are quite distinct from each other,' Trimble (1975: 305) wrote. 'Thus a Sioux is not simply a Sioux despite the generic treatment given in the literature' (306). He even argued that evidence seemed to suggest that there could well be more value orientation differences among members of different American Indian groups than between Indians and Caucasian Americans (Trimble & Fleming 1989).

Despite these assertions, in a series of handbook articles by Trimble (1976, 1981; see also Trimble & Fleming 1989) we see what would emerge as a common feature of much of the cross-cultural treatment literature on Aboriginal peoples, that is, a tension between the need to emphasize cultural heterogeneity and denounce stereotypes, and the need to present meaningful generalizations to the practitioner. Trimble offered 'the next best approach,' which 'would be to list those Indian values that Indians recognize as differing most from those of the dominant culture' (Trimble & Fleming 1989: 208). Hence, Trimble replaced externally generated (etic) lists of values with internal (emic) ones, assuming perhaps that Indian-generated lists would be more authentic.

Unlike Bryde and Richardson, Trimble (1981) based his original discussion of American Indian values and counselling partly on his own
empirical work. In an exploratory study in 1971, he utilized a sentence
completion instrument with a sample of 84 Indians and 137 non-
Indians in southeastern Oklahoma (Trimble 1981). The survey was
designed to assess value preferences and had originally been developed for use with Mexican youths. His Indian subjects were mostly
'mixed blood' individuals from several different tribal groups, including Creek, Cherokee, Choctaw, Chickasaw, and Seminole. They were
not 'reservation types,' and had extensive experience with the broader
American society. Echoing anthropological views of the relative imper-
viousness of values to cultural change, however, Trimble reported that,
'Through all this interaction, a different value system had been retained
somewhat intact in spite of the influence of the dominant culture' (218).
But he further concluded that this value system had probably undergone change from tribal-specific values 'to a more generalized set of
rural pan-Indian values' (218). His statistical analysis indicated that the
Indian students' values were, as a group, separable from those of the
non-Indians, although he did not present a listing of those values. For
Trimble, the important point was that since many of the Indian subjects
did not look Indian but subscribed to Indian values, the integrity of the
therapeutic encounter could easily be compromised.

Trimble's (1981) second empirical study was undertaken in 1973.
Twenty Indian subjects were requested to identify value orientations 'as
conceptualized from their tribal and individual perspectives' during a
roundtable discussion, and content analysis was then used to identify
common dimensions (1981: 214). These were pre-tested on a hundred
Indians in Oklahoma, and the affirmed values were then used in a larger
study of 791 American Indians from five different regions of the country:
an 'Eastern Reservation,' a 'Northern Plains Reservation,' a 'Southwest
Pueblo,' a 'Community College,' and a 'Military Base.' The values identified and tested in this process were: kindness, honesty, self-control,
social skills, social responsibility, reciprocity (altruism), and independence. Statistical analysis determined that there was close agreement
among the five Indian groups on the desirability of the seven values.
Trimble (1981: 214) noted, importantly, that 'While the seven value subscales are broad enough to be generalized to many [non-Indian] subcultures, they contain elements germane to American Indians.'

Can we comfortably conclude from Trimble's experiment that these
seven elements were important American Indian values? If the values

do not differentiate American Indians from other 'subcultures,' of what utility are they? The existence of similar value orientations among groups known to have had very different traditional cultures may provide some support for the idea of underlying common American Indian values. But another possible explanation is evident: the similarity in values could be the result of a more or less uniform process of acculturation to broader American society. Trimble may have been identifying broader American values absorbed by these individuals, or perhaps a merging of American and American Indian values. Are not kindness, honesty, and altruism, for instance, also 'American' values? While at the time Trimble himself was clearly not comfortable with creating 'a generalized Indian value perspective' (210), he appeared to succumb several years later when, citing the work of none other than John Bryde and Kluckhohn and Strodtbeck, he concluded that 'there is some evidence that a generalized value orientation does exist for American Indians and that they do differ, however slightly, from the dominant culture' (Trimble & Medicine 1993: 149).

Delineating the Ethics, Values, and Behaviours of *the* Aboriginal

The issue of values has remained central to much of the Aboriginal treatment literature since the first writings of Richardson and Trimble. Several main themes, often contradictory, appear consistently throughout the voluminous literature.

The cultural diversity of the Aboriginal population is frequently asserted, emphasizing both traditional tribal diversity as well as differences between urban and rural/reservation populations (Youngman & Sadongei 1974; Trimble 1975; French 1979; Edwards & Edwards 1980; Dinges et al. 1981; Katz 1981; Richardson 1981; Trimble 1981; Dillard 1983; Haviland, Horswill, O'Connell, & Dynneson 1983; LaFromboise & Rowe 1983; Trimble & Hayes 1984; Attneave 1987; Darou 1987; Ho 1987; Orlansky & Trap 1987; Tafoya 1989; Trimble & Fleming 1989; Heinrich, Corbine, & Thomas 1990; Herring 1990; LaFromboise, Trimble & Mohatt 1990; Sue & Sue 1990, 2003; Thomason 1991; Dufrene & Coleman 1992; Herring 1992; Ho 1992; Koverola 1992; Renfrey 1992; Dana 1993; LaFromboise 1993; McDonald, Morton & Stewart 1993; Peregoy 1993; Garrett & Garrett 1994; Anderson & Ellis 1995; Duran & Duran 1995; Trimble,Fleming, Beauvais, & Jumpere Thurman 1996; Fisher & Harrison 1997; Sage 1997; Brucker & Perry 1998; Green 1999; Norton 1999; Dillard & Manson 2000). Some have also recognized the existence of intra-community variability (Tefft 1967; Trimble 1975; Dillard 1983; Trimble & Hayes 1984; Trimble & Fleming 1989; LaFromboise et al. 1990; Sue & Sue 1990, 2003; Thomason 1991; McDonald et al. 1993; Garrett & Garrett 1994; Trimble et al. 1996; Sage 1997; Green 1999; Dillard & Manson 2000). It has been suggested that therapists should view the client as an individual first, and an Aboriginal person second, and that it is dangerous to assume cultural and value orientation based on physical appearances or knowledge that a client identifies as Aboriginal (Dillard 1983; Sue & Sue 1990, 2003; Thomason 1991; McDonald et al. 1993; Garrett & Garrett 1994).

Another theme is that some Aboriginal peoples will express non-Aboriginal North American values (French & Hornbuckle 1972; Dillard 1983; Heinrich et al. 1990; Koverola 1992; Renfrey 1992; Anderson & Ellis 1995), and assessing the level of acculturation to non-Aboriginal values is sometimes considered important in treatment (Dinges et al. 1981; Dillard 1983; Trimble & Fleming 1989; Heinrich et al. 1990; LaFromboise et al. 1990; Herring 1990; Sue & Sue 1990, 2003; Renfrey 1992; McDonald et al. 1993; Garrett & Garrett 1994; Trimble et al. 1996; Brucker & Perry 1998). Acculturative stress, expressed as value conflict (being 'caught between two worlds/cultures') is considered to be a particularly thorny problem (French & Hornbuckle 1972; Katz 1981; Dillard 1983; LaFromboise & Rowe 1983; Attneave 1987; French 1989; Trimble & Fleming 1989; Heinrich et al. 1990; Herring 1990; Sue & Sue 1990; Renfrey 1992; Topper 1992; Anderson & Ellis 1995; Trimble et al. 1996; French 1997; Sage 1997).

This nod towards heterogeneity is largely superficial, however, as most discussions tend to proceed quickly from short affirmative statements about diversity to detailed presentations on cultural homogeneity (Youngman & Sadongei 1974; French 1979; Richardson 1981; Trimble 1981; Dillard 1983; Trimble & Hayes 1984; Darou 1987; Ho 1987; Herring 1989; Brant 1990; Heinrich et al. 1990; Sue & Sue 1990; Herring 1992; Ho 1992; Koverola 1992; Renfrey 1992; Brant 1993; Dana 1993; LaFromboise 1993; Garrett & Garrett 1994; Anderson & Ellis 1995; Duran & Duran 1995; Fisher & Harrison 1997; Sage 1997; Brucker & Perry 1998; Dillard & Manson 2000). Some authors have suggested that this commonality is at least partially the product of a contemporary pan-Indian movement which has resulted in the recent convergence of some values across cultural groups, suggesting that to some extent value similarities may be a recent phenomenon (French 1981; Trimble 1981; Attneave 1987; Renfrey 1992).

Finally, most authors have focused narrowly on culture and cultural formations as central to the generation and maintenance of values. Only a few have discussed the role of socio-economic status and class in their construction (Attneave 1982; Dillard 1983; Herring 1990; LaFromboise et al. 1990; Fleming 1992; Herring 1992; Dana 1993). Some authors, such as Ho (1987), have occasionally noted that the values of American society as a whole are those of the middle class, while omitting mention of class when ascribing American Indian values. Hence, non-Indians (usually whites) are deemed to have social class, while Indians have culture.

From the work cited above, it is possible to identify a set of the most commonly declared, universal Aboriginal behaviours, values, and ethics considered relevant for psychotherapy and counselling. The references, including very recent works, clearly indicate the persistence of this core set:

- lack of eye contact (Wax & Thomas 1961; Youngman & Sadongei 1974; Lewis & Ho 1975; Darou 1980; Edwards & Edwards 1980; Attneave 1987; Orlansky & Trap 1987; Tafoya 1989; Sue & Sue 1990; Thomason 1991; Brant 1993; McDonald et al. 1993; Paniagua 1994; French 1997; Brucker & Perry 1998; Dillard & Manson 2000)

- soft handshake (Richardson 1981; Trimble & Hayes 1984; Attneave 1987; Orlansky & Trap 1987; Tafoya 1989; Thomason 1991; McDonald et al. 1993; Paniagua 1994; French 1997)

- reticence/shyness (Wax & Thomas 1961; Youngman & Sadongei 1974; Richardson 1977; Richardson 1981; Dillard 1983; LaFromboise et al. 1990; Brant 1993; Anderson & Ellis 1995)

- emotional restraint (Katz 1981; Brant 1990, 1993; LaFromboise et al. 1990; French 1981, 1997; Ho 1992)

- use of non-verbal behaviour/communication (Youngman & Sadongei 1974; Katz 1981; Richardson 1981; Darou 1987; Herring 1992; Brant 1993; McDonald et al. 1993; Paniagua 1994)

- passivity/submissiveness (Herring 1990; Anderson & Ellis 1995; Still & Hodgins 1998)

- humility (Youngman & Sadongei 1974; Richardson 1977, 1981; Dillard 1983; Heinrich et al. 1990; Dillard & Manson 2000)

- avoidance of personal glory and gain (Youngman & Sadongei 1974; Edwards & Edwards 1980; Dillard 1983; Anderson & Ellis 1995)

- non-competitiveness (Brant 1990, 1993)

- cooperation (Spang 1965; Darou 1987; Herring 1989; Heinrich et al. 1990; Sue & Sue 1990; Ho 1992; Renfrey 1992; LaFromboise 1993; Peregoy 1993; Sage 1997; Brucker & Perry 1998; Still & Hodgins 1998; Green 1999; Dillard & Manson 2000)

- giving/sharing/generosity/kindness (Spang 1965; Zintz 1969; Youngman & Sadongei 1974; Lewis & Ho 1975; Richardson 1977; Edwards & Edwards 1980; Katz 1981; Trimble 1981; Dillard 1983; Brant 1990, 1993; Heinrich et al. 1990; Herring 1990; Sue & Sue 1990; Ho 1992; Renfrey 1992; LaFromboise 1993; Peregoy 1993; Garrett & Garrett 1994; Paniagua 1994; French 1997; Sage 1997; Brucker & Perry 1998; Green 1999)

- harmony (with others)/ avoidance of disagreement (French & Hornbuckle 1972; Lewis & Ho 1975; Richardson 1977; French 1979; Sue & Sue 1990; Koverola 1992; Ho 1992; Brant 1993; Anderson & Ellis 1995; French 1997; Green 1999; Dillard & Manson 2000)

- harmony with nature (Spang 1965; French & Hornbuckle 1972; Youngman & Sadongei 1974; Richardson 1977; French 1979, 1997; Dillard 1983; Ho 1987, 1992; Herring 1989, 1990, 1992; Heinrich et al. 1990; Sue & Sue 1990; Koverola 1992; Renfrey 1992; Dana 1993; LaFromboise 1993; Peregoy 1993; Duran & Duran 1995; Fisher & Harrison 1997; Brucker & Perry 1998; Still & Hodgins 1998; Dillard & Manson 2000)

- present time orientation (Spang 1965; Zintz 1969; Katz 1981; Ho 1987; Herring 1989, 1990; Heinrich et al. 1990; Sue & Sue 1990; Koverola 1992; Renfrey 1992; Dana 1993; Peregoy 1993; Garrett & Garrett 1994; Anderson & Ellis 1995; Duran & Duran 1995; Fisher & Harrison 1997; Still & Hodgins 1998; Dillard & Manson 2000)

- lacking in time consciousness (Spang 1965; Lewis & Ho 1975; Richardson 1977; Darou 1987; Orlansky & Trap 1987; Herring 1989; Brant 1990; Ho 1992; McDonald et al. 1993; Paniagua 1994; Anderson & Ellis 1995; Green 1999)

- respect for age/elders (Spang 1965; Richardson 1977; Darou 1980, 1987; Red Horse 1980; Dillard 1983; Herring 1989, 1990; Renfrey 1992; French 1997; Sage 1997; Still & Hodgins 1998; Green 1999)

- individuality/autonomy/personal freedom (French & Hornbuckle 1972; Lewis & Ho 1975; Edwards & Edwards 1980; Trimble 1981; Herring 1989, 1992; Ho 1992; Renfrey 1992; French 1997)

- non-interference and avoidance of direct questioning (Wax & Thomas 1961; Lewis & Ho 1975; Darou 1980, 1987; Orlansky & Trap 1987; Brant 1990; Sue & Sue 1990; Dauphinais & King 1992; Herring 1992; Renfrey 1992; Fisher & Harrison 1997; Brucker & Perry 1998; Green 1999; Dillard & Manson 2000)

- holism (Heinrich et al. 1990; Koverola 1992; Renfrey 1992; Duran & Duran 1995; Dillard & Manson 2000)

- extended family orientation (Red Horse 1980; Heinrich et al. 1990; Sue & Sue 1990; Peregoy 1993; Garrett & Garrett 1994; Paniagua 1994; Sage 1997; Green 1999)

This somewhat overwhelming list of articles citing essentially the same behaviours, values, and ethics would lead one to conclude, erroneously, that each has been empirically validated, over and over again. But this is not so. A great deal of the 'knowledge' we have of Aboriginal ethics, values, and behaviours is actually the product of authors simply citing earlier works without much concern for the validity of the research base. Herring (1989, 1990, 1992), for instance, relied on the previous work of Richardson (1981), as did Paniagua (1994), Orlansky and Trap (1987), Heinrich et al. (1990), and Dillard and Manson (2000). Koverola (1992), in turn, utilized Herring's work. Renfrey (1992) cited earlier works by Herring (1990), Spang (1965), and French (1989). Trimble's (Trimble 1981; Trimble & Fleming 1989) empirical work, unquestioned, was central to many subsequent articles on values, including Darou (1987), Heinrich et al. (1990), Koverola (1992), Dana (1993), Garrett and Garrett (1994), Sage (1997), and Green (1999). Several authors relied primarily on their own clinical experiences with Aboriginal peoples (e.g., Bryde 1971; Katz 1981; Richardson 1981; Brant 1990; Anderson & Ellis 1995; Sage 1997). Of all those cited, only the work of Trimble appears to have been based on empirical research by the author. The only other empirical studies which were occasionally cited were the work of earlier anthropologists (e.g., Aberle 1951; Kluckhohn & Strodtbeck 1961). An enormous body of stereotypical, even essentialized, traits has been passed down from one generation of scholars to the next largely unchallenged.

The vulnerability of much of the knowledge about Aboriginal values and treatment can been seen through an examination of some of the core works. Miles Zintz (1969), for example, in a volume about cross-cultural education in the American southwest, presented a discussion of the cultures and values of the Navajo and the Zuni. While it is evident that some of his observations were derived from his own personal experiences as an educator and education researcher, the exact source for his value lists cannot be determined. He was certainly influenced by the ethnographic literature, and extensively utilized the works of Elsie Clews Parsons, Edward Dozier, Ruth Benedict, Ruth Bunzel, Fred Eggan, and Margaret Mead, as well as materials generated by the Indian Education Research Project. But his listing of Pueblo values contained no citations whatsoever and no indication to which, if any, specific Pueblo he was referring. Zintz's work was subsequently cited in a discussion of values by several scholars, among them Trimble (1981), Dillard (1983), and Green (1999). In his influential 1981 paper, Trimble faithfully and uncritically reproduced Zintz's comparative list of Pueblo and Anglo values, noting that they compared favourably with Bryde's Sioux-based list. In a subsequent series of revised versions of that paper (Trimble & Fleming 1989; Trimble et al. 1996), Zintz's work was again cited as authoritative for the Pueblo peoples. In his 1983 treatment, John Dillard uncritically cited the Pueblo work of Zintz to support the existence of a set of *universal* American Indian values. In Green's (1999) more recent handbook, at least one of Zintz's specific Pueblo/Anglo value contrasts, that Anglos always prefer to win whereas Pueblo peoples prefer to 'win once, but let others win also' (Green 1999: 244; adapted from Zintz 1969: 210), was transformed into a generic American Indian value! In the course of thirty-five years, this value, originally an undocumented feature of an unidentified Pueblo society, had become a generalized value common to all American Indians.[8]

The vulnerability of the knowledge base can also be seen in work by Wynne Hanson Dubray, a Sioux psychologist who attempted his own empirical study grounded in the work of Trimble, Zintz, and especially Kluckhohn and Strodtbeck. Using the value orientation schedule developed by Kluckhohn and Strodtbeck more than twenty years earlier,

DuBray (1985) interviewed thirty-six American Indian and thirty-six Anglo-American professional mental health workers, all females and all with Masters' degrees. The American Indian subjects were 'randomly' drawn from twenty-eight different tribal groups. DuBray utilized the four categories of value orientations and the four 'life problems' developed by Kluckhohn and Strodtbeck (activity, relational, time, and man/ nature); statistical analysis revealed no difference between the two groups on activity orientation, and a significant difference on relational orientation, time orientation, and man/nature orientation. In particular, the American Indian subjects demonstrated a 'being in activity orientation, collateral in relational orientation, present time orientation, and harmony with nature in man/nature orientation' (35). These findings, given the wide range of American Indian cultures represented, led DuBray to conclude that they supported 'Honigmann's report that American Indians tend to possess a high degree of psychological homogeneity based on common values' (35). Yet he made no effort to explain how groups as culturally diverse and physically distant as the Cree, Hopi, Lakota and Mohawk could share a value orientation, implying instead a psychic connection among the Indian groups. He noted that the American Indian values had remained intact despite years of professional education and social work training, but the Anglo-American social workers presentation of a 'being over doing' activity orientation (a contrast to Kluckhohn and Strodtbeck's 1961 findings) was interpreted as the product of the same training! Apparently, this training had the effect of altering a basic Anglo-American value orientation while having no effect at all on the value orientations of American Indian social workers. Instead, DuBray (1985) argued that the value orientations, as he had measured them, represented a persistence from earlier times, perhaps over centuries, maintained as a form of resistance to assimilationist pressures. There is certainly nothing in his data to substantiate this interpretation.

The conventional wisdom underscored by published values lists has been challenged from time to time. Anthropologist Theodore Graves (1967b), in a comparative study of values among American Indian, Anglo, and Spanish populations in the Southwest, found that Anglos and Indians differed on only one of the three value scales used, the Indians and Spanish likewise differed on only one scale, but the Anglos and Spanish differed on all three. Flores (1986), in a comparative study of value orientations among Papago, Pima, and Anglo-American alcoholics and non-alcoholics, demonstrated that the two Native American

groups were similar in the values they supported and endorsed different values than the Anglo respondents. Anglos placed higher importance on values related to 'societal goals,' such as a world at peace,
equality, and freedom, whereas the Native Americans endorsed more
personal values, such as happiness, self-respect, and a comfortable life.
A strong sense of the Anglos as individualistic failed to emerge from
the study, contrary to common stereotypes held by both Anglos and
Native Americans.

Even these confounding studies of cultural diversity have suffered
from a lack of scrutiny. An example of this process of creating artifacts
is the use of Stanton Tefft's (1967) study of values among an Anglo,
Arapaho and Shoshone sample. Dinges et al. (1981), Trimble (1981),
Renfrey (1992), and Trimble et al. (1996) all agreed that Tefft's work
demonstrated that, 'there is evidence that intertribal differences in values and attitudes are greater among Indians than between Indians and
non-Indians' (Dinges et al. 1981: 245). Yet Tefft's data hardly supports
such a sweeping conclusion. In a study he declared to be of 'limited
scope,' with a small sample, Tefft interviewed 229 white high school
students, 36 Northern Arapaho, and 45 Wind River Shoshone students,
using a modified version of the Harvard Value Study Questionnaire
based, in part, on the work of Kluckhohn and Strodtbeck (1961). All the
students had similar academic records, all were above a C average,
and the Indian students in particular were fluent in English. He concluded that the Arapaho differed from the Shoshone only in terms of
their relational orientation, and that the Arapaho demonstrated less
internal consensus on the rank ordering of the values than did the
Shoshone and the white students. Given the limitations of the data and
the actual conclusions, one cannot sustain the argument that Tefft's
study supported the idea of greater intertribal differences on value orientations than those found between Indians and non-Indians. This key
study in support of the idea of cultural heterogeneity has, like many
others, been misinterpreted and overgeneralized.

Essentializing the Aboriginal/Non-Aboriginal Dichotomy

The stereotypes generated in values studies appear as classic, essentialist tropes. 'Like others living in close harmony with nature,'
Mohawk psychiatrist Clare Brant (1990: 536) has written, 'the Native
person has an intuitive, personal and flexible concept of time.' *The
Aboriginal person is one who lives in harmony with nature*, unre-

Table 10.3
'Selected Cultural Contrasts' (J.W. Green, 1999)

Native American	White American
Cooperation and sharing are highly valued; individualism, assertiveness and impulse are discouraged	Early displays of individualism and lifelong care for the needs of the self are considered normal and even healthy
Noninterference and respect for the rights and choices of others are highly valued. Confrontation is rarely appropriate	Assertive (but not aggressive) speech and behavior styles are favored. Leadership and individual achievement are honored
Pacing the activities according to the needs and expectations of others is more important than observing clock time and abstract schedules	Punctuality, promptness, and adherence to abstract time schedules are critical to success
Elders have important ceremonial and sometimes political roles; their views count	Elders usually live apart and are not expected to exercise political, ceremonial, or financial control over others

stricted by the bonds of Western notions of time, free to move unencumbered with the seasons. Aboriginal peoples have a primal, holistic world view, embodied in the wisdom of the elders. They are natural people, who relate to each other in natural ways. They listen before they speak; they do not threaten or act aggressively. They share. They have a 'Harmony Ethic' (French 1981: 144).[9] They are a humble people. They are a *cultural* people.

Values do not exist in isolation, however, and are most frequently contrasted with other, less desirable values, especially those of other, less desirable groups. This underscores the importance of comparative lists of values, which serve to highlight difference rather than similarity. With Aboriginal peoples, the favoured contrasting group is the non-Aboriginal or 'white' individual, and, as for Aboriginal peoples, stereotypes of white values pervade the discourse. This is not simply a remnant of an unsophisticated scholarly past, either. Consider Table 10.3, a partial list of 'selected cultural contrasts' between 'Native American' and 'White American' communities offered by anthropologist James Green in 1999 (242).

The language may be different, but Green and E.H. Richardson are both saying the same thing about Indian and Anglo-American cultures. Green's disclaimer (1999: 242) that 'this list of statements may or may not apply to any specific individual' only muddles the picture: of precisely what utility is a list that 'may or may not' apply in the absence of criteria to determine its applicability? Little changed as we entered the new millennium. Dillard and Manson's (2000) treatment expressed the whole range of ethics, values, and behaviours listed earlier, citing the works of Richardson (1981) among others without critical assessment.

Most reported Aboriginal values are really expressions of essentialist non-Aboriginal oppositions, even when, typically, little effort has been made to define who these mysterious non-Aboriginals are: where Aboriginal peoples value generosity and sharing, non-Aboriginals value greed and accumulation; where Aboriginals are present-time oriented, non-Aboriginals are future-time oriented; where Aboriginals show emotional restraint, non-Aboriginals are assertive. The tone of the literature frequently disparages non-Aboriginal values. And the Aboriginal values of old are seen as persisting even today, as having withstood the onslaught of Europeans despite the other cultural damage that many argue has ensued (e.g., Red Horse 1980). Paniagua (1994: 75) has insisted that 'many of the [contemporary] American Indians' rules, roles, values, and beliefs were developed during the precontact period.' Attneave (1987: 137) suggested that 'the unconscious persistence of tribal values, customs, and ways of relating are still very strong' even where conscious recall is problematic. Similarly, Brant (1990: 534) argued that certain values, ethics, and rules of behaviour 'persist in disguised form as carryovers from the aboriginal culture and ... strongly influence Native thinking and action even today.' Specific ethics, values, and behaviours are apparently embedded within the very essence of the Aboriginal.

The suggestion of a kind of psychic unity among North American Aboriginal peoples continues to loom large in this discourse, a reflection of earlier anthropological ruminations on personality and culture (as found in Honigmann, for instance). Garrett and Garrett (1994: 135) explained that 'a prevailing sense of "Indianness" based on a common world view seems to bind Native American Indians together as a people of many peoples.' French (1980: 76) has written that 'Social, physical and linguistic differences aside, North America's indigenous people possess a similar psychocultural orientation, at least in their traditional aboriginal heritage. It is a cultural philosophy tailored to the cooperative lifestyle of these aboriginal societies, one where interpersonal and environmental harmony were important survival norms.' According to

McDonald et al. (1993: 4), Indian psychology 'is virtually unchanged and springs from the very earth itself.'

Remarkably, we find little attempt to critically orient this psychic unity to contemporary times. There is little discussion in the literature of the ways in which a common, relatively recent colonial history, combined with the dominance of a Western European colonizer, may have had a uniform effect on formerly disparate Aboriginal cultures. Could intertribal similarities be the result of such cultural convergence, especially in the direction of a broader Euro-American culture?[10] Even extensive experience in non-Aboriginal society cannot eliminate these apparently innate cultural traits. The 'ancestral cultural values [of Indian children in white foster homes] are very strong and they permeate the family, social, vocational and sexual lives of the adolescents,' according to Katz (1981: 458). Even where an individual had assimilated, suggests Norton (1999: 83), somehow 'there are likely to be issues in the assessment that are linked to aspects of traditional American Indian cultures.' How this can be is not explained. Kirmayer, Brass, and Tait (2000: 611) have suggested that the very creation of an ethnic identity requires the elevation of certain beliefs and practices to the status of 'core values' which are claimed as shared experiences, and which obscure individual variation. 'A shared history invests ethnic identity with social value and contributes directly to mental health,' they claim. It is possible that this 'shared history' is a relatively recent phenomenon, a reaction of Aboriginal peoples to the effects of generations of colonialism, and not the persistence of an innate psychic unity. Yet shared values do not necessarily follow a shared history, and scholars rarely point out the problematic nature of ascribing sets of values to specific Aboriginal populations or communities. Adelson (2001) described the conflict that emerged in one James Bay Cree community when, faced with a general desire to reinvigorate indigenous values, residents discovered that opinions actually varied on what these were. In the end, the idea that pre-contact, unconscious, and disguised cultural and psychical formations persist today despite centuries of contact is largely a matter of rhetorical faith, not empiricism.

Values and Treatment

In much of the literature there is little explication of the reasons why ethics, values, and behaviours are important in psychotherapy and counselling. Value conflict has been seen by some as a major contributor to emotional and psychological problems. Trimble (1981: 221), for instance, suggested that a client's problems could be prompted by an issue of value conflict, which could 'contribute to feelings of inadequacy and diminished self-worth' (221). Some of his later work (e.g., Trimble et al. 1996: 190) recognized that value loss and conflict were not inevitable, even in problematic contexts such as relocations from the reservation to the city. But even here it was noted that 'the conflicts surrounding movement between cultures may be what brings them into counseling' (204). Early work often emphasized the need to find ways to alter Aboriginal values which inhibited acculturation. This was the emphasis of Bryde's (1971) work to some extent, and it was clearly articulated by Spang (1965: 13) when he wrote, 'How does one encourage an Indian student to become competitive when it is not in his value system to be so?' Later work reversed this pattern, emphasizing the need to enhance and restore Aboriginal values. French (1989: 161) has written that 'the therapeutic effort should be first and foremost the challenge of enhancing the client's Indianism' regardless of his/her actual cultural heritage or experience. Aboriginal values are inherent and need only to be coaxed out of remission.

A belief in the existence of authentic Aboriginal peoples and an authentic Aboriginal culture, an ethnographic 'pure product' (cf. Clifford 1988), is central to much of the work on Aboriginal values. Paniagua (1998: 76) bluntly advised counsellors to ask, 'Is the client an authentic Indian?' Authentic culture is located on the reservations, according to many commentators, and off-reservation Indians can be expected to suffer the most from value conflicts. For Anderson and Ellis (1995: 185), the reservation was 'the physical embodiment of the tribe and for an individual to leave the reservation that individual must, in a sense, reject the tribe and the values it represents.' Such individuals must adopt the values of the non-reservation world if they are to be successful, and this often leads to conflict and trauma. French (1981, 1989) has suggested that many 'marginal' Indians are still enveloped in the values surrounding the warrior ethos, and are still trying to 'count coup,' but in a contemporary sense: they drink, they fight, and they break the law because these are the only avenues open to them. 'The warrior psychology remains essentially the same,' but efforts to achieve that exulted status have been thwarted in today's society. Denied 'access to a significant rite of passage,' Indians acquire 'a dependent/adolescent status, regardless of their chronological age' (1989: 163).

For those Aboriginal clients who exhibit cultural orientations that are different from those of the clinician, the need to adapt counselling and psychotherapy is seen as a necessary precondition for successful treatment (Trimble & Fleming 1989). Darou (1987: 33), for example, simply stated that, 'To be effective, counselling [sic] must fit with certain Native values.' The failure to achieve this fit, he contended, would lead to 'a considerable amount of hostility' among clients. Sue and Sue (1990: 186) explained why: 'Much of what we do is based on Western values and influences.' The counsellor brings to the clinical encounter an expectation of normative and appropriate ethics, values, and behaviours based on his or her own culture. 'We expect clients to establish good eye contact, to discuss inner feelings, and to verbalize concerns.' 'American Indians,' they continued, 'will not display these behaviors.' In other words, Aboriginal peoples may not make good clients as defined by the therapist. Trimble and Fleming (1989: 191) suggested that a lack of solid grounding in American Indian values may contribute to 'identity problems' and 'feelings of marginality' that are brought into the clinic, and value conflicts between the American Indian and the Anglo-American cultures played out in the clinic are problematic. A value-free counselling environment, presumed to be typical of many conventional approaches, might need to be replaced with one in which certain 'traditional' values were asserted by the counsellor (LaFromboise et al. 1990: 633).

Two issues in particular have dominated discussions of conflict between Aboriginal clients and Western-trained clinicians and therapists. The first pertains to the cultural compatibility of the caregiver with the client, the second deals with the particular approach to therapy utilized. In each instance, appeals to Aboriginal values have been made to bolster claims for one position versus the other. It is to these issues I now turn.

The Issue of Counsellor Affinity

Should an Aboriginal person have an Aboriginal therapist? Is an Aboriginal therapist better positioned to be helpful and to understand an Aboriginal client than a non-Aboriginal therapist?[11] Much of the argument in favour of cultural affinity (or 'ethnic matching'; see Littlewood & Lipsedge 1997) between therapist and client is predicated on the assumption that Aboriginal peoples currently underutilize and avoid mental health services, a product of the alleged existence of differing value systems and negative experiences with non-Aboriginal counsellors (Sue & Sue 1977; Sue, Allan, & Conaway 1978; Dinges et al. 1981; Trimble et al. 1984; Trimble & Hayes 1984; Trimble & Fleming 1989; Trimble 1990; LaFromboise 1993; Manson 2000).[12]

The conviction that Aboriginal counsellors are more effective for Aboriginal clients exists almost as a matter of faith in much literature (e.g., Darou 1987; Dufrene & Coleman 1992; Herring 1992; Renfrey 1992; Brucker & Perry 1998). Richardson (1977: 13) argued axiomatically that 'Indians will trust a fellow Indian where they are naturally suspicious of the white professionals.' Much of the support for the affinity case comes from studies of therapist preference. Some, such as Ho (1987: 86) have simply asserted that 'American Indian families prefer American Indian workers.' An empirical study published in 1983 by Haviland, Horswill, O'Connell, and Dynneson, based on interviews with sixty-two Native American college students indicated that they expressed a 'strong preference for Native American counselors' (1983: 267). Johnson and Lashley (1989) employed a 'cultural commitment' scale in their work, and suggested that those 'with a strong commitment to the Native American culture place a greater importance on the ethnically similar counselor than do participants with a weaker commitment' (1989: 120). Similarly, Price and McNeill's (1992) study of eighty American Indian college students from forty-six tribes also utilized an instrument which measured 'cultural commitment,' and determined that those with the strongest commitment were most hesitant to make use of conventional counselling resources. The expression of preferences is very different from actual work with a therapist, of course. It is not necessarily indicative of therapeutic efficacy, and may constitute expressions of political or ethnic alliance which illuminate little about the therapeutic encounter. Even Haviland et al. (1983: 267) cautioned 'that indications of likely counseling center use do not necessarily mean students will actually seek counseling if they experience real-life problems of the sort described in this study.'[13]

Contradictory arguments on the question of therapist affinity have certainly been made, however, and the matter is far from resolved. Devereux (1942: 83) argued many years ago that Aboriginality per se was not important in understanding treatment effectiveness. It was his view that 'the fact that one is a Sioux Indian does not qualify one to do social work among the Navajo Indians,' and that putting a Sioux therapist on the Crow reservation, the Sioux's traditional enemies, would be folly. He also argued that working within one's own community created peculiar kinds of strains and problems. A study undertaken by LaFromboise, Dauphinais, and Rowe (1980), a survey of 150 Indian and 50 non-Indian high school students in Oklahoma, was discouraging for those promoting the 'culture-is-essential' perspective. They noted that 'the findings of this study fail to substantiate that it is perceived to be important that an effective helping person be professionally trained, be able to "analyze" people, be knowledgeable about personal cultural matters, or, even, be an Indian person' (1980: 15). Similarly, Lewis and Ho (1975: 382) warned that 'the Native American social worker [or therapist] who has assimilated the white man's culture to the extent that he no longer values his own culture could do more harm than good.' The effect of professional training on Aboriginal therapists, within the context of their supposed cultural affinity with Aboriginal clients, is underdeveloped in the literature. In 1981, Dinges et al. (271) concluded that 'there is precious little empirical basis for claims of superior therapeutic effectiveness of the Indian versus the non-Indian, or the interculturally trained versus the noninterculturally trained therapist.' By 1989, Trimble and Fleming (1989: 185) were cautioning that the literature was somewhat ambiguous, that while some argued that Indian counsellors were more likely to be effective, others were suggesting that characteristics such as 'warmth, genuineness, respect and empathy' were more important. Anderson and Ellis (1995) suggested that the American Indian client might be reluctant to openly disclose to a professional from the same community, for fear of a breach of confidentiality, and that a non-Indian counsellor might be preferred. As Kirmayer, Brass, and Tait (2000: 613) have recently reminded us, 'Aboriginal heritage is ... no guarantee that a professional will be culturally sensitive, both because of the diversity of traditions encountered and because of the implicit cultural values and assumptions of psychiatry' (613).

Individual and Group Approaches to Therapy

There is also a clear tension in the literature on the relative utility of individual versus group-oriented approaches to therapy; not surprisingly, the advocates for each have employed their own conceptualization of the essentialized Aboriginal to support their arguments. The common view in much contemporary psychological research, that societies can be characterized as either 'individualist' or 'collectivist' (Triandis 1996), or egocentric versus sociocentric, has been criticized by some anthropologists as too simplistic (Bock 2000). Nevertheless, it has retained considerable influence in psychology, and the notion that Aboriginal peoples were and remain inherently collectivist has clearly had an impact on the forms of treatment deemed appropriate.

Recalling that a strong extended family orientation is considered a core Aboriginal value by many, it is not surprising that family therapy has received considerable attention (Tafoya 1989; Marín & Gamba 2003). Sutton and Broken Nose (1996: 33) stated boldly that 'The Indian Way consists of families working together to solve problems' [capitalization original]. Paniagua (1998: 81) has even suggested that 'among the American Indians, the extended family has primacy; the self is secondary ... The family and the group take precedence over the individual.' Families, especially those considered more traditional, tend to keep their problems within their bounds, according to Trimble and Fleming (1989), and therefore family approaches to therapy make sense (see also Lewis & Ho 1975; Atkinson, Morten & Sue 1993; Peregoy 1993). LaFromboise et al.'s (1990) articulation of network therapy similarly suggested that the family network, involving upwards of forty to seventy people, emphasizes the historic use of consensus in decision making among American Indians (see also Attneave 1969). LaFromboise and Jackson (1996) would include as part of this network not just family members but 'respected community leaders, traditional leaders [and] elders.' Family therapy is particularly appropriate because it is deemed to mimic more traditional Aboriginal healing approaches in which the healers were often family members (Brucker & Perry 1998).

It is easy to agree with Trimble's (1992) assertion that psychotherapeutic intervention in Aboriginal communities cannot focus solely on individuals; family and community influences are too strong. But one potential problem with family therapy approaches is the fact that many Aboriginal families are considered to be dysfunctional. 'Family function,' Red Horse has cautioned (1980: 466), 'should not be taken for granted.' Attneave (1969: 196) acknowledged the existence of 'socially deteriorating and disorganized tribes' in her discussion of network therapy, concluding that pathologies may be perpetuated by existing social structures. She described the case of one individual, a key member of an extended family network wracked with episodes of murder, suicide, and assault, who was himself suffering from depression and was suicidal. Paniagua (1998: 88), touching only briefly on this, noted that the therapist in such circumstances needs to work with the family first to ensure 'basic needs' are being met before therapy can proceed. Topper and Curtis (1987: 341) have gone so far as to suggest that 'the extended family can also be manipulated by the patient, and vice versa, to create a long-standing pattern of pathological maladaptation.' Much of the literature on Aboriginal family therapy seems to eschew these warnings, preferring an Arcadian model of the fully functioning, harmonious and traditional Aboriginal family.

Group therapy is different from family and network approaches in that all members of the group themselves have identified psychopathology for which they are being treated, and rarely are those members related. There was a time when group therapy approaches were deemed to be too culturally inappropriate to be useful with Aboriginal clients (Neligh 1988). Underscoring this viewpoint was the blind acceptance of Aboriginal ethics, values, and behaviours which worked against the demands of the group therapy process: Aboriginal peoples were stoic, silent, shy, humble, and reluctant to talk about themselves, especially with strangers; and the ethic of non-interference would prevent them from interacting with others in the group (Archibald 1974; Manson, Walker, & Kivlahan 1987). Some still argue for the inappropriateness of group therapy (e.g., Reimer 1999 for Inupiat).

Others have suggested that group approaches are particularly well-suited to Aboriginal peoples, because of their traditional, collectivist philosophy (expressed, for example, through group decision making), an ethos that the group (i.e., tribe or family) is more important than the individual, and a view of traditional Aboriginal healing that involved individuals other than patient and healer (Lewis & Ho 1975; Edwards & Edwards 1980; Manson et al. 1987; Ashby, Gilchrist, & Miramontez 1987; Peregoy 1993; LaFromboise & Jackson 1996; Trimble et al. 1996; Dillard & Manson 2000). Neligh, Baron, Braun, and Czarnecki (1990) have pointed out the apparent similarity between group approaches to traditional healing characteristic of many American Indian societies and conventional group therapy processes. In essence, an appeal to cultural tradition has often been made. Gustafson (1976), in a study of Plains Indians in Wyoming and Montana, for instance, argued that these individuals did not seek out individual therapy because they felt a need to transcend the ego and connect with the community. Edwards and Edwards (1984: 7) argued that, for the treatment of alcohol abuse, group approaches had become 'the treatment of choice for a number of agencies with programs serving American Indians.' Manson et al. (1987) and Neligh (1988) have also suggested that there has been a productive increase in the use of group therapy approaches, especially in the area of alcohol treatment. Collective approaches to treatment are seen as important in lifting direct blame from the shoulders of the individual and recentring the troubled person in a community as a socially responsible being (LaFromboise 1993; Waldram 1997).

Assessing the utility of group therapy approaches is difficult given the lack of clarity in the literature on key variables. Frequently missing are clear descriptions of the purposes and constituents of groups (in the case of the latter, gender and cultural background are examples), the political-legal context (e.g., whether participants are voluntarily undergoing treatment or whether it has been mandated), the racial and cultural backgrounds of the therapists leading the groups, and the values and lessons being communicated. Implicit assumptions that the Aboriginal participants are culturally homogeneous or that cultural differences are not relevant are apparent though rarely detailed.

The composition of the groups themselves is obviously important. Several researchers have described problems in the group process that were related to the differing cultural backgrounds of participants (Wolman 1970; McDonald 1975; French 1989; Waldram & Wong 1995). The cultural background of the therapist leading the group is also an issue. Some (Koverola 1992; Paniagua 1998) have suggested that, where a non-Aboriginal person is the group leader, an Aboriginal co-therapist be brought in, particularly to introduce a cultural component. The integration of Aboriginal history, culture, and approaches to therapy into group experiences is frequently advocated though rarely analysed (e.g. Weibel-Orlando 1987; Dufrene & Coleman 1992; Waldram & Wong 1995; Trimble et al. 1996; Waldram 1997; Paniagua 1998). Descriptions of community-based programs exist (e.g., Wolman 1970 with Navajo, Kahn, Lewis, and Galvez 1974 with Papago), and the most effective would appear to be those involving all-Aboriginal participants linked to singular communities, where there is increased likelihood that participants will share a common language and history. But, even here, the relative cultural homogeneity does not eliminate problems, as Kahn et al. (1974) found with Papago adolescents who were reluctant to speak openly in front of their peers about many topics. Anonymity and confidentiality evaporate with familiarity in group contexts.

Those advocating for individualist approaches to treatment base their arguments on the the same fertile soil of essentialized Aboriginal and non-Aboriginal culture as the collectivists employ but they have called upon their own Aboriginal to offer a contrasting position. Edwards and

Edwards (1980: 503) have written that, 'because of the Indian's belief in the value of individuality, some of them will consider it inappropriate to discuss the problems of other members of their families in meetings with social workers.' 'The value of individuality,' they suggested, 'also dictates to some Indians that they must resolve individual problems on their own' (503). Many of the scholars cited above have attested to the trait values of individual autonomy and non-interference. Kline and Roberts (1973: 864) have applied to this the primitivist-sounding label 'psycho-social nomadism,' and the legacy of the construct of the atomistic, hyper-individual Aboriginal of psychological anthropology looms large. But the individualists remain a clear minority in the discourse and are accused of promoting an oppressive, culturally inappropriate model. Collectivists like LaFromboise and Jackson (1996: 195) have continued to argue that, 'unlike the Eurocentric value placed on individualism, in many American Indian tribes, identity is not defined apart from the group but rather in relation to community, family, or clan.' Similarly, LaFromboise et al. (1993: 148) argued that 'there is considerable evidence to support the view that counseling services designed around a conventional individual therapy regime are indeed inappropriate for service deliveries in Indian communities.' Treatment, therefore, should extend beyond the one-on-one relationship of therapist to client to include 'respected community leaders, traditional leaders, and elders and larger social units such as the extended family and other relevant groups' (195). LaFromboise et al. (1990: 639) have criticized therapies which emphasize 'one-on-one interaction, outside the context of family and community,' and Paniagua (1994, 1998) has suggested that individual-oriented therapy may conflict with family and tribal goals and hence cause disharmony.

There is also disagreement over the use of directive versus non-directive approaches in individual psychotherapy. Herring (1990: 136), for instance, argued that 'Many Native Americans do not respond sincerely or voluntarily to nondirective leadership.' Spang (1965), Trimble (1976), Dillard (1983), and Tafoya (1989) have also argued in favour of directive approaches. Others, such as Koverola (1992), Herring (1992), and Paniagua (1994), disagree. Koverola (1992: 350) likened directive approaches to broader colonial processes in which non-Aboriginal ways have been imposed on Aboriginal peoples; directive approaches, to her mind, represent another form of oppression. LaFromboise et al. (1990) would concur. Lewis and Ho (1975) have suggested that a major stumbling block to the utilization of directive approaches is the traditional value of non-interference. Richardson (1981: 239) straddled the fence on this issue, arguing in his characteristically forthright prose that 'Prodding and slapping around the American Indian to motivate him or her does not work.' He added, however, a 'caution that a completely permissive atmosphere is interpreted by the American Indian as another write-off.' 'The Indian,' he concluded, 'expects direction.'

For Sue and Sue (1990: 187) the disagreement over directive and non-directive approaches is in part a 'matter of timing.' 'American Indians cannot be expected to talk about issues in a meaningful manner until trust has developed,' they suggested. The issue is more fundamental than that, however. Clearly there is a more basic conflict within the literature centred on questions of essentialized Aboriginal culture. One perspective argues that Aboriginal peoples require direction; the other suggests that an active therapeutic approach will be rejected as an external cultural imposition, or because it violates the value of non-interference. Both arguments are based on faulty assumptions regarding the uniformity of Aboriginal cultures in the contemporary context.

Assertions about the usefulness of individualist or collectivist approaches to mental health treatment are rarely grounded in empirical research. Rather, most are based on predetermined assumptions with respect to Aboriginal cultures and individuals as they exist today. Trimble and Fleming (1989: 196) have argued that 'an Indian client's responsiveness to counseling is not necessarily a function of where he or she was raised,' but 'rather it would appear that the acculturation of the client is a potent contributor to a client's receptivity to counseling in a conventional sense.' Sue and Sue (2003) recently reminded us that many American Indians adhere to 'mainstream,' as opposed to Indian, values. The actual cultural orientation of the individual, however, is frequently lost despite the attention devoted to developing both cultural competence among therapists and culturally appropriate approaches for Aboriginal clients. How easily is this lost? Very easily. Attneave (1982: 57) has written that 'Probably 50 per cent of the [American Indian] cases that arrive on the therapist's doorstep will be well-educated, typically middle-class people with similar problems and similar attitudes as the rest of their clientele. The underlying racial and cultural characteristics make no more or no less difference than those of a migrant family of any type that has acculturated itself to the United States for several generations.' But then, ignoring her own insight, she proceeded to present readers with a table contrasting 'Traditional Cultural Value Preferences for U.S. Middle-Class' with 'American Indian/Alaska Native Populations' (63), 'based on traditional values as observed and discussed in about 50 tribal groups,' without being more specific. According to Dillard and Manson (2000: 243), 'Given the lack of outcome studies with this population as well as considerable diversity between and within tribes and groups, it is not surprising definitive guidance is lacking in regard to effectiveness of one treatment approach over another.' Indeed, why should the question of a single approach for such a diverse population be an issue at all?

Conclusion

Assertions that there are core, essential Aboriginal ethics, values, and behaviours, resistant to change and sometimes buried deep within the Aboriginal psyche, are pervasive, yet the empirical base for these assertions is uniformly weak. While the attempt to locate Aboriginal culture, and to bring culture into the clinic, is certainly laudable, the difficulties in operationalizing the concept have clearly confounded scholars and clinicians. Much of the literature cautions against over-generalizations and stereotypes, yet these cautions are typically followed by detailed lists of generalized Aboriginal traits which clinicians are to consider carefully in order to provide culturally competent care. So, while Dillard and Manson (2000: 245) have warned that 'the current state of knowledge as well as the diversity among Indians and Natives currently preclude a "standard" approach to assessment or treatment,' most of the guides and handbooks designed to assist clinicians consistently present stereotypical lists, including Dillard and Manson! What can the clinician take away from such material if not recollections of neatly packaged ethics, values, and behaviours to be invoked at the moment an Aboriginal patient walks into the office?

There is also considerable confusion in the literature on the nature of ethics, values, and behaviours, and the relationship between the three is not well developed. The values underlying actual behaviour may be very different from those endorsed in research. Anthropologists Bradd Shore (1996) and Charles Nuckolls (1998) have theorized these concepts in a manner that lends important insight to the work presented in this chapter. They have argued that societies characteristically contain sets of competing, conflicting, and even dialectically contradictory values, and these are often activated in specific contexts. Value expectations for individuals may change over their lifetime, and individuals may occupy culturally sanctioned roles which promote specific values over others, or exhibit conflicting values. Nuckolls believes that cultures are deliberately ambivalent with respect to values, and Shore

(1996: 304) has written that 'culture can orchestrate alternative justifications for contradictory positions to be invoked by competing interest groups or by a single group on different occasions.' Furthermore, Shore (1996: 305–6) makes the crucial distinction between 'private and subjective experience' in the expression of values, which 'is apt to be experienced as ambivalent and ambiguous,' and their 'public representation,' which 'is more likely to be framed as categorical and absolute.' Finally, Shore (1996: 286) has noted that 'Societies seem to reveal their value systems most clearly to outsiders when these values are represented as coherent models that contrast maximally with the ethical models of another society.'

There are several basic reasons why Aboriginal values have been presented as 'categorical and absolute' despite evidence of extensive ambivalence, ambiguity, and contradiction. First, the values are clearly charged with post-colonial political symbolism, in that they purport to contrast Aboriginal peoples with the colonizers. In this sense they are culturally constructed, but in a purposeful way to deal with contemporary realities, and Aboriginal peoples, including Aboriginal scholars, have played an active role in promoting them. Second, our discussion of primitivist discourse suggests strongly the need for non-Aboriginal peoples to construct, for Aboriginal peoples, a finite set of ethics, values, and behaviours that contrast maximally with those purported to characterize the decaying, decadent Western lifestyle. Third, such stereotyping makes it easier, in the minds of therapists (and the public), to deal with the complexity of culture in general, and Aboriginal cultures in particular. Ethics, values, and behaviours are particularly amenable to superficial operationalization in cross-cultural research, and therefore to the exaggeration and stereotyping of difference. Simply put, culture, when operationalized in terms of values, is easy to investigate; by extension, this version of culture, especially for the cultural others, is easy for clinicians to learn. But as this chapter demonstrates, the attempt to become culturally sensitive, especially within the clinical setting and within the context of the therapeutic relationship, has led inevitably down the dead-end road of quick-fix cultural handbooks that perpetuate stereotypical values and behaviours and serve only to cement the culturally different client in a fully constructed cultural quicksand.[14] As I said earlier in this chapter, and with a nod to Foucault, such a constructed Aboriginal individual appears to be everywhere, and yet nowhere.

CHAPTER ELEVEN

Healing the Traditional Aboriginal

I should like to show with a few curious examples that among primitive mankind a surprisingly deep understanding is possessed for the hidden meaning of certain manifestations. His unconscious hears and understands here with sensitive ear the for-help-calling voice of the unconscious of suffering persons, and equally discovers in a sensitive and instinctive manner exactly proportioned psychotherapeutic precautions. (Pfister 1932: 234)

Historically, Native Americans had a limited range of labels for causes of distress. (Dana 1993: 86)

Two quotations some sixty years apart. One suggests the existence of individuals capable of astounding therapeutic insight, both 'sensitive and instinctive,' reflective of well-developed, complex psychomedical thought tinged with a primal intuitivism. The other posits the opposite, suggesting an intellectual simplicity that frequently characterizes notions of the 'primitive.' How do we make sense of this?

In this chapter, my aim is to examine critically how scientific conceptions of Aboriginal conceptions of mental health, illness, and 'healing' have been constructed. I will do this in several ways. First, I will explore Aboriginal theories of mental health and illness as they have been articulated by scholars. Then I will examine the argument that, unlike the Westerner, in whom mind/body dualism is axiomatic, the Aboriginal is holistic in approach to mental and physical health. Aboriginal understandings of mind and body, health and illness, order and disorder will be critically examined. Finally, I will turn my attention to the contemporary uses of culture, tradition, and 'healing' in selected treatment programs. My basic argument here is twofold: that Aboriginal thought, as demonstrated in the literature, appears considerably more complex than the holism paradigm would suggest, and that when operationalizing 'traditional Aboriginal healing' in a contemporary context, little attention has been paid to comprehending precisely what 'Aboriginal,' 'traditional,' and 'healing' actually mean.

Aboriginal Theories of Mental Health and Illness

A fairly defined and limited set of medical 'beliefs' is said to be characteristic of most Aboriginal groups. That this idea has underscored discussions of non-Western peoples is evident from attempts to develop globally relevant conceptual categories. The most influential early attempt was that of Forrest Clements (1932), who offered a pioneering scheme of global theories of disease causation which included eighty-nine Aboriginal groups from Canada and the United States.[1] Utilizing ethnographic and historical sources, Clements generated five categories of causation that would prove to have great resilience: sorcery, breach of taboo, disease-object intrusion, spirit intrusion, and soul loss. Clements only rarely made mention of specific psychiatric conditions in his work, although he occasionally offered the insight that many societies thought of mental problems as somehow separate from physical ones.[2] Spirit intrusion, as an example, was suggested to be a cause of insanity among the eastern Cree, and 'mental suggestion' was considered to be important in both causing sickness and effecting cure among many societies (191). But one must work hard to tease these data from Clements's presentation. The casual reader is left with the overall impression that the mental and the physical were not meaningfully separate in the illness world-views of the globe's 'primitive' peoples. This would prove to have an enduring legacy.

After the publication of Clements's (1932) schema, several critiques emerged. Hallowell (1935) was perhaps the first out of the gate, arguing that Clement's categories were too broad and noting his uncritical use of sources and his failure to take into account intracultural variation within the sampled societies (likely, in part, the product of the data sources themselves). Hallowell also stated that he had never found among the Saulteaux a belief that spirit possession caused insanity, thereby committing the same fallacy as Clements (i.e., believing that any singular study proved the presence or absence of a trait).

Rogers (1944) argued that the five categories were 'neither mutually exclusive nor parallel in significance' and that Clements failed to note that dreams were a common cause of sickness among many of the peoples in his sample.

Despite these critiques, which were more concerned with fine-tuning than outright rejection, Clements's (1932) ideas persisted and made their way into many introductory anthropology textbooks as explanations for how 'primitives' thought about health and disease. George Murdock (1980), a leader in cross-cultural ethnographic research, undertook a reanalysis of sorts, using a better organized database and including some twenty-two Aboriginal societies from Canada and the United States. The Human Relations Area Files, a collection of global ethnographic texts organized by theme, allowed Murdock to produce a more sophisticated schema, but one which still included many of Clements's basic categories, such as soul loss and object intrusion. As recently as 1996, one renowned anthropologist still employed Clements's work to argue that while 'non-Western disease constructs and treatment techniques also include "empirical" causes ... critical weight is given to transempirical causative factors' (Hughes 1996: 136).

Clements's (1932) and Murdock's (1980) work also served as the foundation for another influential work on conceptualizations of Aboriginal sickness in Canada and the United States, a seminal article by Trimble, Manson, Dinges, & Medicine (1984). In their examination of indigenous notions of mental health, they focused on six 'tribal-specific' concepts of disorder: windigo psychosis, *pibloktoq*, ghost sickness, soul loss, spirit intrusion, and taboo breaking. The first three, as we have seen in the earlier discussion of culture-bound syndromes, remain problematic; the remaining three demonstrate an intellectual debt to the work of Clements. The authors went to some length to stress that each of these conditions represented an external, even biased, view that was not entirely informed by the specific sociocultural context in which they were found, that they were not necessarily characteristic of other Aboriginal groups, and that Aboriginal societies in which they were found were undergoing cultural changes, including a trend towards an emerging pan-Indianism. These were solid critiques, and, absolutely necessary to place these six in context. Why, then, were these indigenous notions presented at all, given these caveats? Unfortunately, many subsequent commentators used Trimble et al. (1984) as authoritative, while failing to mention the limitations cited. And these ideas diffused throughout the literature over time to the extent that they came to be characteristic of virtually all Aboriginal societies, even within the contemporary context (e.g., Neligh 1988; Renfrey 1992; Dana 1993; Trimble & Medicine 1993).

The role of the spiritual or supernatural in understandings of sickness may inadvertently have been exaggerated in much work, as is commonly done in most treatises on Aboriginal healing (which tend to ignore more pedestrian and less exotic theories of natural causation and practical treatment strategies, such as splinting broken bones and suturing wounds). Some took the basic ideas to an extreme, arguing, as did Miles (1967: 430), that 'the primitives saw all disease, from furuncle to psychosis, essentially as the manifestation of a single etiological agent - the supernatural.' Miles's perspective, surprisingly, is not that dated, and the sentiment has persisted.[3]

These etiological explanations were appealing because they characterized the primitives' propensity for 'magical' thinking, what the West would decry as non-positivist and irrational thinking. Many years ago, anthropologist A.L. Kroeber (1923), exhibiting long-standing Victorian attitudes, characterized entire societies according to the extent to which they employed magic and superstition as explanatory factors; the more these factors were employed, the more 'primitive' the society. Civilized societies, he argued, no longer held such beliefs, although individuals within such societies might. Reflecting a recognizable theme, these deviant Western individuals were those 'whose social fortune is backward or who are psychotic, mentally deteriorated, or otherwise subnormal' (298).[4] Employing the metaphor of societies as stages of human development that we touched upon in an earlier chapter, Kroeber, like Freud, suggested that advanced, more civilized cultures were 'psychologically more adult,' and 'primitive' or, in his words 'retarded' cultures, were more 'infantile' (301). These were harsh observations, to be sure, laden with the language of the cultural evolutionism that ruled in Kroeber's day. The fact that 'civilized' people could believe in 'God' and not be accused of magical thinking was only one of several obvious contradictions. But, as I noted earlier, surprisingly similar language surfaced decades later in DSM-III in 1980, and again in DSM-III-R in 1987, where 'magical thinking' as a pathological condition was said to be characteristic of schizophrenics, children, and 'primitive' peoples (American Psychiatric Association 1980, 1987).[5] Underlying the suggestion that Aboriginal peoples' medical and psychological thought was based on a foundation of magic, superstition or, more generously, spirituality, was a parallel view that

Aboriginal societies did not distinguish between mind and body, what I refer to as the 'holism thesis.

The Holistic Aboriginal

The belief that Aboriginal North Americans were, and remain, a 'holistic' people is widespread and tenacious. We saw earlier that 'holism' has been pegged as a core value for Aboriginal peoples, said to characterize them in a way that suggests a world-view very different from that of Europeans. This idea is represented in the literature by the argument that Aboriginal peoples believed, and still believe, that the mind and the body, as well as extra-body entities such as the environment, society, and the cosmos, exist as an integrated whole, a system that is simultaneously physical and metaphysical. Ronald Lewis (1980: 458) succinctly defined this view: 'Their [Native Americans] basic orientation toward mental health and physical health (which are not seen as separate entities) is the reflection of an unseen harmony between an individual and his environment. It includes three areas: the natural living world, relationships with fellow human beings, and the mystical. Mental illness indicates an imbalance between man and any of the three above areas or all of the above areas (Native Americans approach this matter in an holistic manner).'

Silver and Wilson (1988: 340) expressed the same view: '... American Indians do not separate religion from psychology, and within the psychological healing practices, there is no separation of body and mind. Further, American Indian psychology tends to blend cognitive, emotion, behavioral and existential orientations. If nothing else, it is a holistic and integrated approach to understanding behavior.' Such a view is, more generally, said to be characteristic of 'primitive' peoples. Ackerknecht (1943: 60), for instance, suggested that 'the primitive not only in his medical concepts does not separate diseases of the body and the mind, but also does not produce such disparate units,' adding that researchers may well have missed this connection between 'body ailments' and 'mental elements' in their work. Morley (1978: 16) argued that 'in traditional societies medical knowledge is far more closely integrated with the institutions and all encompassing cosmology of the society as a whole than is the case in more differentiated industrial societies.' Price-Williams (1975: 87) more broadly argued for 'the fact that in cultures other than our own, psychotherapy is marked by a unity of the medical, the psychological and the spiritual.' Hughes

(1996: 136) would concur, arguing that 'overwhelmingly non-Western, indigenous medical systems – those not based on Western science–derived concepts and techniques – are holistic in scope. Not for them the seductive Cartesian division between body and mind.' Trimble et al. (1984: 201), respected scholars of American Indian mental health, spoke broadly of the philosophical perspective of many American Indians, in which 'subject and object are unified and holistic.' 'States of mind and body, social roles, family and community, and the like,' they added, 'are functionally interrelated and virtually inseparable.' Aboriginals are, one might conclude, both spiritually and secularly 'collectivist.'

It has so commonly been asserted that religion, psychology, and medicine are intertwined and inseparable among Aboriginal peoples that assertions of holism occur like a mantra (Locust 1988; Silver & Wilson 1988). Fleming (1992: 160) has provided a succinct set of statements which characterize this mantra: 'Illness affects the mind and spirit as well as the body'; 'Wellness is harmony in the body, mind, and spirit'; and 'Unwellness is disharmony in body, mind and spirit.' Jilek-Aall (1976: 355; see also Jilek 1978, Jilek & Jilek-Aall 1978) argued boldly and unequivocally that the 'non-western patient,' including both Coast Salish and Navajo, makes 'no essential distinction ... between physical and mental illness,' in contrast to the western psychiatrist who conceptualizes these as distinct entities. This viewpoint has been reiterated over the years largely without question (e.g., Silver & Wilson 1988; Abbott 1998). Duran and Duran (1995: 15) were similarly unequivocal. 'In Western experience,' they wrote, 'it is common to separate the mind from the body and spirit and the spirit from mind and body.' 'Within the Native American worldview,' they continued, 'this is a foreign idea.' Among the Navajo, Csordas (2000: 463) has recently asserted, 'religion and spirituality are intimately entwined' with healing. This fact is seen as an extension of the holism thesis, an epistemological point which establishes an essential, and I would argue essentialized, distinction between Aboriginal peoples and European settlers of this continent.

The discourse of holism is rooted in a perceived, and constructed, dichotomy between European and Aboriginal thought. While this dichotomy has often been employed to argue for a view of 'primitives' as intellectually inferior to Westerners, it has also fuelled notions that these peoples remain privy to a pristine mode of thought which has been distorted, corrupted, and even destroyed by Western civilization.

Table 11.1
Jilek-Aall's (1976) 'Classical Western Psychiatrist' and 'Non-Western Patient'
(selected items)

Classical Western Psychiatrist	Non-Western Patient
Inner-directed orientation	Tradition-directed orientation
Belief in individual solutions	Belief in collective solutions
Intrapsychic conflicts seen as most relevant	Extrapsychic (social) conflicts seen as most relevant
Emphasis on scientific knowledge (rational)	Emphasis on magic knowledge (arational but not irrational)
Disease primarily seen as phenomenon of nature, devoid of moral implications	Disease frequently seen as phenomenon of the supernatural, full of moral implications
Physical and mental illness seen as distinct entities	No essential distinction made between physical and mental illness
Treatment viewed as 'profane' and 'scientific'	Treatment seen as 'sacred' and 'magic'
Tendency to explain the incomprehensible by psychopathology	Tendency to explain the incomprehensible by supernatural powers

The intellectual heritage of this discourse of dichotomy has influenced how some scholars perceive 'primitive' populations even today. It is found, for instance, in the suggestion that despite centuries of cultural change these primal, even instinctive, abilities to connect with the metaphysical realm remain innately embedded within the Aboriginal. Jilek-Aall (1976: 355) exemplified this belief in her presentation of a comparative listing of traits of the 'Classical Western psychiatrist' and the 'Non-Western patient,' a list which was based to a large extent on her research and clinical work with Coast Salish. Some of the items in her list are presented in Table 11.1.

This dichotomous perspective received a revitalizing boost when anthropologist C.R. Hallpike (1979) published *The Foundations of Primitive Thought*, a throwback to early-twentieth-century ruminations on the nature of uncivilized man. In a volume which was soundly criticized by other anthropologists (Shweder 1982) as well as psychologists (Jahoda 1982), Hallpike (1979: 491) synthesized earlier thought on the mind of the 'primitive' and presented a list of traits contrasting the 'rational' with the 'non-rational' mind. While several of the items in his list of non-rational traits were suggested to be characteristic of 'an educated and intelligent member of our society' as well, the majority distinguished the 'primitive' from the 'civilized,' including the following:

Rational (i.e., 'Civilized')	Non-rational (i.e., 'Primitive')
sanity	insanity/absurdity
wisdom	folly
objectivity	subjectivity
articulate	inarticulate
discussion	violence

Hallpike's schema was built on an intellectual tradition which had pervaded all aspects of social thought for a very long time, and it found its way into the Aboriginal mental health discourse with relative ease.

The tendency to view Aboriginal peoples and Europeans in terms of contrasts or opposites invariably led to the construction of certain fixed, essentialized images which were considerably more dogmatic than they were empirical. These contrasts were also secured in a timeless present, as if not only had neither society experienced any cultural change, but, more importantly, they had also never contacted or influenced each other. And, as dogma, they required only assertion, not investigation. This is seen clearly in the recent special issue of *Medical Anthropology Quarterly* on Navajo healing, in which Begay and Maryboy (2000) employed the concepts of 'holism' and 'wholeness' no fewer than nine times in just one section of the paper. A mantra indeed.

Re-opening the Mind/Body Debate

Are Aboriginal North Americans really holistic? More specifically, are mind and body, the mental and physical, truly an integrated whole within Aboriginal thought? When we look closely at the ethnographic data in particular, we discover a great deal of evidence that, if it does not challenge the holism perspective directly, certainly undermines its pivotal position in the mental health discourse.

The question of the cultural relativity of notions of normality and abnormality was raised very early in the twentieth century by individuals such as Ruth Benedict (1934a), who, we saw in an earlier chapter, built extensive theory on culture and personality upon her work with

American Indian groups. Devereux (1940, 1942), in his work with the Mohave, argued that 'primitive' peoples certainly conceptualized abnormality and pathology, although these conditions were culturally constructed and not necessarily compatible with Western understandings. His work on Mohave 'ethnopsychiatry' was pioneering and certainly among the most comprehensive. Devereux presented detailed evidence of various Mohave psychiatric and psychological states, including some very esoteric ones, such as '*Hiwa:Itck*,' or 'heartbreak,' which was characterized by psychotic episodes and which referred specifically to a condition of older men whose younger wives had left them. Insanity was seen by the Mohave as a serious problem, Devereux argued, and they had a variety of practices designed to eliminate this condition. Devereux (1969: 490) believed that the Mohave had the ability to distinguish between 'the psychiatric sequelae of organic illness and the organic sequelae of psychiatric illness,' even though they had not developed an explicit theory of psychopathology. Likewise, in a history of Aboriginal and western medicine in Canada, Margetts (1975: 404) argued that 'all indian [sic] and eskimo [sic] tribes have equivalent or descriptive names for discrete mental illnesses such as "madness," "confusion," "epilepsy," etc., and they have crude nomenclatures.' Is it true, then, as Dana (1993: 86) asserted in the opening quotation of this chapter, that Aboriginal peoples were characterized by a simplistic understanding of mental phenomena?

The Navajo, as perhaps the most researched and documented Aboriginal North American group, have provided much evidence of psychiatric sophistication. Kaplan and Johnson (1964: 207) noted that traditional Navajo medical treatments often concentrated on the specific, afflicted body parts, implying a capacity to focus on and differentiate the part from the whole. They also commented that there was 'an astonishing variety of recognized causes of mental illness among the Navajos,' and while noting that many of the Navajo theories of illness were equally applicable to mental and physical conditions, there remained 'a large number of quite specific behaviors that lead to mental illness,' especially where the illness was a consequence of bad or inappropriate behaviour. For example, 'moth craziness' was caused by brother-sister incest: it was believed that a moth entered the body and, by flying about, caused 'crazy' behaviour. Luckert (1972: 96) argued that many Navajo ceremonies were 'cures for anti-social tendencies,' perhaps personality disorders in current DSM language, and 'that their varying symbolism reflects various forms of the mild or serious neuroses produced by family life.' Levy, Neutra, and Parker (1987) provided a more detailed study of 'moth madness' and other Navajo mental disorders, and they noted a tendency to somatize disorders which had as their origin, or were related to, the mind. Navajos, they suggested, exhibited a reluctance to talk about mental conditions, preferring instead to indicate physical disorders. 'The mind is thought to control the body,' they have written, and 'weakness of the body implies a mental disturbance' (95). Hence, they concluded that the fact 'that Navajos find it preferable to refer to somatic symptoms suggests that the interaction between mind and body is not reciprocal but that the mind takes precedence' (95). They determined that Navajos distinguished depressed individuals from those suffering from other problems, making a distinction between emotion and intellect. The Mountainway healing ceremony, according to these authors, was particularly useful in the treatment of anxiety, nervousness, delirium, and insanity, while the Evilway ceremony was employed in the treatment of depression.

The Inuit data are equally compelling. Murphy and Leighton (1965: 79; see also Murphy 1964), accepting Clements's (1932) schema, argued that Eskimos viewed insanity as caused by spirit intrusion, and that while there seemed to be no equivalent in Inuktitut for 'psychiatry,' 'they have notions about a variety of behaviors, emotional states, and thinking patterns which they recognize as "something being wrong" and which they clearly distinguish from purely organic disorders.' Furthermore, they suggested quite clearly that 'the two elements,' mind and body, 'were at times conceived separately' from each other (80). Disorders recognized by biomedicine as psychiatric were described by Eskimos as either 'psychologically expressed,' such as those having to do with personality characteristics (e.g., what the Eskimos called 'out of mind' or 'too much nervous'), or 'psychologically derived,' those having to do with physical sensations or mood disturbances (e.g., 'heart beating too hard' caused by 'too much worry') (80–1). Murphy (1964) continued the analysis by arguing that, within the contemporary context of her research, the Eskimos sought out physicians for physical problems but the shamans for psychiatric ones. Vallee (1966: 58), in a description of eastern Arctic Eskimo theories of mental illness, suggested that these people had Inuktitut glosses for such English terms as 'crazy as a loon' and 'simpleton,' and even a gloss for mental illness: 'niaqureriyuq,' or 'he has illness of the head.' He also found terms approximating epilepsy, extreme sadness, and depression. Jean Briggs (1970), in her classic study of Eskimo emotional life in northern Canada, demonstrated the complexity of Eskimo thought through linguistic analysis. These Eskimo utilized a term, *ihuma*, or 'reason' as she glossed it, to 'refer to all functions that we think of as cerebral: mind, thought, memory, reason, sense, ideas, will' (359). Ihuma could disappear in individuals, resulting in 'sick people who are unconscious or delirious, unaware of their surroundings,' as well as insane or psychotic behaviour, all caused by the intrusion of evil spirits (362). Alternatively, having 'too much *ihuma*' was also a problem, as it could result in prolonged anger or brooding (362). Briggs also identified at least three different types of loneliness recognized by her informants.

Kirmayer et al. (1997) presented a somewhat different, though no less intriguing, picture of the Inuit. While arguing, in contrast to Vallee (1966), that there was no Inuktitut equivalent for 'mental illness,' these authors did determine that two terms were used to describe mental problems. The first one glossed as 'too much thinking,' 'having heavy thoughts,' and 'being worried,' and described, in the authors terms, mild to moderate forms of depressed or anxious mood. The second term described more severe problems and glossed as 'crazy' or 'doesn't know what's going on around him,' generally indicating an inability to think properly (32). Kirmayer et al. (1997) also uncovered a term for 'going crazy,' as well as a class of unnamed disorders recognized by the Inuit, which looked to the researchers to be similar to personality disorders. Depression was viewed as a mental problem, although not necessarily an illness, while mental retardation and seizures were viewed as physical problems. Despite the existence of these terms and recognition of these conditions, however, the Inuit did not view mental health and illness in terms of a system of classification and categories, but rather as lived, somewhat individualistic experiences. Nevertheless, Kirmayer et al. (1997: 65) noted that the evidence supported a notion of an Inuit 'ethnopsychological model of the workings of the mind (*isuma*) as the cause of emotional and behavioral problems.'

Another kind of distinction in states of illness has also been identified for several specific Aboriginal groups; this distinction identifies certain problems as having their genesis exclusively within either the Aboriginal or non-Aboriginal population, a dichotomy that is clearly a reaction to colonialism. Jilek (1982) described spirit sickness among the Coast Salish as an 'Indian sickness' which afflicted only the Indians and which only they could treat. Linda Garro (1990) documented the distinction between 'Anishinaabe' (Ojibwa) and 'Whiteman' sickness in a Manitoba Indian community, and noted that a behaviour pattern characterized by 'acting abnormally/crazy' was an Anishinaabe sickness, thereby implying that it predated colonization. Adelson (2000) has noted among the James Bay Cree a similar propensity to distinguish Cree sickness from Whiteman's sickness. Adelson goes further than Garro in suggesting that the Cree see the genesis of 'Whiteman's' sickness in the process of colonization, which reflects the development of 'Whiteman' as a metaphor for a whole range of negative consequences, from environmental disruption to political oppression. Berry and Bennett (1992), also working with the Cree, solicited words in their language for items like 'stupid,' 'crazy,' and 'backwards knowledge,' and came up with terms that were semantically close to the Cree words for 'Whiteman'! The existence of categories of 'white' sicknesses within Aboriginal thought suggests that much of the recent discourse on holism (and all the evidence seems to suggest that 'holism' as an Aboriginal concept is a post-1960s creation) can be related to ideas of contact, cultural change, and oppression. It is possible, in other words, that the concept of holism has been embraced by many Aboriginal peoples and their supporters, including many scholars, as a counterpoint to the supposed dualistic nature of non-Aboriginal thought. Holism, as a value, sets Aboriginal peoples apart and, in some minds, renders them more sophisticated in their approach to health and wellness.

There are many reports of similar intellectual complexity among other Aboriginal groups, and there is no need to present data group by group to make the case for such sophistication. Beiser (1985) has asserted that what the West called psychosis, that is, behaviour that was unpredictable and required controlling, was recognized and labelled an illness in all cultures. Hahn (1978: 32), while suggesting that few Aboriginal societies harboured an equivalent to the West's notion of psychiatry, believed nevertheless that 'rich evidence of psychiatric theorizing' could be found in many of them. Manson (2000) has argued cogently that Aboriginal peoples have rich lexicons for describing varying emotional states, and his work on Hopi depression, discussed in a previous chapter, supported this belief with empirical data (Manson, Shore, & Bloom 1985). But Manson has also suggested that Aboriginal thought works along different lines from that of non-Aboriginal, that the experience of emotions and psychiatric distress may be more than just intra-psychic phenomena. I agree that the available evidence supports this assertion *for some Aboriginal peoples, and within specific spacial and temporal contexts.* Context is everything, yet, as I have demonstrated repeatedly, it is frequently ignored in favour of essentialized portraits of Aboriginality.

The evidence that Aboriginal peoples were not actually holistic in their thought (as the concept is employed today) is compelling, and much more work needs to be done in this area. But my discussion of the literature is not presented as unequivocal evidence that Aboriginal North Americans had complex understandings of the mind and body, and of mental and physical health, as both separate and integrated phenomena. All of the studies cited need to be carefully scrutinized, conceptually and methodologically, just as I have done elsewhere in this book. My tack here is different. Looking at these studies uncritically – which, by and large, is the norm – one wonders how the holism perspective so easily gained a foothold, for there is ample evidence of ideas about the mind and the body as distinct, and of complex lexicons describing various states of mental normality and abnormality. The notions of dualism and holism are both reductionist and overly simplistic, and in adopting them European and Aboriginal societies have each established the other as, indeed, the 'other.' The empirical work clearly leans in the direction of the dualism proposition, at least in suggesting the existence of knowledge regarding the mind as, in some ways and at some times, separate from the body; the more polemical work, it seems, advances the holism proposition.

As Csordas (1994: 7) has suggested, 'It appears at times that there is, among champions of the body in contemporary human-science theorizing, a tendency to vilify what is usually called "Cartesian dualism".'[6] But it also seems as though, in the process of vilification, champions of the holism thesis have lost their empirical edge. In many ways, the assertions of holism over the years have remained unsubstantiated, frequently rendered in the absence of empirical support. Hahn (1978) noted this problem more than two decades ago, when he lamented the lack of research into the mind/body issue, a matter he related to the difficulties of learning the complex indigenous languages wherein would lie the linguistic codes that would inform the issue. Assertions of holism escalated throughout the 1960s and 1970s, as the so-called counter-culture took hold and embraced the idea that under every cactus sat a personal Don Juan of Carlos Castenada's imagination.[7] Angst over the apparent dualism of Western societies also emerged at this time; it is my argument that the rise of the holistic Indian and the dualistic whiteman are not unrelated phenomena. Seminal works (e.g., Kirmayer 1988; Lock & Scheper-Hughes 1996) have dissected biomedicine's propensity towards the Cartesian separation of mind from body, the psyche from soma, and mental from physical illness. The very existence of psychiatry in part suggests the dominance of the Cartesian model (Gaines 1992b), but the tension within this field between the biological and social factions emphasizes the contested nature of the model.

While these critiques have been both thoughtful and warranted, they have been concerned with one particular aspect of western *intellectual* history and professional discourse, and their focus has been on biomedicine as a system of knowledge. The implication is that Western society as a whole is characterized by mind-body dualism, and that people employ a fractured conceptualization of the self in distress. Yet the evidence for this supposition is circumspect, and even the DSM-IV-TR has challenged the dualism inherent in the concept of 'mental illness' (American Psychiatric Association 2000: xxx). In one study which challenged the appropriateness of the dualism model at the level of the individual, Angel and Guarnaccia (1989: 1229) explored the issue of somatization among Hispanics in the United States and argued that 'distinctions between the psychological and the physical are more the conventions of the scientific discourse than representations of the ways in which individuals experience their phenomenological realities.' Similarly, Jackson (1994: 208) described the experiences of chronic pain sufferers which 'confound' the Cartesian dualism of 'mind over matter' and 'matter over mind.' With respect to Aboriginal peoples, Levy, Neutra, & Parker (1987: 3–4) argued for a need to investigate 'actual patients as opposed to relying solely on normative statements elicited from knowledgeable informants.' In this light, Jilek-Aall's table, reproduced above, clearly confuses apples with oranges: it would make the most sense to compare the views of psychiatrists with indigenous healers, or Western patients with non-Western patients. When we look carefully at the issue of holism versus dualism, we discover that the assertions of dualism in the West are rooted in the highly specialized knowledge contained within science and the biomedical system, knowledge that is not necessarily known or readily available to non-specialists. Assertions of holism within Aboriginal societies have come primarily from a few intensive and questionable studies of singular, idiosyncratic healers or elders such as the Lakota Black Elk, and tomes produced by New Age raconteurs like Hyemeyohsts Storm, Sun Bear, and Rolling Thunder.

This fact has not escaped comment. Indeed, some have posited a fairly precise connection between the New Age movement and the rise of the holism thesis. Kehoe (1990: 198), in a scathing critique of New Age 'Indian' healing, argued that an 'unbridgeable difference between

Indians and Europeans' had been constructed, including the premise of two very different 'mental workings.' Part of the cultural primitivist discourse, she suggested, is the view that Indians, as 'natural people,' know the secrets of health and have access to both spiritual insight and natural medicines, in contrast to the 'coldly rational' physicians of biomedicine. Kunitz and Levy (1994: 218) argued even more specifically for a connection between the holism paradigm and the New Age movement: 'The traditional cultural values that Indians invoke, especially those having to do with holism, bear an uncanny resemblance to New Age ideas as well as to alternative traditions within orthodox medicine. This is not simply because New Age ideas and psychosomatic medicine reflect Indian cultural beliefs, but because many Indians, like many non-Indian Americans, have absorbed these ideas as part of the ambient cultural atmosphere. More specifically, some contemporary Indians working in health and social service bureaucracies have accepted as an accurate rendering of their traditional culture the picture painted by non-Indian New Age savants and psychosomaticists.' Such views frequently generate vociferous opposition because of the clear suggestion that 'traditional' Indian is in fact 'invented tradition,'[8] and more importantly, that these traditions often have a European origin, or at least influence. American Indian scholar Gerald Vizenor's critical (1994) work on cultural 'simulations,' which suggests the reality of European-influenced invented tradition, demonstrates that it is not only non-Aboriginal scholars who are thinking this way.

There are two ways to look at the dualism/holism debate. Holism can imply a sophisticated mode of thought, conceptualizing the mind/body more completely as an integrated system and therefore providing a more truthful understanding of the human experience. This is precisely the interpretation offered by the advocates of holism, and not infrequently it is contrasted with a reductionist, fractured biomedicine which, it is suggested, has lost sight of the human while bogging down in the organs. Holism, then, becomes a tool of an Arcadian post-colonial discourse. Alternatively, holism can be seen as primitively simplistic, the thought pattern of Barbarian peoples who lacked the ability to conceptualize how the various parts of the body work both as separate organs and as an integrated whole. Hence, the concept of holism can be used to represent both advanced thinking as well as backward thinking, depending on one's inclination. Once again we are faced with the two pillars of the primitivist framework.

The Use of Culture and Tradition in Treatment

In recent years, scholars have devoted increasing attention to the revitalization of Aboriginal cultures and, more specifically, to the use of 'traditional' Aboriginal healing methods in mental health programs (Jilek 1971). The reification and reinvention of Aboriginal 'culture' as a treatment modality has been a fascinating process, and one in which an unconscious essentialist, and even primitivist, agenda appears to have been at work, even where Aboriginal peoples themselves have been actively involved in the process. Lucas and Barrett (1995: 301) have suggested that, within the Arcadian tradition of primitivist discourse, the harmonious relationship of 'primitive' peoples with the environment has been interpreted as inherently therapeutic, including 'a certain protective capacity ... in respect of mental illness' (p.302). Furthermore, 'In the Arcadian tradition the healing properties of traditional societies are seen to flow from their close relationship to nature. Primitive peoples are more attuned to their bodies ...' (303). That Aboriginal healing has been characterized as a form of 'natural healing' (Silver & Wilson 1988) explains the attention it has received in these disaffected times. The Aboriginal shaman 'appears in Arcadian images as a seer, visionary, poet, artist or innovator, but most of all as a healer' who can only heal (Lucas & Barrett 1995: 312), ignoring the view within many Aboriginal societies that those with the power to heal are also capable of causing illness, and frequently do – this is not compatible with the views of New Age philosophers.[9] Few scholars have written about these programs in this manner, but it is not difficult to tease out these underlying notions through an examination of some of the reports of traditional healing projects.

How 'traditional' is contemporary traditional healing? In many instances, programs look suspiciously like conventional programs with some feathers and beads thrown in. Navarro, Wilson, Berger, and Taylor (1997) recently described a substance abuse program for thirty-five Native American students called 'The Natural Connection,' which emphasized the supposed connection between mind, body, and spirit characteristic of Aboriginal peoples. The program involved presentations by traditional healers and spiritual leaders, and the students constructed both a sweatlodge and a medicine wheel (the stone style).[10] The authors noted that the students came from a variety of tribal backgrounds, which they did not describe, and that this complicated their 'search for spiritual commonalities' (7). But the sweatlodge ceremony and smudging were acceptable to most students, because they were seen as 'near-universal expressions of present-day Native American spirituality' (8). The authors seemed aware of some of controversies regarding New Age appropriation of Aboriginal traditions, and the issues surrounding the authenticity of elders and healers. However, in addition to these traditional healing approaches, the students also took classes (and wrote exams!) involving readings of 'classics in Native American literature' (4), many of which were written by authors such as Ed McGaa ('Eagle Man') and Hyemeyohsts Storm, individuals who have been at the forefront of the New Age movement and whose authenticity has been challenged on many fronts.

In another recent piece, Fredericks and Hodge (1999) described a cancer intervention program for American Indian women in California which was 'culturally designed.' The program was based upon the value of sharing in the 'talking circle,' which, they suggested, had historically been utilized by most tribes for discussing important matters (316). The program also involved 'traditional tribal tales,' 'storytelling,' and 'respected members of the Indian community' (316). The way in which the program operated indicated the extent to which the design deviated from what one might think a 'traditional' program would look like. The talking circles were rigidly scheduled, once a week for sixteen weeks, and of one hour duration. There were 'rules' that were explained to the participants at the outset, and a 'talisman,' in this case a feather, was employed to empower the speaker. There was also a set curriculum, based on 'chapters' that provided 'essential background information for successfully implementing the talking circles' (p.319). Flip charts were used. Thus, while emphasizing the importance of stories and the oral tradition, a great deal of the program was in fact text based and highly structured. And even though it was presented as a traditional program, one that was 'culturally appropriate,' no mention was made of the cultural or tribal backgrounds of the participants. Despite acknowledging that intertribal variability created a challenging dilemma in terms of which specific traditional treatments to provide, the authors reverted to an essentialized portrayal of '*the* American Indian worldview' (emphasis added).

Even where researchers have recognized the influences of non-Aboriginal culture and conventional approaches to therapy, the tendency to ignore or downplay these in favour of a more strictly defined Aboriginal healing tradition is profound. This often leads to some absurd contradictions, as in the case of a study by Watts and Gutierres

(1997: 10) to identify cultural themes and 'fundamental traditional Native American beliefs and values' related to alcohol and substance abuse. This project involved fifty-eight individuals from three residential treatment facilities in Phoenix, who were involved in traditional treatment practices such as sweatlodge ceremonies and talking circles. 'What emerged' from their research, they argued, 'represents a *Native American-based* cultural model of substance dependency and recovery' (10; emphasis added). 'These Native American respondents referred particularly to alcohol as having agentive, animate potency,' which, they suggested, 'may reflect traditional cultural conceptions about natural forces and supernatural agencies as inherently capable of exerting both beneficial as well as potentially dangerous influence on humans' (12). The researchers noted that a sense of powerlessness or lack of control over alcohol was a common response to addiction, that the philosophy of Alcoholics Anonymous was clearly embedded in the perspectives of many of their respondents, and even that the main narrative offered to support the agentive theme was 'nearly a verbatim quote from the Big Book' of AA (13). But rather than acknowledging the role of AA in shaping both individual and program perspectives, they preferred to suggest that the theme represented commonalities in traditional Native American cultures, a 'culturally constructed common sense' (13). Yet once again we remain in the dark about the specific cultural backgrounds of the respondents, learning only that they were from fifteen different tribal groups and that most had extensive off-reservation experience. Nevertheless, Watts and Gutierres (1997: 13), ignoring the AA program's use of a deity figure as penultimate master, concluded that 'the notion of "dependency" as a relinquishment of personal autonomy and control to an overpowering non-human agency appears more culturally relevant to these Native American respondents than the disease-centered, Western concept of "addiction".'

'Traditional healing practices involve local contexts of power that should not be immune from critical examination,' according to Kirmayer, Brass, and Tait (2000: 614). To this end, however, only occasionally does a report surface that does more than pay lip service to the idea that not all Aboriginal individuals are equally interested or involved in traditional healing. Tension and conflict can occur. Scurfield (1995), in an examination of the treatment of American Indians with post-traumaic stress disorder, provided a glimpse into the broader political implications of Aboriginal healing. By adding a spiritual and cultural component to a conventional eleven-week PTSD program, the treatment staff hoped to make the program more culturally appropriate and, therefore, more successful. Several complex issues emerged when activities such as sweatlodge ceremonies, powwows, and spiritual/healing services were offered. The first issue pertained to who was eligible to participate as an 'American Indian,' as issues of bloodedness and cultural experiences were bandied about, suggesting that this program was not going to avoid controversy. With twelve veterans from ten different tribal groups and nine states involved, plus a reservation-urban split, the specifics of the various traditional treatments were hotly contested, and Scurfield (1995) documented an emerging division between the 'traditionals' and 'assimilated' clients, and between the 'bloods' (full-bloods) and 'breeds' (mixed Indian or Indian/non-Indian heritage) over what traditional services were to be provided, and how and when they were to operate. For their part, the staff were puzzled and overwhelmed by these complex issues, and, perhaps fearful of acting in a culturally inappropriate way, they were hesitant to set limits on behaviour or to confront Indian clients in situations where they would have confronted non-Indians. And, more interestingly, despite the fact that most clients had both an American Indian and non-American Indian heritage, the staff tended to overlook the non-Indian component: the clients were treated as if they had only one salient cultural heritage and identity, that of American Indian.

Similar issues were uncovered in my prison research (Waldram 1997). Aboriginal inmates from a variety of cultural heritages were offered 'traditional' spirituality and healing programs as part of their rehabilitation. The form of the services offered was determined by the cultural tradition of the provider, and therefore it was common for individuals to experience some degree of cultural dissimilarity or incompatibility with the program's content. Some were reluctant to participate because the ceremonies and spiritual symbolism were different from that of their own cultures. Others had been warned by their own elders that prison was an inappropriate place for things spiritual and that harm would likely befall any one who participated. Christian Aboriginal inmates viewed the spiritual services as Satanic. And those individuals who had been more or less fully acculturated, often as a result of adoption into non-Aboriginal families, sometimes saw no relevance whatsoever in traditional Aboriginal healing. Constant controversy, centred not only on the cultural form of the services but also on their very existence, dogged every institution studied.

Prison staff, hoping to be supportive by facilitating the programs, were understandably perplexed by this disunity.

The simple fact that there is considerable variability even within Aboriginal communities is not lost on some scholars, fortunately. Linda Garro (1990) was hard-pressed to uncover any meaningful consensus concerning the identities and expertise of traditional healers in a Manitoba Anishinaabe community. Similarly, Mohatt and Varvin (1998) described the case of an Ojibwe woman whose family appeared to disagree with broader community views of traditional healers. Csordas (2000: 463), in an overview of his Navajo healing project, declared that 'life in Navajoland today proves the outdatedness of any simple dichotomy between tradition and modernity/postmodernity,' and explicitly recognized three healing traditions, the 'traditional,' the Native American Church, and Navajo Christian faith healing, with the latter two clearly incorporating elements from non-Aboriginal society. Not surprisingly, his research discovered that there was no distinct line between the three and, in conjunction with biomedicine, they represented options of which Navajo freely availed themselves. Adelson (2001) described how many contemporary Aboriginal communities are divided by differing interpretations of culture, tradition, and belief. In the case of the James Bay Cree, she documented that, while health was inseparable from 'being Cree,' there was no single way to 'be Cree,' and disagreements between Christians and traditionalists, for instance, were profound.

Underscoring the Aboriginal healing revival, and implicit in much of the work discussed so far, is the fact that many Aboriginal people have little or no knowledge of the general philosophical approaches to healing or the specific healing ceremonies, symbols, or practices commonly employed, in part because these ideas are actually foreign to their communities and cultural heritages, and in part because culture change has eliminated this knowledge. In prison, it is crucial for healers to first educate inmates about the symbols and their meanings, which necessitates broader cultural education, before healing can ensue (Waldram 1997). This process involves the reinterpretation and selective presentation of 'traditional' culture. Education for healing, as distinguished from broader cultural education, is difficult to discern, and this has led to the view of some that 'culture heals.' Parker (1990: 257), in a study of thirty-four Narragansett Indian adolescents in Rhode Island, explicitly examined the hypothesis that 'the teaching of cultural traditions is preventive of alcohol and drug abuse by incorporating cultural materials into a standard prevention approach.' These cultural traditions did not, in and of themselves, appear to have anything to do with healing per se. These adolescents' cultural education consisted of 'learning handicrafts, such as beadwork and moccasin making, listening to traditional songs and "lore," and learning traditional subsistence patterns and the prehistory of the region' (259). They were also encouraged to explore their identities as American Indians, undertook field trips to museums and archaeological sites, and discussed political issues such as land claims. One cannot escape the sense that these students were receiving a variation of an introductory Native American Studies course. But the program demonstrated a 100 per cent retention rate, in comparison to half that for a control group, which the author attributed to the cultural education component. Insightfully, she noted, 'the specific mechanism by which making moccasins, visiting museums, or participating in pow-wows serves to decrease drug and alcohol use is still to be discovered' (Parker 1990: 265).

Cultural education is linked to ideas, discussed in previous chapters, that many Aboriginal people who have problems suffer from identity confusion or, even more seriously, lack any identity at all. How one can completely lack an identity is another of those puzzles that scholars generally rush past. Hughes and Sasson (1990) described one such identity-less individual in their case study of an Ojibway youth diagnosed with paranoid schizophrenia. He lacked 'a sense of self' in their view, and was not able to 'pick up' an identity while residing in a predominantly non-Aboriginal psychiatric hospital. Their task 'became aiding him in consolidating a sense of who he was and where he belonged' (185).

As we saw earlier, related to the idea that an Aboriginal person can lack an identity is the idea that he or she can lack a culture, or at the very least that the European elements of their cultural orientation have overwhelmed and subordinated, if not oppressed and repressed, their inherent Aboriginal cultural elements. This is sometimes even seen as a primal process: the Aboriginal person raised in a non-Aboriginal home needs to 'return' to his or her Aboriginal culture in order to heal. Many years ago Weibel-Orlando (1984: 66) described 'one argument gaining some credence among Indian alcoholism treatment groups ... that to be truly Indian one must return to traditional social forms ...' But of course these 'traditional' forms no longer exist, if in fact the term is taken to mean *pre-contact* forms. Variations of these forms certainly exist, but these have characteristically been altered by culture contact and several centuries of change. 'Traditional' as an adjective has changed from a descriptor of a particular kind of ancient cultural formation or individual cultural orientation/lifestyle into a metaphor, and an oppositional one at that, for a particular kind of very contemporary lifestyle and identity, in which culture is no longer as much a lived experience as it is a practice or even a performance.

The reification of Aboriginal culture as a treatment modality is clearly intertwined with broader concerns over identity, themselves a product of an emerging Aboriginal consciousness in reaction to a colonial legacy. In the treatment of Aboriginal offenders (Waldram 1997), the issue of identity was of central concern in the minds of those Aboriginal inmates involved in traditional healing programs, and while for some this issue was personally meaningful, for others it appeared as a manufactured, broadly political us-versus-them dialectic employed to challenge the prison hierarchy and authority. So, while Jilek (1982: 111) described the attractiveness for young people of Coast Salish spirit dancing as anchored in their linguistic disenfranchisement and desire to return to the 'old Indian ways' as the 'hallmark of Indianness,' others, such as Adelson (2000, 2001) have once again suggested that healing is, to some extent, political in the contemporary context. Translating the James Bay Cree expression for 'health' as 'being alive well,' she argued that this notion 'ultimately transcends the individual, and as part of the realm of "being Cree" is linked to a larger strategy of cultural assertion and resistance in a dynamic balancing of power between the State, the disenfranchised group, and the individual' (Adelson 2000: 9). Grobsmith (1989) and I (Waldram 1997) both documented how involvement in Aboriginal programming in prison, including traditional healing, was in part a political act of solidarity, a way of expressing separateness and politically opposing both the non-Indian inmate population and the prison officials who regulated inmate behaviour. The demands for traditional healing, it would seem, were as much about power as they were about rehabilitation. Traditional healing, then, in the eyes of critical observers, is only partly about health and illness in the biomedical sense and, it would seem, also only partly about 'healing' in the sense of contemporary Aboriginal discourse. Only occasionally has this broader dimension to traditional healing been recognized by those scholars who, according to Weibel-Orlando (1989), have become 'hooked on healing.'

Many mental health professionals argue for collaboration between

Aboriginal healing and biomedicine. Inevitably, as more and more calls for collaboration have rung out, there has been a dramatic – although in some ways fairly quiet – transformation in the traditional healing practices themselves. In most programs involving traditional healing, syncretism of healing systems is the norm, and traditions are often either revived or imported. Prison-based alcohol programs that Grobsmith and Dam (1990) examined differentially incorporated traditional healing into conventional programming, often relying on Alcoholics Anonymous and similar biopsychosocial treatment regimes. Most programs were hesitant to offer traditional treatments that were too tribal-specific for fear of alienating individuals from different tribes. Hence, a kind of pan-tribal approach was the norm, frequently centred on the ubiquitous sweatlodge which, it is clear from the literature, has become the most common component of Aboriginal traditional healing, even where it was not characteristic of the tribal group in the past. Hall (1985: 135; see also Hall 1986) has explained that the sweatlodge 'has become a concrete symbol for Indian persons concerned with practicing their traditional culture. Its simplicity and power have made it accessible and attractive to persons with minimal traditional experience as well as to groups composed of native [sic] persons with diverse tribal backgrounds.' What this means, of course, is that the 'traditional' sweatlodge ceremony is an imported and/or invented tradition for many Aboriginal groups. But not everyone accepts such imported traditions. Anderson (1992), in a study of an alcohol program among the Nuu Cha Nulth in British Columbia, noted that the sweatlodge fell into disuse because it was not a local tradition, and that sweetgrass ceremonies, also not local, were attended primarily by the non-Aboriginal staff.

Collaboration between biomedicine and Aboriginal healing has had the effect of bureaucratizing the latter. Kunitz and Levy (1994) described how a more formalized approach to Navajo healing, in effect its acceptance *as* a comprehensive therapeutic approach by biomedicine, led to the more thorny issue of codifying specific practices and, especially, billing services. They described how some twenty-two 'client service codes' were generated for reporting various components of a tradition-based alcohol treatment program, and the rigid scheduling of healing activities that became necessary to integrate them with biomedical approaches. I described a similar situation in prison: traditional healers were expected to sign contracts outlining specific 'deliverables,' including spiritual and healing services, and their activities were regulated by prison officials (Waldram 1997). Traditional Aboriginal healers now frequently have offices, fax machines, and voice mail, and even occasionally malpractice insurance (Waldram, Herring, & Young 1995). Of course, in most types of collaboration or formalization, the issue of payment arises, and there has been enormous controversy regarding the question of paying healers for services rendered. It is an interesting debate, in that it is assumed by opponents of fee-for-service or contract arrangements that *real* healers are not paid, because *traditionally* they were not paid. This is an indigenous essentialism of its own, for ethnographic and historical sources make it clear that remuneration of some sort was common to most healing systems; certainly the healers I have worked with over the years do not see the current system as anything more than a modernized, more practical implementation of a traditional practice. The Arcadian tradition, in this instance, seeks to confine the healers to a mythical, altruistic bygone era in which, in the absence of remuneration of some type, presumably they would have starved!

Collaboration has also brought Aboriginal healing more clearly within the gaze of the medico-legal systems of Canada and the United States. The use of peyote by members of the Native American Church represents one of the best-known cases of conflict over the issues of religious freedom and healing activities (Aberle 1966). Jilek (1982) cited several cases in the 1970s in which participants in the Coast Salish healing practice of spirit dancing were injured or died during the ceremonies. After much negative publicity, including accusations that the ceremony was 'demonic and satanic' (127), a judicial inquest was held which determined that there was no basis for charges to be laid. The issue resurfaced again in 1992, when an individual who had been forced to participate in the spirit dancing ceremony successfully sued several healers and was awarded damages for 'assault, battery and false imprisonment' (Waldram et al. 1995: 223; Waldram 2000). Generally, however, there has been little analysis of the complications caused by the application of Western notions of legal medical practice to Aboriginal healing.

Defining 'Traditional Aboriginal Healing'

What precisely is 'traditional Aboriginal healing'? The literature, not surprisingly, offers no clear definitions. The issue is rarely addressed, perhaps because of the complexities involved, but more likely as a result of a certain naiveté among researchers. Breaking down 'traditional Aboriginal healing' into its constituent parts provides only a little more insight.

'Traditional' clearly infers something old or perceived as continuous with the past. Lewton and Bydone (2000: 477), in the Navajo Healing Project, described traditional Navajo healing as having 'roots extending deep into Navajo history,' a clear affirmation of the past as the source of knowledge and expertise. But 'tradition' as a cultural construction 'is a selective representation of the past, fashioned in the present, responsive to contemporary priorities and agendas, and politically instrumental,' suggested Linnekin (1992: 251), and not simply the handing down of culture from one generation to the next. And what constitutes the 'traditional' is not fixed in time but changes. It is, to quote Darnell (2001: 16), 'a moving target': individuals, both patients and healers, adopt new knowledge from other societies, including biomedical knowledge and elements of European religious traditions, and these are incorporated into the 'traditional' (Waldram 2000). In the Navajo project, Milne and Howard (2000) noted that people tended to explain how their traditional healing worked by using biomedical equivalents, for instance, comparing diagnostic procedures such as hand trembling to X-rays.

'Aboriginal' is likewise an ambiguous and ill-defined category, as we have seen throughout this text. At first blush the concept alludes to the pre-contact period, when things were still entirely 'Aboriginal.' Does this notion preclude the infusion of any European influence? If so, then the Native American Church would certainly not be 'Aboriginal.' Nor would a sweatlodge ceremony I once attended which, along with various songs and Aboriginal prayers, included a recitation of the Lord's Prayer. And how should we view a healing ceremony which is borrowed from one Aboriginal group by another? Should we be thinking on a continent-wide scale, affirming trends towards the deployment of pan-Indian practices and beliefs? Or perhaps we should be thinking globally, since certain North American Aboriginal practices have spread as far as Aboriginal Australia (Brady 1995). Issues of authenticity are also pertinent; there have been many critiques of the New Age appropriation of Aboriginal healing symbols and ceremonies, and of the work of both non-Aboriginal and 'charlatan' Aboriginal healers, underscoring the notion that not only can *only* Aboriginal people be 'healers' – although it is clear that non-Aboriginal people are often welcomed as patients – but only a certain *authenticated* Aboriginal person can be a healer (Brave Heart & DeBruyn 1998). The process of authentication is, needless to say, both informal and ambiguous, but it appears to be a negative process in which accusations of involvement in 'untraditional' activities (such as selling healing services) result in ostracism and, in some instances, public labelling of charlatanism (see, e.g., Churchill 1994).

And what of 'healing?' For decades it was assumed by scholars that Aboriginal medicine in all its manifestations was primarily psychotherapeutic. 'The main area of traditional [Coast Salish] healing,' explained Jilek and Todd (1974: 353) 'is conditions in which psychoreactive and psychophysiologic mechanisms are prominent.' More recently, scholars have come to think of healing as something considerably broader than the notion of 'curing' within biomedicine, although emphasis on psychotherapeutic components remains strong, as can be seen in collaborative programs generally (Waldram 2000). The Aboriginal healing discourse situates 'healing' as something that falls partly, and sometimes primarily, outside the physical body of a singular individual, a human 'patient.' Healing, of course, is 'holistic.' It is also social, more so than many have been willing to admit. 'The aim of healing for First Nations people,' McCormick (1996: 164) has written, 'is concerned with attaining and maintaining balance between the four dimensions of the person: physical, mental, emotional, and spiritual ... connecting with family, community, culture, nature, and spirituality all seem important in successful healing.' Healing is also undertaken 'to reaffirm cultural values' and to 'consider the individual within the context of the community' (McCormick 1997: 174). Adelson (2001: 123) attributed to the James Bay Cree the idea that 'healing is never simply a personal phenomenon. While it implies a process of recuperation and recovery from personal or social traumas, healing always, by definition, takes place in a particular historical and social context.' And it cannot be understood separately from indigenous notions of health which, admittedly, often suffer in the translation. Adelson (2000) struggled to explain the Cree's extra-body conceptualization of health that related to hydroelectric dams and the environment.

Healing, it would seem, eludes definition. It should come as no surprise, then, that several scholars have lamented the lack of scientifically based empirical studies of the efficacy of traditional healing (Grobsmith 1989; Waldram 2000; Weibel-Orlando 1989). There is a marked tendency in the reports of traditional healing programs to present them in a favourable light, to avoid critical assessments of efficacy and, more generally, the asking of hard questions (Weibel-Orlando 1989). Opportunities to uncover patient and family perspectives on efficacy are all too frequently missed, as in the case described by Mohatt and Varvin (1998) of an Ojibwe woman who consulted a second healer after what appeared to be an unsuccessful encounter with one from a different cultural heritage. Not only did the second healer disagree with the first (an intriguing suggestion of variability if not professional disaffinity), but the authors of this DSM-style cultural formulation did not appear to investigate the link between the patient's increasingly psychotic behaviour and the sweatlodge therapy she had received from the first healer only two days earlier.

Part of the problem is related to the assumed interrelationship between healing practice and culture, such that criticism of the practice is interpreted as criticism of all things Aboriginal, another attack on indigenous integrity by the colonizer. Investigation of any type is often assumed to be the precursor to either derogation or banning of the practice. The problem can also be related to a profound inability of non-Aboriginal people to understand the linguistic and cultural traditions of Aboriginal peoples; they seek rote equivalents in their own cultural experience as a means of understanding. Manson et al. (1996: 275) argued that healing ceremonies have been defined as such 'probably because that was the best available metaphor by which non-Natives could describe and understand ... what was happening.' Further, they stated that 'these ceremonies greatly exceed that which is commonly understood as healing by the biomedical perspective, and can have a positive social effect far beyond the individual who is the focus of the healing ritual' (275). Many studies of traditional healing have tended to use methods appropriate for biomedical, clinical studies, but not appropriate for the particular, unique exigencies of traditional forms of healing. Science is clearly not sure what 'traditional healing' means and therefore reverts to the default position of assuming that it pertains to *medicine* in the scientific sense, perhaps only more primitive. We might even say that healing is deliberately ambiguous, and therefore can serve many different purposes. This ambiguity in meaning is found not only in the work of those scholars who study it, but also in the explanations offered by Aboriginal peoples. We are no further ahead when Aboriginal scholars such as Duran et al. (1998) adopt avowedly contemporary discourse to refer to traditional Aboriginal healing as 'post-colonial.'

Fundamental to contemporary conceptualizations of traditional

Aboriginal healing, then, are ideas of power and resistance, of employing Aboriginal culture to consciously reject European culture and its attendant values. Aboriginal culture has been reified and essentialized into a tool of change as well as therapy; as Brady (1995: 1490) has suggested, 'culture has become a "thing" that you either have or you have lost,' and those who are without culture are prone to alcohol abuse and other mental health problems. This view of culture is overly simplistic, as Brady noted, and it has become synonymous with 'tradition,' or culture as it is perceived to have existed in the past but which remains embodied in elders and can still be recovered by others. An authentic culture is promised, but what is frequently delivered in mental health programs is a limited set of pan-Indian ceremonies, invented traditions, and commodified and fetishized products representing the past but attached to contemporary values (such as capitalism). Indeed, there are many examples of the contemporary use of healing metaphors which may well represent invented traditions. This is not to suggest that these healing metaphors fail to achieve therapeutic success, however defined. I wish only to draw attention to the overall lack of critical insight which has been brought to bear on the issue of traditional healing, a kind of hands-off approach that has been recognized by only a few scholars (e.g., Edgerton 1992; Eisenberg & Kleinman 1981). As Gilbert Lewis (1993: 193) has argued, perhaps 'we are too ready to credit the mysterious powers of psychological and psychosomatic forces when the cases come from distant places and are about Aborigines or Africans.' He continued: 'The readiness goes with a certain romanticism about exotic people and a set of attitudes or beliefs attributing emotional liability or oddness to other people, especially those called primitive, simple, or oriental.' These critiques have been primarily concerned with the lack of studies of efficacy, however, and not with the lack of critical examination of the conceptualization and use of 'culture' and 'tradition' in contemporary healing programs. These are two separate issues, although the underlying primitivism to which Lewis alluded is equally pertinent.

Conclusion

Scholars frequently lament the difficulties involved in studying traditional Aboriginal healing, and the fact that some aspects have been declared secret and off limits for researchers. Critical scrutiny has often been interpreted as a sacriligious 'defacement' of sacred knowledge (cf. Taussig 1999). And as *Aboriginal* knowledge, its conceptualization as a kind of spiritual or intellectual property that can be owned is conditioned by contemporary political relations with the colonizing societies. That there is a political dimension to healing today is without question. There is a deep-seated fear on the part of researchers that any kind of challenge to the assertions made regarding healing and its effectiveness will result in charges of intellectual imperialism and even racism. This is an unfortunate situation, especially since these forms of healing appear to have positive benefits. It is equally apparent that, in the absence of solid empirical studies, a wealth of claims, some fantastical, have been made about the nature and effectiveness of indigenous treatment modalities.

The scholarly discussion of traditional Aboriginal healing clearly suffers from some conceptual underdevelopment, leading to ambiguities that challenge our ability to know much about it. The very notion of 'traditional healing' as presented in the literature appears to represent an internal tension or conflict in meaning and constitutes a 'moving target,' shifting from place to place, context to context, and from time to time. Within the healing discourse, 'tradition' appeals to the glory of the past and exists today as a metaphor for an uncontaminated pre-contact culture that is the property of Aboriginal peoples, a 'thing' that can be owned, practised, and lost, a thing that can heal. But 'healing' seems to be a metaphor for socio-political change as well as personal recovery and includes both processes of cultural repatriation or revival and political self-determination. Tradition looks to the past, healing looks to the future, yet they are combined in often clever and dramatic ways to construct Aboriginal peoples in the present as both different from, and perhaps more advanced than, non-Aboriginal peoples in the curing/healing arena. Underscoring this is a primitivist view of Aboriginal holism versus European dualism. But are we not simply replacing one dichotomy, that is, mind/body, or physical/mental, with another dichotomy, *dualism/holism*? Does this not appear to be the essence of primitivist discourse, with its parallel appeal to the broader nature/culture, savage/civilized, or Aboriginal/non-Aboriginal dichotomies? Those who argue for Aboriginal holism, especially given the empirical data on the topic, appear to be replacing one rigid construct with another, and are doing so largely as a matter of affirmation and not empiricism.

CHAPTER TWELVE

Conclusion: The Windigo's Revenge

There is increasing recognition that we have failed to see others clearly but have instead treated their cultural worlds like funhouse mirrors that hold up distorted reflections of our own cultural preoccupations. (Kirmayer & Minas 2000: 439)

The study of Aboriginal mental health in the fields of anthropology, psychology and psychiatry has been at heart the study of both cultural difference and cultural marginality, yet the way in which Aboriginal culture has been shaped, constructed, and individually personified has varied through time. At the turn of the twentieth century, the view that Aboriginal peoples were primitive and childlike, with a simplistic form of 'natural' culture, prevailed and intruded into scientific thought. This view guided a great deal of research throughout the century. While remnants of this sentiment remain today, contrasting interpretations of this cultural condition can be discerned. For the sciences, Aboriginal North Americans continue to exist in a timeless, eternal past as both the primitive Barbarian and the simplistically civilized Arcadian, both conditions maladapted to modern times. These funhouse images reflect far more of the nature of European intellectual traditions than they do of Aboriginal societies. Despite the enormous amount of research undertaken on Aboriginal peoples, we have consistently failed to comprehend the meaning of contemporary Aboriginality for mental health and illness. In this concluding chapter I wish to identify several common themes which have been developed in the text as I address the two questions posed in the introduction: what do we think we know about Aboriginal mental health, and on what basis do we think we know it?

Disturbed, Disordered, and Dysfunctional

What emerges from my analysis is a constructed Aboriginal, a simulation that reflects back upon the scientific lens which has been used to observe, measure, assess, and treat. This lens has hardly been uniform, however, and has shifted across time, and from discipline to discipline, to mirror both intellectual tradition and excitement over new, emerging theoretical and methodological ideas. All research must, in the first instance, be seen within its own historical and intellectual context, and we can judge work by current standards only with great caution. However, it is abundantly clear that old ideas are not simply replaced by new ones, with the former forgotten in the mists of intellectual time; rather, ideas are carried forward into subsequent generations as part of scholarly deliberations, homages to tradition, as well as the building blocks of new knowledge. Our intellectual past remains an integral part of our intellectual present, and we must adopt a diachronic perspective if we are to fully assess our current state of knowledge about Aboriginal mental health.

I began my analysis by looking at constructions of Aboriginal personality, a logical starting point given the importance of early psychological anthropology within the Americanist anthropological tradition. Anthropological efforts to understand the link between culture and personality, and to define the normal and the abnormal, found North American Aboriginal populations to be fertile fields of data waiting to be harvested. Ethnographic observation and some nascent psychological tests were employed in generating cultural profiles, an early example of the potential for collaboration among anthropology, psychology, and psychiatry. The Aboriginal initially emerged from this gaze in a somewhat favourable light, troubled by the advances of civilization and in need of assistance in making the transformation to the modern era, but not inherently pathological. Indeed, much of the work in the Indian Education Research Project flattered the intellect and abilities of the Indian, and defined an individual well-adapted to functioning in pre-contact Aboriginal society. The problem, at least from the point of view of administrators, was one of maladaptation to changing circumstances, an inability to adapt to cultural change if you will (ignoring, for the moment, that the change process was foisted upon Aboriginals), a theme that would dominate a great deal of subsequent analysis. Thus began the interest in Aboriginal culture among mental health researchers, an interest initially shaped by the interdisciplinary collaboration of pioneering theorists and methodologists. The partnership would ebb and flow over subsequent decades.

The introduction of psychoanalytical frameworks into Aboriginal mental health research, including the development of the Rorschach and other projective tests, encouraged the assessment of personality on an unprecedented level, and direct comparison among Aboriginal and non-Aboriginal groups. However, this inadvertently contributed to emerging portraits of Aboriginal cultures and individuals as inherently pathological. Northern Aboriginal social organization, for instance, was determined to be atomistic, with social relations governed by suspicion, invidiousness, and tension. Atomism, in itself, created a variety of personality disorders. The concept of atomism also played into the hands of those who saw assimilation as the only proper goal of Aboriginal policy. The types of behaviours exhibited by the sober atomistic individual were largely contrary to North American norms for behaviour, which emphasized individualism and assertiveness. Aboriginal peoples all over the continent were painted with a broad brush: they were stoic, quiet, shy, non-confrontational, and uncommunicative, and these personality traits bedevilled professionals and administrators trying to help them to cope with modern problems. But the implications of the atomistic personality exploded into view with the European's introduction of alcohol which, it was suggested, provided the release mechanism that allowed for culturally repressed tensions to rise to the surface. Aggression and violence were frequently the result. The Aboriginal was thus a problem either sober or drunk.

Concern about the cultural appropriateness of more contemporary research and diagnostic instruments, such as the MMPI and Wechsler, has consistently been raised, yet these tests have been employed on a regular basis, and portraits of individual personalities and abilities have been presented for our consumption even by those who were unconvinced that the instruments were valid. The utilization of these intelligence and personality tests has been extensive, underscoring one of the pervasive problems in psychological research with Aboriginal peoples. By transforming the lived experience of culture into a variable, especially one marked solely by alleged membership in a particular category, such as 'Indian' or 'white,' researchers pushed these tests forward and employed them in situations where their interpretations must be suspect. Aboriginal understandings of intelligence and competence were supplanted by Euro-North American standards, complete with validity and reliability protocols and testing manuals.

While colonization stands as a symbolic benchmark in almost all considerations of Aboriginal mental health, only a relatively small number of researchers have recognized that the Aboriginal of Columbus's time was not the Aboriginal they were studying, or felt the need to develop concrete ways to measure the effects of that colonization on Aboriginal cultures and individuals. The need to separate cultural survivals from newly introduced European cultural elements became a concern, and some researchers began to see the assessment of cultural orientation, in particular acculturation to the dominant European settler society, as crucial to determining the validity and interpretation of psychological tests. Attempts to measure acculturation or cultural orientation were largely unsuccessful, however, mostly because they were guided by a fractured understanding of Aboriginality and by underdeveloped models of culture that assumed the limited capacity of the individual to absorb new cultural ideas. Only recently have more sophisticated approaches to the measurement of culture, which emphasize culture's multi-dimensional and contextual nature, been developed. Measuring culture was difficult, and most researchers ignored the question of acculturation altogether, content with their assumptions that the Aboriginal was and remained, in his or her essence, a distinct primal cultural being.

The premise that Aboriginal peoples were ill-equipped to adapt to the arrival of Europeans has fed into a notion of acculturative stress, a powerfully appealing conceptual framework which has contributed to a view of Aboriginal peoples as 'caught between two worlds,' struggling with some kind of cultural liminality, lacking both coherent cultures and coherent self-identities. Very little empirical work has been done to substantiate these ideas, however. In fact, almost all the research has been based solely on a theoretical and even ideological foundation, with researchers assuming a priori that Aboriginal individuals must be experiencing psychic distress because of colonialism and its after-effects. The discovery of distress of any kind by researchers has served to reinforce the currency of the caught-between-two-worlds explanation.

Given that so many studies have assumed that Aboriginal peoples were inherently disordered, culturally maladapted to modern times, or succumbing to acculturative stress, it is not surprising that contemporary epidemiological studies have tended to find widespread psychopathology. The rates of pathology are alarmingly high, suggesting that contemporary Aboriginal peoples live profoundly dysfunctional lives.

While considerable energy has been expended in trying to understand the reasons for this lamentable situation, only rarely have researchers looked critically at their own assumptions and methods and asked themselves if, in their work, they were creating artifacts rather than uncovering supposed facts. A reluctance to challenge their own work has been buttressed by what appears to be a strong inclination to find pathology. Occasionally, when the appropriateness of specific research methods has been challenged – as in the case of post-traumatic stress disorder (PTSD) – the challenge has ensued because researchers were puzzled by apparently *low* rates of pathology, betraying once again an underlying assumption of widespread dysfunction among Aboriginal peoples.

The study of alcohol perhaps best encapsulates the essential debates of Aboriginal mental health discourse. Competing theories for the supposed problematic relationship between alcohol and Aboriginal peoples initially focused on biological explanations, the apparent susceptibility of Aboriginals to the effects of alcohol. Several influential and problematic studies perpetuated this myth, and the notion of biological susceptibility, reinforced by anecdotal evidence, emerged among both Aboriginal and non-Aboriginal peoples as a popular and widespread explanation of alcohol-related pathology. Many continue to believe this explanation today, underscoring dramatically how erroneous propositions of the past can be sustained well into the future. Researchers generally posited sociocultural explanations as well, one based on the assumption that alcohol problems were related to pre-contact cultural patterns, another that these problems were related to contemporary sociocultural disorganization. No matter what the explanation, there remained a sense that Aboriginal peoples drank the way they did, and experienced related problems, because of their differences from, and not their similarities to, white people.

In order to ease therapeutic tensions, the developing notion of cultural competence was embraced, and handbooks were designed to provide the well-intentioned therapist with the necessary information to treat Aboriginal patients. Given the enormous complexity of Aboriginal cultures, it was inevitable that distillation would occur, that neat cultural cheat-sheets would be produced to assist the busy therapist. This is a logical extension of a research literature which has consistently treated Aboriginal cultures as if they were homogeneous. The singular Aboriginal that originally emerged from the work of Hallowell, Honigmann, Barnouw, and others found a new home in these professional self-help manuals, with their lists of the ethics, values, behaviours, and personality traits of *the* Aboriginal individual as he or she might present in the clinical setting. While researchers have interpreted these Aboriginal culture traits in various ways to support their own particular contention regarding the most appropriate modes of therapy, as evidenced in the debate over individual versus collective therapeutic approaches, all have appealed to an essentialized Aboriginal.

For many scholars, the only way out of the psychopathological morass of Aboriginal existence is through a return to 'traditional Aboriginal healing.' Seen as the way to correct the ills wrought by Western civilization, this appeal is predicated on a challengeable construction of the Aboriginal world-view as holistic, in contrast to the fractured, anti-therapeutic Cartesian dualism said to characterize Western society and biomedicine. Ironically, while there are some treatment programs in which non-Aboriginal content is barely discernible (these, it seems, are rarely documented), many of the contemporary approaches to healing appear to borrow as much if not more from non-Aboriginal treatment modalities as they do from traditional ones, shrouding mainstream therapy in the discourse of Aboriginality, introducing sweatlodges into twelve-step programs. While the incorporation of different treatment modalities within the contemporary context may make a great deal of therapeutic as well as political sense, frequently a very modern and discursively moulded form of 'traditional' healing is being advanced. That it may well be therapeutically effective simply confounds our inclination to construct simplistic analytic frameworks.

The sum total of the Aboriginal mental health literature is a series of conflicting and contradictory portraits of seriously disturbed individuals living disordered lives in dysfunctional communities, suffering from cultural anomie, marginality and maladaptation, yet continuing to bask in the warm, inherently therapeutic glow of historical cultural traditions, psychically brought forward even by individuals without any experience whatsoever of these traditions. These two portraits do not mesh, and I would suggest that neither is accurate, yet their coexistence is easily predictable from the perspective of primitivist discourse. Aboriginal peoples have clearly experienced the 'overpathologizing bias' said to be characteristic of minority groups more generally (Good 1997: 239), and have persisted despite this alleged psychiatric chaos. Is something missing from the research literature? Has the penchant of scholarly research to focus on the sensational, the problematic, and the dysfunctional elements of human existence, especially of cultural 'others,' overwhelmed the pragmatic and positive aspects of that very existence? How have Aboriginal individuals continued to find meaning in their lives? How can they still laugh and play, raise families, teach their children? Why do scholars appear so desperately to need Aboriginal peoples to be either 'at one with nature' or totally dysfunctional? These questions have only rarely been addressed.

Problems of Culture and History

Things Aboriginal, including mental health, were once predominantly the scholarly domain of anthropologists. For many decades, Aboriginal peoples served as important sources of data and experience as anthropologists sought to develop both theory and methodology, and to construct and apply models of culture to the people they studied. The contribution of the 'Americanists' to broader disciplinary trends is beyond question (Darnell 1998, 2001), but the extent to which they realized their goals is debatable, and the knowledge they gained is uneven at best. The knowledge generated about the Aboriginal mind and mental health cannot be divorced from the major trends in the development of anthropological theory which influenced this knowledge, nor can it be isolated from trends in the fields of psychology and psychiatry that interacted with this anthropology. Fundamental ideas which shaped all of these twentieth-century disciplines can be traced back through the Victorian era and Darwin to the Enlightenment, if not further.

In the twentieth century especially, some very influential work, often involving collaboration between anthropologists, psychologists, and psychiatrists, established both an empirical baseline and broader methodological approaches to the problem of studying the Aboriginal. More recently, however, anthropological interest in the mind and mental health of North American Aboriginal peoples has waned somewhat; the anthropologists seem to have moved on to other topics as the first North Americans, coming to look and act so much like later European settlers, perhaps lost their exotic lustre.[1] But psychologists and psychiatrists, having discovered culture for themselves, moved quickly to assert their authority. As the idea of culture became more acceptable as an element of study in both of these disciplines, the search for cultural 'others' to test the cross-cultural applicability of accumulated psychological and psychiatric knowledge led invariably to the conveniently located North American Aboriginal. But, while the Boasians often focused on cultural reconstruction, generating portraits of cultures as if Europeans had never colonized, and subsequent anthropological research seemed directed toward documenting the 'traditional' rather than the contemporary, the psychologists and psychiatrists could not easily evade the consequences of colonization or ignore the contemporary context in their work. By concentrating on contemporary conditions, these professions simply accepted, uncritically, that anthropology had done its part by accurately constructing Aboriginal cultural pasts, and that these pasts informed the present in meaningful ways. They also deferred to what they believed were accepted ideas of 'culture' emanating from the one discipline claiming scientific authority to its study.

In recent decades, anthropology has moved into a reflective, critical phase and culture is now conceptualized as a constructed, negotiated, and contested entity. The discipline has become embroiled in debates over the veracity and validity of its own concepts, methods and ethnographic portraits, and the idea of anthropology as a science has been challenged from within by those with a more humanist bent. Psychology and psychiatry have remained largely aloof from these debates, firmly ensconced within the embrace of the earlier, now disputed 'truths' of a once avowedly scientific anthropology, what can be seen today as anthropological anachronisms. These anachronisms include the following:

1 There are discrete cultural and biological populations, and these can be delineated and bounded conceptually and geographically.
2 Cultures can be aggregated into larger units, culture areas, on the basis of trait similarities, and these larger units can in turn be conceptualized as essentially culturally homogeneous.
3 Biological heritage, community, nationality, and self-identity are synonymous with culture.
4 Cultures are internally consistent and all culture-members know their culture in exactly the same ways.
5 Cultures can be conceptualized as either 'collectivist' or 'individualist' in terms of their social organizations, and these orientations are largely impervious to change.
6 Cultures can be categorized by perceived levels of socio cultural integration which, in turn, reflect an inherent pattern of cultural evolution.
7 Culture contact and subsequent cultural change inherently cause disruption, stress, and mental health problems.

8 An individual's capacity for culture is severely limited, and individuals can exist in a culture-less state.

For the most part, then, psychology and psychiatry avoided the more complex and uncomfortable challenges being experienced within anthropology and sought refuge in the simpler tenets of historical particularism, diffusionism, culture, and personality, as well as acculturation and evolutionary theories, to explain the contemporary problems they were studying. Psychologists and psychiatrists were more interested in methodologically circumscribing culture than understanding it, and ethnographic approaches were too time-consuming, too particularistic, too 'unscientific,' and too prohibitive of comparative analysis to be useful. The experimental and quasi-experimental approaches of psychology and psychiatry, and the population health perspective of epidemiology, merged to create a new form of cultural essentialism, the reduction of culture to the status of variable in 'cross-cultural' research, something that could be measured in one or two items, or at best with a singular instrument, to be scored and then entered into multi-variate analyses (Cole 1996). Even the most basic, core assumption that there was a meaningful and singularly identifiable Aboriginal Canadian or American Indian population was largely unquestioned. 'By itself, the term *American Indian* is vacuous and provides little in the way of cultural specificity,' Trimble and Medicine (1993: 149; emphasis original) once warned. 'Furthermore,' they continued, 'when data gathered on American Indians are compared with those from other ethnic populations the meaninglessness of the findings are enhanced.' Yet the persistence of *the* Aboriginal as a meaningful population unit has remained largely unchallenged by researchers, perhaps the most fundamental of all the conceptual flaws that has characterized the mental health research.

What is missing from the recent turn to the clinical and epidemiological approach is any kind of coherent theory, or even a working model, of culture. Theorizing about culture, more generally, is largely absent as well. Culture is treated as a given and not something to be problematized. Yet both culture and, in the specific case of Aboriginal peoples, history, are central to explanations of Aboriginal mental abilities and mental health, and hence how they have been conceptualized and operationalized is crucial to understanding the legitimacy of the conclusions rendered. These conclusions are often confusing and contradictory, and there is a tension in the mental health discourse between conceptualizations of cultural continuity and discontinuity, and cultural homogeneity and heterogeneity.

The idea that Aboriginal peoples suffer primarily from *modern* problems of maladaptation, related mostly to colonialism and its attendant stresses and cultural changes, has certainly dominated the contemporary mental health discourse. That the Arcadian Aboriginal is deemed to have lived a utopian existence in a perfectly balanced society, free from mental health problems, is a clearly discernable theme in the literature. There is such strong support for this romantic essentialism that it presents as one of the foundational truisms of the Aboriginal mental health field. Contemporary mental health problems are frequently viewed in relation to the complete lack of experience of Aboriginal peoples with disorder and distress, a 'virgin soil' framework reminiscent of that offered to explain the damage caused by European diseases (Waldram, Herring, & Young 1995). But the Barbarian has not disappeared, and the idea that contemporary problems are sometimes related to inherently dysfunctional, even 'primitive' cultures, or cultures which are not equipped to adapt to modern times, is also visible. The persistence of Aboriginal culture, vaguely conceived, becomes the problem, as evidenced in the continued existence of maladaptive personality traits, social atomism, and collectivism. Cultural continuity presents in its most fantastic form in the suggestion that certain culture-bound syndromes have survived (gruesomely Barbaric, of course!), and continue to plague magical-thinking Aboriginal peoples today. But there are also suggestions that indigenous understandings of mental disorders such as depression and suicide also exist and challenge the Arcadian view of a disorder-free paradise.

The notion of problematic, psychopathological, cultural persistence is accompanied by another, just as tenacious, view that Aboriginal 'culture' has largely disappeared, that individuals suffer from problems related to cultural loss, and that one can even become 'caught between two worlds.' Marginalization has been largely conceived in terms of this cultural loss, rather than in socio-economic terms. 'Aboriginal' culture, its persistence, its absence, or its disappearance, is invariably seen to be at the root of most mental health problems.

However, particularly in the discourse of treatment, we also find the idea that there are certain positive cultural survivals with the potential to effectively eliminate contemporary mental pathology. Discussions of the solutions to current mental health issues involving appeals to 'traditional' culture and 'healing' have become pervasive, as if these represent unchanged cultural elements which provide millennia-old solutions to contemporary problems. Aboriginal peoples, allegedly lacking in true Arcadian fashion a pre-contact history of mental disorder and emotional distress, or having fallen into the culture-less abyss, have nevertheless inexplicably retained ancient approaches to treat disorder and distress, one of those awkward contradictions that remains uninvestigated. Missing from the debate has been any kind of theoretical reasoning to explain why some cultural elements appear to have remained intact while others have been lost altogether, or why some are the problem and others the solution.

At the base of the understanding of Aboriginal cultures throughout the years has also been the competing models of cultural heterogeneity and homogeneity. We see this at many levels in the Aboriginal mental health discourse, and like the tensions between the Barbarian and Arcadian, often contradictory perspectives have been offered. While assertions of the heterogeneity of Aboriginal peoples have consistently been made, testaments to their vast cultural differences and warnings to novice therapists not to assume too much when encountering an Aboriginal client, there has been a parallel and stronger tendency to treat them as essentially all alike, to dig as deeply as necessary to find that common, inner Aboriginal. Indeed, the heterogeneity argument is frequently given short shrift, as if paying homage to the idea is an intellectual (and perhaps politically correct) prerequisite but not scientifically useful. Only the relatively small number of scholars interested in acculturation have given heterogeneity concerted attention.

Aboriginal cultures have usually been portrayed as easily bounded units that harbour consistently uni-cultural citizens, 'hermetically sealed beyond the reaches of time and the world system' (Keesing 1990: 53). Until recently, anthropology as a field had continued, at least surreptitiously, to imply that discrete cultures existed, that cultures were homogeneous entities and that culture members were all equally 'culturally competent' (Greenfield 2000). And anthropology is still vexed by the essentializing and homogenizing of its subjects (Vayda 1994). An assumption of cultural homogeneity continues to guide much research within the fields of anthropology, psychology, and psychiatry, and the sense that there are strong cultural similarities among contemporary Aboriginal individuals, regardless of their traditional heritages and post-contact experiences, that there is a singularly cultural Aboriginal, is pervasive.

The cultural homogeneity perspective is expressed through two explanatory frameworks. The first posits the existence of a kind of primal culture, an Aboriginal psychic unity, that has not only characterized all Aboriginal peoples in the past, because of their collective Aboriginality (despite evidence that pre-contact Aboriginal populations represented different bio-cultural populations), but which has also proven to be resilient in the face of the cultural change caused by the arrival of Europeans and others. Even the interbreeding of Aboriginal with non-Aboriginal peoples has been deemed, by and large, to be inconsequential, with the essentialized Aboriginal somehow managing to suppress even a more substantial non-Aboriginal biological presence. Fundamental ethics, values, and behaviours have persisted, for instance, even in the face of a much larger, dominant society allegedly promoting their direct opposites.

The second explanatory framework is the idea that, separate from the question of pre-contact diversity or homogeneity, the arrival of the Europeans set in motion certain historical forces which have had the effect of culturally homogenizing Aboriginal peoples, with a strong suggestion that this process represents one of pan-Aboriginal convergence. If, however, we are going to invoke history as an explanation we need also to problematize it. Cultural convergence must remain an empirical question. There has not been a uniform process of cultural change in North America, and colonial experiences were not identical. Some Aboriginals quietly became integrated into the fur trade, others were ruthlessly uprooted and marched across the continent, and still others engaged in prolonged campaigns of armed resistance. Some inter-married so extensively with Europeans and Africans that eventually they ceased to exist as separate populations. Others, through inter-marriage, produced a new mestizo society unique and separate from the donor cultures. Some Aboriginal communities, located at the edge of major urban centres, have struggled to preserve any semblance of an indigenous language, while others, located in remote areas of the north, have maintained their indigenous language as the lingua franca. It is possible that more recent government legislation and policy in Canada and the United States, such as the establishment of reserves, has sparked a process of homogenization of Aboriginal cultures, but even this needs to be exposed to critical investigation. Further, we need to consider if the product of that cultural change represents the emergence of a new, still distinct but more or less singular Aboriginal culture, or whether it represents a convergence with the dominant culture within the state itself.

One must question if a colonial paradigm is the best one for comprehending the position of Aboriginal peoples in North America today, or if, after several centuries of significant changes for both the Aboriginal peoples and the settlers, a new paradigm is needed. This is not to deny the importance of history for Aboriginal peoples, or the importance of history for understanding contemporary contexts. But the colonial paradigm, linked as it is not only to historical processes of European commercial expansionism and settlement, but also to more fundamental scholarly ideas of cultural exoticism and primitiveness, is perhaps no longer a useful means through which an understanding of contemporary Aboriginal mental health can be achieved. The 'determinants' of Aboriginal mental health might be best located in the same place as those for non-Aboriginal peoples. Are the Sioux still best understood as 'warriors without weapons,' for instance? At what point are Aboriginal peoples better culturally conceptualized as contemporary Aboriginal *North Americans*, for whom the 'harder issues of class, economic disadvantage, racism, and power' are more pertinent (Mezzich et al. 1999: 462)?

Defining the Aboriginal

Cross-cultural research is based on an assumption of a priori cultural difference, that, for instance, a registered or self-declared Indian *is* culturally different in meaningful ways from a non-Aboriginal person (Trimble 1975). Researchers have rarely explored this as an empirical question. Further, while researchers often seek to 'validate' research or diagnostic instruments for an Aboriginal population, only occasionally do they define this group. The vast majority of scholars engaged in cross-cultural research have failed to question the extent to which the individuals in their sample were actually culturally similar enough to be considered members of the same culture. When they have found that there are differences in some clinical dimension, the prevalence of a specific pathology as measured by a standardized instrument, for example, the argument has logically followed that this must be due to cultural differences. Observed differences in psychopathology between research populations presumed to be internally homogeneous and distinct have been explained in terms of cultural differences precisely because of pre-existing assumptions that they are culturally different. Characteristically, no other explanations for the observed differences are explored. Both the heterogeneity and homogeneity perspectives assume difference, creating arbitrary boundaries around research populations for purposes of comparison. The only real distinction between the two positions is where they draw the boundaries: *among* Aboriginal groups, for example, comparing presumably homogeneous Navajo to presumably homogeneous Lakota, or *between* a singular, presumably homogeneous and ubiquitous Aboriginal group and a contrasting equally homogeneous and ubiquitous non-Aboriginal one. Regardless, the key issues remain not only how one determines the culture of an individual in order to slot him or her into the appropriate category of the cultural variable, but whether culture is even operative as an explanatory device of significant power. A vague conceptualization of culture that is supposed to encapsulate difference eclipses the cultural specificities of class, race, and gender that surely exert an influence on Aboriginal peoples, just as they do for everyone else on the continent.

The simplistic approach to culture characteristic of much research allows for the unquestioned use of pre-existing cultural markers, regardless of their empirical base, theoretical heritage, or contemporary relevance. The continued utilization of culture area models as sampling frames, and broad cultural or tribal affiliations, stand as important examples of unquestioned cultural markers. These are both convenient and entrenched in a long scientific history, but as representations of *culture* they are woefully inadequate. Culture areas represent an antiquated, ecologically based schema which was specifically designed to anchor individuals in the past, to cement them into a way of life that, in the Boasian tradition, was seen to no longer exist. Culture areas were a means to study the past, not the present, and represented a conceptualization of cultures as geographically circumscribed entities. First Nation or tribal appellations are equally useless: first, singular 'tribes' or 'bands' as political entities are often composed of several different historic Aboriginal populations; second, membership in the political unit is usually based on geneology and not cultural affinity; and third, self-declaration of First Nations or tribal membership may be inaccurate. The First Nation or tribe exists today largely as a political, not cultural, unit of citizenship, as a marker of certain rights, and/or as a legal distinction; it is a mistake to simply impute culture from such an entity. In both Canada and the United States, increasingly large numbers of First Nations or tribal members are residing off-reserve, and whole generations are growing up in the complex cultural arenas of our cities. That such individuals remain members of specific First Nations or Tribes makes using citizenship or culture areas as unequivocal cultural markers problematic.

Reliance on vague notions of culture also appears, somewhat para-doxically, in the use of racial criteria, such as blood quantum, to deter-mine tribal membership and occasionally even the degree of 'Indian-ness.' The confusion of race and culture is a characteristic theme of much of the research examined in this book. In addition to being avow-edly racist, blood quantum says nothing about culture, despite euphe-mistic appeals to the contrary. Yet the notion that bloodedness and cultural orientation are positively correlated underscores many con-temporary views on Aboriginality. Bloodedness also remains as per-haps the purest example of Aboriginal essentialism, through the implication that Aboriginality is inherently a biological phenomenon, a construct which has continuously challenged itself as measures of bloodedness have become increasingly diluted in response to increas-ing intermarriage. What constitutes a sufficient amount of Aboriginal blood to be 'Aboriginal' is a hopelessly ambiguous, confused, and ever-changing matter. Further, despite the discourses of bloodedness (and its implied biology), most measures of blood quantum have actually been based on self-reported family geneology, a social and cultural construct. Blood quantum as a measure of Aboriginality employed in determining citizenship or membership in an 'Aboriginal' research cat-egory is, therefore, problematic.

Identity self-declaration, a common strategy for generating samples, is similarly problematic. Declarations of self are notoriously reactive to broader social, cultural, and political trends as well as the specific con-texts in which such declarations are rendered. Cultural identities are also multifaceted. Any cultural declaration may represent a wish rather than a reality, a pining for a 'culture' one does not actually know and which is likely romanticized. It may also represent a political state-ment, a declaration of otherness to be contrasted with the colonial oppressor. According to Keesing (1990: 48), 'our conception of culture almost irresistibly leads us into reification and essentialism,' and the construction of culture as 'thinglike' has created 'an ideal rhetorical instrument for claims to identity, phrased in opposition to modernity, Westernization, or Neo-colonialism.' Not surprisingly, Aboriginal peo-ples in Canada and the United States have embraced certain symbols, from 'traditional' values to medicine wheels, in an effort to 'other' themselves, to create a contradistinction to the settler society even as they become more indistinguishable from it. Aboriginal culture has become intertwined with matters of politics, race and biology, and, in Wikan's (1999: 57–8) terms, a 'thing with a fixed and revered existence,

– like a holy cow' that is 'amenable to use in defense of all kinds of special interests.' Individuals, especially cultural 'others,' have become culture-bound, their individuality and actual cultural orientations obliterated by their perceived membership in a cultural group, a membership that they often claim when it is not ascribed to them; that they have in turn come to manipulate this in their own interests is of little surprise. These are the new cultural facts, the facts of globalization and post-coloniality, and they should cause any researcher bent on employing a simplistic conceptualization of culture to shudder. Individuals, research subjects, do not walk about displaying their cultural orientations like a feathered war bonnet; indeed, an individual wearing a Plains Indian war bonnet today is just as likely to be a Mohawk steelworker from Manhattan or a German 'hobbyist' as he or she is to be an elected Plains Cree politician. So, just as it is wrong to assume that a self-declared Gitksan and a self-declared Cree are culturally similar because they are both Canadian Indians, it is also absurd to assume that they are culturally different because they are from different culture areas or are enrolled members of different tribes, or because they claim to be different. Both could have been born and raised in the same Vancouver suburb, speaking only English and with no personal knowledge of the reserves of their relatives.

Of course, the 'Aboriginal' of scientific construction has a foil: the non-Aboriginal or, more colloquially, 'white man.' My interest in this book has been with the Aboriginal, but it has been difficult to resist at least a cursory excursion into the construction of this ubiquitous bogeyman, the real-life colonizing windigo who is characteristically located in contradistinction to the Aboriginal. A great deal of research has compared specific Aboriginal populations with an allegedly comparable white sample (or 'national'data). Since the focus has invariably been on the Aboriginal, even less has been written on who, specifically, these 'white' people were. The same issues hold in the dissection of this category as in that of the Aboriginal: how is 'whiteness' defined, and how are subjects determined to be 'white' for purposes of recruitment? Perhaps more importantly, what does 'whiteness' mean in mental health research, for psychological testing, or in understanding specific disorders? In this sense, white people are just as essentialized as are the Aboriginals, and not always favourably. In the eyes of many scholars, the European settlers lack both history and culture, as neither seems pertinent to understanding their psychopathology. Socio-economic status, poverty, and homelessness are the focus of most of the explanatory work for white people, as even a cursory examination of health determinants models would demonstrate. The comparative mental health literature, then, may well be doubly meaningless, as both categories, the Aboriginal and the white, may be nothing more than 'simulations' (Vizenor 1994). Our pronouncements of the comparative mental health status of Aboriginal peoples, by definition, can be no more valid than our conceptualization of the contrasting non-Aboriginal or white study populations.

There is no question that Aboriginal mental health has been dominated by non-Aboriginal researchers, and that some clear biases have consequently intruded into the discourse. However, despite considerable criticism to the effect that non-Aboriginal researchers have failed to understand the cultures and mental health issues of Aboriginal peoples, the growing number of American Indian and Canadian Aboriginal scholars, in the fields of psychology, psychiatry, and anthropology have not really approached mental health differently. Many continue to employ conventional theoretical frameworks and methodological techniques, often treating culture as a variable, and some Aboriginal scholars are as prone to the primitivism and essentialism I have documented throughout this book as are the non-Aboriginal scholars. This forces us to question the privileging of *any* perspective over any other on the basis of supposed or asserted racial or cultural affinity.

Contemporary Aboriginal Cultural Realities: Creolization and Beyond

Clearly, attempts to understand the Aboriginal population, both from a research perspective and within the context of the clinic and treatment, have not been particularly fruitful. For the most part, we have failed to comprehend the contemporary cultural reality of Aboriginal peoples in North America, and we have failed to grasp the meaning of Aboriginality in an ever-changing world. Cultural understanding remains as elusive as ever, despite the centrality of culture in the appeal of Aboriginal peoples for researchers. We remain unsure as to what culture is, and when and in what contexts it is important, and as a result there is too great a reliance on vague, poorly conceived notions of culture in our research. As psychological anthropologist Bradd Shore (1996: 315) has written, 'Any powerful theory of cultural knowledge must clarify not just the power of culture to explain how we make meaning but also the limits of culture as an explanatory device.' Culture should not be taken 'too seriously,' in other words (Christopher 1998: 40). Alarcón, Wester-meyer, Foulks, and Ruiz (1999: 468–9) have recently cautioned that 'a clinically relevant cultural psychiatry should warn the clinician against the "overculturalization" of the clinical phenomenon (i.e. notions such as "cultural perculiarities" or "respect for the uniqueness of human groups") that might trivialize true clinical situations and thus deprive individuals and groups of an appropriate diagnostic assessment and treatment.' Further, they have argued that 'When evaluating any patient, the clinician must attempt to delineate the extent to which culture can explain the behavior being examined or, conversely, contribute to the production of symptoms, and to their accurate diagnosis, treatment and overall management' (469). These concerns read as an indictment of the search for, or creation of, cultural difference in those who, for a variety of reasons (such as physical appearance), are a priori assumed to be culturally different. Yet it is also necessary to guard against underculturalization, the failure to see culture or, worse, to oversimplify it, thereby creating the illusion of cultural understanding.

The task of conceptualizing culture for research purposes is enormous, for culture 'has the same ubiquity and transparency as water' in the words of Kirmayer and Minas (2000: 438). George Devereux (1971: 23) was not exaggerating when he wrote of culture that 'anyone who understands it may be said to possess the open-sesame' of anthropology. Unfortunately, none of the disciplines of anthropology, psychology, and psychiatry have yet to develop the tools to properly assess culture either in research or in the clinic. But rendering culture convenient by simplifying and essentializing it is not the answer, and since these disciplines have largely ignored each other with respect to the culture concept, theoretical advances have been fleeting. While reducing culture to a set of variables is questionable from an anthropological perspective, it is entirely reasonable within the framework of cross-cultural psychology and psychiatric epidemiology. Clearly there needs to be some reconciliation among the disciplines.

What it all adds up to, in the end, is a great deal of questionable social science and medical research concerning the mental abilities and mental health of Aboriginal peoples. The assumptions are frequently problematic, the methods are frequently faulty, the interpretations are frequently unjustified, and the results frequently over-generalized. The science upon which portraits of Aboriginal mental health have been constructed represents a proverbial house of cards, and a close look at this construction reveals just how tenuous our scientific knowledge is in these areas. Scholars cite earlier work, which cite still earlier work, and so on, with the result that old ideas, sometimes little more than audible ruminations of spelunking commentators, become reified as scientific fact. Each citation, each uncritiqued idea, like each card, builds upon that which came before. The house of cards grows, becomes immense, but remains fragile. All the while, based on this 'knowledge,' real Aboriginal individuals are categorized, studied, analysed, and treated.

The culture of science is powerful, and challenging its basic premises, its theories and methods, frequently comes at some cost. Certainly science has delivered to us immense knowledge which has reshaped the world and how we view it. But the culture and power of science is also its Achilles heel when we assume too readily that previous research is sound and build from it without question, when we take for granted that acquired knowledge is accurate and truthful. This is ironic, given that science is supposed to be a sceptical intellectual tradition, one that challenges with relish existing theories and methods, which picks apart published studies and attempts to replicate them. Something was clearly lost in the adoption of a unifying scientific model by those who seek to understand human culture and behaviour. Rather than challenging and restudying, fields such as anthropology and psychology have too readily accepted past work as accurate and sound. For its part, psychiatry, in so far as it pays any attention to social science research at all, seems similarly disinclined to question social science data and interpretation, perhaps erroneously assuming that the findings and interpretations have been subjected to the same kind of critical scrutiny and restudy as medical research.

Readers might well be frustrated by an apparent lack of 'solutions' to the problems of culture and mental health outlined in this book. Frankly, at this stage I do not have any easy answers, but I believe strongly that a critical re-reading of the field is the first logical step and a legitimate goal in itself. A blanket condemnation of science and Western culture, however, is neither pertinent nor fair. Kirmayer and Minas (2000: 444) have cautioned that a cultural critique of psychiatry 'and the concern to hear the voices of others, does not mean abandoning scientific empiricism or clarity of thought. The effects of racism, imperialism, and systematic suppression of others' cultures will not be counteracted effectively by a wide-eyed naïveté that sees in anything non-Western a better form of medicine.' I agree. But perhaps these authors are viewing oppression too narrowly, as historic, political, and economic. A postcolonial perspective challenges us to critically examine scientific hegemony, as science has certainly been one of the agents supporting the oppression of others. While the *truths* generated by science and accepted faithfully in the development of mental health knowledge have frequently been little more than poorly conceived artifacts passed down from generation to generation, they have contributed to the creation of a formalized, official knowledge about Aboriginal peoples that guides government policy, public attitudes, treatment approaches, and research. Many Aboriginal peoples, in turn, have embraced these truths, and the science behind them, and act to manipulate them in their own interests. Unravelling this 'knowledge,' then, becomes risky but crucial.

Anthropologically derived definitions of culture as *shared* necessarily imply generalization and the existence of a cultural core, and have led inadvertently to a discursive trimming of variability. Seeking only the prototype, or even the archetype, for culture has inevitably taken us down the road of over-generalizing, stereotyping, and essentializing. The discipline of anthropology, for one, has entered an era in which some of its practitioners appear to be trying to make amends for steering us in the wrong direction. 'A more critical cultural theory,' Keesing (1990:57) has written, 'would make no assumptions about closed boundaries within which cultural meanings hold sway: a "culture" as a bounded unit would give way to more complex conceptions of interpretation, superimposition and pastiche.'

In which direction should we now turn? Should we abandon attempts to theorize and, even more problematic, measure culture? Is the world too complex for these efforts? Is *culture* too complex for these efforts? Bibeau (1997), Kirmayer and Minas (2000), and Alarcón (2001) all speculate on the importance of developing a 'creolizing' cultural psychiatry, one that recognizes and can handle the apparent cultural changes wrought by processes of globalization. Cultural change appears to be proceeding at an unprecedented rate, and simply drawing boundaries around cultures, defining them as discrete entities, no longer makes sense (if it ever did). The existence of specific cultures must remain an empirical question, and it is time to adopt a different perspective entirely. Perhaps creolizing has been with us much longer than the fashionable idea of globalization would lead us to think. As psychologists Herman and Kempen (1998: 1113) have argued, 'cultural mélange typically precedes the present era in which many social scientists often discuss Western and other cultures as if these were pure in their origin and development.'

I find the suggestion that anthropology (and, by extension, other disciplines) should abandon the concept of culture (e.g., Abu-Lughod

1991; see also Borofsky, Barth, Shweder, Rodseth, & Stolzenberg 2001) vacuous. We need to continue to develop theories of culture from which scholars can derive working models to guide their research. Much of the scholarship on Aboriginal mental health has suffered from underdeveloped and fractured theory, and hence dysfunctional models of culture. Abandoning the culture concept is not the answer to this problem. But neither is leaving cultural theory to wallow in its current fragmented state. Perhaps a 'distributive' model of culture, which focuses more on semantic meanings shared by populations which are unbounded, might be the answer, a framework that seeks to study the 'cultural' without studying 'cultures' (Keesing 1990; Rodseth 1998).

The question of what we think we know about Aboriginal mental health is tied to the question of how we think we know it. My analysis suggests that, conceptually and methodologically, much work is problematic and, therefore, our knowledge about Aboriginal mental health should be suspect, particularly if we are assuming that in some way Aboriginality is relevant. Anthropology, psychology, and psychiatry continue to conceptualize Aboriginal peoples as different, and this is why special attention is often given to them in mental health research and clinical practice. We hunt for difference, and when we cannot find it, we construct it, even 'overstate' it (Keesing 1990: 48). If we are going to treat Aboriginal peoples as different, in research or in the clinic, then we must understand how and why they are different, and in which contexts the difference is relevant. Despite assertions of marginality, this difference is only occasionally conceived of in contemporary economic and political terms. Most frequently, it is represented as one of historical experience, cultural distinctiveness, and cultural marginalization, but rarely are such presentations accompanied by theoretically or methodologically rigorous intellectual supports. Just as we have diagnosed the windigo psychotic without seeing the patient, so too have we imputed culture without seeing it, without understanding or conceptualizing it. The windigo's revenge is not its return to eat us in the embodied sense, but rather the persistence and tenacity with which we cling to ill-conceived ideas as truths, the ways in which we are consumed by the very knowledge that we trust to guide us. Having given life to the psychotic cannibal, inadvertently unleashing its primal forces into our ethnographies, our psychiatric textbooks, our clinics, and even our popular culture, we must now find a way to finally terminate it. Otherwise, the windigo will continue to return, perhaps in the guise of an Ojibwa patient in a Toronto mental health clinic. Hungry.

Notes

Chapter 1. Introduction: Monsters and Mental Health

1 The concept of post-colonialism is itself contested, and not all will agree with my, or Bhabha's, use of this one aspect.

2 The terms 'Barbaric' and 'Arcadian' are both derived from Greek epistemology. Barbaric described an individual who was inherently animalistic; Arcadian referred to individuals living a life of idyllic simplicity. See Lucas and Barrett (1995) for a more elaborate discussion.

Chapter 2. Constructing Aboriginal Personality: The Early Years

1 The concepts of Apollonian and Dionysian were borrowed by Benedict from Nietzsche's study of Greek tragedy.

2 A subsequent chapter will look more closely at the work and impact of the acculturationists.

3 Some of these individuals wrote little or nothing on the project, acting mainly as consultants. Others continued to publish data based on the project for many years, or else went on to refine their work. I have not attempted to develop a comprehensive bibliography for all of these individuals as it pertains to the Indian Education Research project.

4 These included works by Macgregor (1946) on the Dakota Sioux; Joseph, Spicer and Chesky (1949) on the Papago; Thompson (1950) and Thompson and Joseph (1965) on the Hopi; Leighton and Adair (1966) on the Zuni; and Leighton and Leighton (1949) and Leighton and Kluckhohn (1969) on the Navaho. I will deal primarily with the Hopi and Sioux studies here.

5 By the mid-1970s a new method for employing and analysing the Rorschach test, known as the 'Comprehensive System,' had been adopted

throughout much of the world as a standardized technique. By this time, use of the Rorschach with American Indians had declined substantially.

6 Not every portrait of the Hopi at this time was as flattering. Dorothy Eggan, who undertook field research with the Hopi commencing in 1939, was struck by the 'mass maladjustment of these people, maladjustment being here defined as a state in which friction predominates in personal relations, and in which the worst is anxiously and habitually anticipated' (Eggan 1943: 357).

7 In contrast to my views on this issue, Kracke (1987: 39) has suggested that Erikson's brief research with the Sioux must be placed within proper perspective, in that anthropologists 'of the time,' such as Ruth Benedict and Esther Goldfrank, often spent only a few months in the field. Overall, Kracke presents a much more sympathetic portrait of Erkison's work than I have done.

Chapter 3. The Psychoanalyst's Aboriginal

1 Some of Hallowell's best work on the Saulteaux and his use of the Rorschach can be found in a compilation called *Culture and Experience* (Hallowell 1955).

2 Hallowell also continued to present Rorschach-based papers to the American Anthropological Association (e.g., Hallowell 1942).

3 Hallowell also employed the Thematic Apperception Test, but he is most celebrated for his pioneering Rorschach analysis.

4 I will critically examine the culture area concept and its use in research later in the book.

5 The concepts of atomism and the ethic of non-interference will receive critical review in subsequent chapters.

6 Others, such as ethnographer and psychoanalyst George Devereux (1951) in his report of psychotherapy involving a Plains Indian, argued for the persistence of a basic personality which continued to exist in the unconscious despite extensive cultural change.

7 Hallowell's interpretations of the problems at Lac du Flambeau were subsequently 'confirmed' by Caudill (1949) using the TAT.

8 It should be noted that various other societies around the world were also labelled 'atomistic' by proponents of this concept, as Honigmann discussed in his article (1968).

9 Another critic was anthropologist Harold Hickerson (1960, 1962, 1967).

10 Honigmann (1968) noted that many views of the atomistic society accepted the basic premise of George Foster's 'image of limited good' concept, in

which peasants, competing for resources which they see as inherently limited, assume that any personal gain is achieved at the expense of others. This creates a wariness in social relations, since friends and even kin are also competitors.

Chapter 4. Measuring the Aboriginal

1 As I note in a subsequent chapter, however, some scholars have suggested the existence of a primal Aboriginal culture buried within the assimilated body.

2 Attempts at measuring cultural orientation or acculturation for other groups have also been made. Inkeles and Smith (1974) have dealt with this issue cross-nationally; Doob (1967) for Africa; Dawson (1969) and De Lacy (1970) for indigenous Australians; and Olmedo, Martinez, and Martinez (1978), Olmedo and Padilla (1978), and Cuellar, Harris, and Jasso (1980) for Mexican Americans. Berry, Trumble, and Olmedo (1986) and Zane and Mak (2003) provide good introductions to the issues involved.

3 Some tests I will not discuss but which have been employed with the Aboriginal population include: the Eysenck Personality Questionnaire (Hurlburt & Gade 1984); the Rotter Locus of Control Scale (Hurlburt, Gade & Fuqua 1983); the California Psychological Inventory (Mason 1967, 1968, 1969, 1971; Davis, Hoffman, & Nelson 1990); the Social Readjustment Rating Scale (Liberman & Frank 1980); the Piers-Harris Self Concept Scale (Long & Hamlin 1988); the Differential Personality Inventory (Hoffman & Jackson 1973); and the Raven Matrices (Wiltshire & Gray 1969; MacAvoy, Orr, & Sidles 1993). For a review of intelligence and personality tests used with Aboriginal North Americans, see Dauphinais and King (1992).

4 Some, such as French (1993) continued to work on adapting projective tests for use with American Indian and other minority populations

5 The 'F' scale is designed to examine the subject's attitude towards the test. If attitude is determined to be acceptable, the F scale also serves as a good indicator of psychopathology. High F scores are often associated with high scores on the clinical scales (Graham 1990).

6 An excellent source on nineteenth-century science and Aboriginal North Americans which speaks to this and the related issue of blood quantum is Bieder (1986). See also Gould (1996).

7 Comparisons between American Indians and Negroes was common in the late nineteenth and early twentieth centuries as a means of elevating the status of the former (Harris 1968).

8 While I am going to focus the remainder of my discussion on the Wechsler

tests, readers should be aware that many other kinds of intelligence tests have been employed with North American Aboriginal peoples. See, for instance, Havighurst and Hilkevitch (1944), Snider and Coladarci (1960), West and MacArthur (1964), Wiltshire and Gray (1969), as well as the other literature cited in this section. Several reviews of the use of intelligence tests for Aboriginal peoples can also be consulted, including Dana (1984), McShane and Berry (1988), and Dauphinais and King (1992).

9 Several commentators have even suggested that from a psychometric perspective the differences are slight. For instance, Beiser and Gotowiec (2000) note that Wechsler cited WISC-R as part of the evidence for the validity of WISC-III. See also McShane and Plas (1984).

10 Performance on some items of the Wechsler tests is evaluated, in part, on the speed of execution.

11 The concept of blood quantum per se is not a predominant method of assessing Aboriginality in Canada, and the expression is rarely heard.

12 As I embark on this critical examination of the use of the culture area concept, I confess to having used it myself as a means of framing pre-contact Aboriginal cultures in a volume intended, in part, to inform psychologists and psychiatrists (see Waldram, Herring, & Young 1995).

13 In some instances, there can be important differences among communities – such as among the Navajo and Sioux – that could suggest somewhat different cultural orientations; mixing of research subjects should therefore be avoided. In the Arctic, however, research lumping several Inuit villages together may not be problematic because of strong cultural similarities (e.g., Wilgosh, Mulcehy, & Walters 1986).

Chapter 5. The Construction of Aboriginal Psychopathology

1 Ackerknecht (1943), in the article I have referenced here, was one of the few to challenge the idea that 'primitive' societies were inherently psychopathological.

2 Hippler (1976) provided a good review of the controversy surrounding the mental status of shamans.

3 Certainly there were those who argued differently. A minority viewpoint was offered by Chance and Foster (1962) and Chance (1965), in a study of Alaskan Eskimos. Utilizing a variety of indices and instruments, including the Cornell Medical Index, they determined that both male and female Eskimos were adapting to Western-influenced rapid cultural changes quite well. This appeared to be the case for a variety of reasons: as a product of a traditional cultural pattern supporting adaptation rather than entrench-

ment; because the change was largely voluntary; and because these people seemed to have ready access to the means to achieve new goals through employment. Barger (1977) described the differential adjustment of Inuit and Cree to the town of Great Whale River, noting that the Inuit were better integrated within town life, but that there were no significant differences between the two groups in terms of mental illness and deviancy. However, these perspectives on the impacts of cultural change are relatively rare, and most research has been based on the assumption that, for Aboriginal peoples, cultural change since the arrival of Europeans has had negative consequences for mental health.

4 Berry, Wintrob, Sindell, & Mawhinney (1982) acknowledged the existence of Hudson's Bay Company and other stores in the Cree communities.

5 The experiences of North American–born ethnic minority individuals have more recently been described as qualitatively different from those of recent migrants, which confounds acculturation studies in which individuals from each group are combined into a single category (Zane & Mak 2003). Theorizing about how Aboriginal peoples might experience acculturation differently from either new immigrants or members of other resident ethnic minorities has been lacking, and is sorely needed.

6 The Cornell Medical Index (CMI) was a 195-question instrument detailing past and present health status, moods, feelings, and so forth which required simple 'yes' or 'no' answers by self-reporting respondents. It was highly popular in the 1960s and 1970s.

7 The authors did cite work by Hollingshead and Redlich (1958) as the source for this method.

8 See, for example, the studies many consider to be classics of psychiatry: *My Name Is Legion* by Alexander Leighton (1959b) and *The Character of Danger* by Leighton, Harding, Macklin, Macmillan, and Leighton (1963).

9 Those few studies which have attempted to consider class have characteristically failed to theorize the concept and have instead usually employed a variation of the concept of 'socio-economic status.'

10 Rodgers (1974) similarly noted that, in a study of psychopathology among the Inuit, new housing and infrastructure combined with a campaign against tuberculosis resulted in a decline in psychiatric referrals.

Chapter 6. The Alcoholic Aboriginal

1 In an interesting twist on this argument, Boyer (1964b: 218) suggested that the Apache believed that 'an immoderate tendency to drink is inborn,' and that they understood this to be the result of the actions on a previous gener-

ation of 'witches, angry "power," and the schemings of whites' who sought to destroy the people. The tendency was then passed on through the generations.

2 Several influential studies which have combined elements of both the paradigms I will discuss here include: Whittaker (1963); Hurt and Brown (1965); Ferguson (1968, 1970, 1976); Jilek-Aall (1974); Cooley (1980); and Jones-Saumty, Hochhaus, Dru, and Zeiner (1983).

3 Horton (1943) did not suggest that all 'primitive' societies were incapable of controlling individual behaviour, and cited the Hopi and Zuni as examples of those that seemed to have little interest in alcohol.

4 Stratton, Zeiner, and Paredes (1978) found a similar phenomenon among various Indian tribes in Oklahoma: the tribes that had been most acculturated, those originally in the east, had fewer alcohol problems than those more connected to their traditional cultures, the Plains Indians.

5 The idea of levels of sociocultural intergration has been employed with some frequency in alcohol studies. Stratton, Zeiner, and Parades (1978: 1175), for instance, argued that North American Indian tribes with a hunting-gathering tradition would have more serious drinking problems than tribes with an agricultural tradition, because of the emphasis on communal values and ceremonies in the latter. The individualistic behaviour characteristic of those at the 'band' level of sociocultural intergration was thought to be somewhat of a risk factor for alcohol, according to May (1982, 1996), which for him explained high rates of alcohol abuse in the Plains and low rates among the Pueblos. The nature of band societies was also seen as rendering them more vulnerable to externally generated processes of cultural change.

6 On this point, Kunitz and Levy (1994: 234) have written that they were accused of falsifying the data on the Hopi because the speculation that many were solitary, non-public drinkers 'flew in the face of what everyone knew to be the truth about Hopi behavior.'

7 Interestingly, Jilek (1982) subsequently described the spirit dance as an integral mechanism in the sobriety movement on the northwest coast.

8 Longclaws, Barnes, Grieve, and Dumoff (1980) speculated that among the Brokenhead Ojibwa in Manitoba, young people were attracted to cannabis because it provided a spiritual outlet which filled the void caused by the decline in traditional beliefs.

9 Lamarine (1988) refers to this as the 'historical theory' of Indian alcohol use. In a reaction to this idea, John Price (1975) argued that alcohol was indigenous to much of Mexico, and therefore the fact that the people had quite a bit longer to develop norms for drinking failed to explain the high rates of alcohol consumption there.

10 I am not suggesting that such studies are irrelevant, however, since they demonstrate a great deal about lifestyles of individuals. Perhaps the best study of this type, by Jarvis and Boldt (1982), examined 'death styles' among Aboriginal people in Alberta by interviewing families and friends of individuals who had died from accidents, violence, and suicide, and they were able to demonstrate the paramount role that alcohol played not only in these deaths but in the lives of the ill-fated individuals leading up to the moment of death.

11 The most influential epidemiological studies would appear to be: Whittaker (1962), Westermeyer (1972a), Kline and Roberts (1973), Shore et al. (1973), Gracia (1976), Streit and Nicolich (1977), Beltrame and McQueen (1979), Kraus and Buffler (1979), Manson et al. (1992), Kettl and Bixler (1993), and Barker and Kramer (1996).

Chapter 7. The Depressed Aboriginal

1 I have chosen to discuss suicide primarily in conjunction with my discussion of depression. Much research suggests that the link between suicide and alcohol abuse among Aboriginal peoples is quite strong, however, and therefore a discussion of suicide in chapter 6 (alcohol) would also have been appropriate.

2 This may not be entirely accurate, however. Medicine (1982: 204), a Lakota anthropologist and native Lakota speaker, has argued that this interpretation is off-base, and that the expression 'ta watl yesni' actually means 'tiredness,' as in tiredness of a specific obnoxious situation.

3 This notion of loss is also well-developed in Willms et al. (1992) for Nishnawbe (Ojibwa) people in northern Ontario.

4 Most of the epidemiological evidence does suggest some fairly broad patterns in suicide, however, including the propensity for Aboriginal suicides to be young, male, under the influence of alcohol or another drug, and for the suicide to be a spontaneous act involving a more or less instantaneously lethal method.

5 Readers are best directed to the relevant report for a full discussion of the methodology (Manson et al. 1985).

6 Despite her concern with the appropriateness of the DSM framework for the Flathead, O'Nell nevertheless attempted to fit one case study into DSM-IV's cultural formulation as part of the series of such exercises ('clinical case studies') published in the journal *Culture, Medicine and Psychiatry* (O'Nell 1998). Her treatment is actually one of the best, but this is because of her rich and detailed knowledge of these people, which grew out of her fieldwork. In these circumstances, the cultural framework becomes redun-

dant. What is frightening is the possibility that individuals with relatively little knowledge about a given culture will utilize the formulation and generate ill-informed interpretations.

7 Elsewhere, I have described this process as the biomedicalization of indigenous medicine and suggested that a superficial focus on English language terminology often results in inappropriate judgments regarding efficacy (Waldram 2000).

8 O'Nell was not opposed to the use of DSM in cross-cultural research, however, but believed it needed to better capture the essence of culturally meaningful syndromes. I, on the other hand, am less convinced that it is possible to use DSM meaningfully in cross-cultural research, at least for the foreseeable future.

Chapter 8. The Culture-Bound Aboriginal

1 Windigo is also spelled 'witiko' and 'wittiko' in the literature, often in reference to the Ojibwa ('windigo') and Cree ('wiitiko'). I will use 'windigo' generically in this chapter, except when citing specific literature.

2 Other explanations posited for windigo psychoses are centred more directly on environmental stresses and nutritional deficiencies. See Marano (1985) for a review of these.

3 Similar to windigo psychosis (see note 2), environmental and nutritional explanations were also offered for *pibloqtoq*. See Wallace (1961), Foulks (1972), and Dick (1995).

4 The Hmong are a southeast Asian people. Their experiences in the United States as immigrants have been well documented; one of the more engaging accounts is Fadiman (1997).

5 There is one other mention of American Indians in DSM IV-TR. The Navajo are presented as exhibiting a variant of the disorder known as amok, 'a dissociative episode characterized by a period of brooding followed by an outburst of violence, aggressive, or homicidal behavior directed at people and objects' (American Psychiatric Association 2000: 899). Amok was originally identified among Malaysians, and its facile extension to the Navajo perhaps underscores DSM's problem with conceptualizing cultures and culture-bound syndromes.

6 This symptom list for ghost sickness is taken almost verbatim from Kaplan and Johnson (1964: 212) without attribution. Further, note how the ethnographic detail from Navajo, Mohave, and several Apache groups has been converted into 'many American Indian tribes.'

7 Interestingly, this was the only version of the Merck Manual to discuss cul-

ture-bound syndromes; the subsequent seventeenth edition did not mention them and has even eliminated the discussion of cross-cultural issues. However, new exotic disorders such as chronic fatigue syndrome and Gulf War syndrome have been added (Beers & Berkow 1999).

8 This website is maintained by Parkhurst Publishing, a Canadian company that produces two periodicals for medical professionals, *Doctor's Review* and *Parkhurst Exchange*.

9 See, for instance, 'Spider-Man,' volume 1, no. 10 (May 1991), published by Marvel Comics.

10 Rogler (1996) accurately noted that many scholars have suggested that anorexia nervosa should be defined as a culture-bound syndrome; however, he also noted, tellingly, that it is *not* included as a culture-bound syndrome in DSM-IV. Mezzich et al. (1999), scholars who were active in providing advice on culture for DSM-IV, imply in their discussion of DSM-IVs glossary of culture-bound syndromes that anorexia nervosa, among other 'Western' disorders, was included when in fact it was not; a discussion of cultural considerations for anorexia nervosa appeared within the text of DSM IV itself but the condition is not identified as a culture-bound syndrome.

11 According to Martínez-Hernáez (2000: 68), the DSM has been translated into twenty languages and is used worldwide, even though it was originally intended only for use in North America. On this latter point, I would note the assumption that 'North America' was obviously viewed as culturally homogeneous.

12 Interestingly, while DSM-IV contains a definition of 'disorder,' it does not define 'syndrome.' In an excellent review of these concepts, Kirmayer and Young (1999: 447) defined syndrome to mean a condition in which 'certain signs and symptoms (experiences and behavior) are found to frequently co-occur and thus form a recognizable pattern that, through naming the syndrome, is given the status of an entity.' They argued that 'The notion of disorder attempts to go beyond the notion of syndrome by implying that there is some distinctive underlying disturbance of functioning that characterizes these syndromes' (448). DSM-IV defines a medical disorder as 'a clinically significant behavioral or psychological syndrome or pattern ...' The implication of all this is that culture-bound syndromes exist in a kind of liminal or tenuous position between 'real' psychiatric disorder and something else, perhaps artifact or fabrication. When the concept of culture-boundedness first arose these states were often conceptualized as culture-specific illnesses; they were then elevated to disorders (e.g., Foster & Anderson 1978; Kleinman 1980), but recently lost this status as they were bumped to syn-

330 Notes to pages 209–33

dromes. It would seem that, at least in some circles, there is considerable apprehension about their existence, yet this sentiment is rarely communicated directly in the psychiatric literature.

Chapter 9. The Traumatized Aboriginal

1 Kirk and Kutchins (1992) and Kutchins and Kirk (1997) have done an excellent job in demonstrating the social and political underpinnings of the DSM.
2 Manson (1996) has also published a report on one veteran diagnosed with PTSD utilizing the DSM-IV cultural formulation. Like many of the 'cultural formulation' case studies published in the journal *Culture, Medicine and Psychiatry*, very little actual cultural information was provided; under the section on 'cultural identity' we learned only that the patient was a 'fullblood' who was enrolled in 'a southwestern American Indian tribe residing largely in Arizona' (492) and who spoke his Indian language fluently. It is also noteworthy that, unlike many other PTSD conceptualizations with regard to Aboriginal peoples, little historical analysis was presented in the case. O'Nell's work, discussed in the chapter on depression, demonstrates that DSM clearly does not encompass historical dimensions of disorders, and Manson, who has written of this history, was obviously unable to find a way to work it in.
3 Indeed, *Native American postcolonial psychology* is fraught with the kinds of contradictions one might expect in the presentation of ideas which are still under development. For instance, the authors anchor their psychology in the work of Jung while criticizing the whole psychology framework, advocating for a move away from 'linear' thinking, and arguing for an 'indigenous' perspective.
4 Elsewhere in the volume, Duran and Duran (1995: 52–3) again criticized the DSM and its ever-evolving nature, while advocating for the inclusion of this new disorder. Since the DSM aspires to be a global nosology, they were in effect accepting that psychiatrists and psychologists without any knowledge of the American Indian history or situation would be applying the criteria for this diagnosis.
5 Gagné (1998) has done a similar thing for the Cree of James Bay, utilizing a dependency theory perspective.
6 Chrisjohn and Young (1997: 31–3) presented a considerably more detailed listing of abuses. My abbreviated list is intended only to give the reader an introduction.
7 The focus of the Aboriginal Healing Foundation also includes healing projects not directly related to residential schools.

8 At the time of writing, the Aboriginal Healing Foundation maintained a website which documented the projects they have funded. The web address is *www.ahf.ca*.

9 This individual refused to let me see a copy of the instrument, but its existence was advertised in an Aboriginal newspaper, *Windspeaker*.

10 I realize that this will be a contentious point for many, as it implies some people are simply faking. Having spent seventeen years in a Native Studies department, I can attest to the existence of these stories as they circulate informally or are raised in the classroom by Aboriginal students, many of whom feel that these charlatans are damaging the case of the real survivors of the schools. As one student once told me, any Indian in western Canada can find a relative who was in a residential school, and then scream 'intergenerational residential school syndrome!'

Chapter 10. The Clinician's Aboriginal

1 The Harvard (University) Values Project, for instance, attempted to look at values within the context of cultural change in several American Indian communities, and generated a great deal of data (Honigmann 1961b).

2 Wax and Thomas (1961) were influenced by Freudian psychoanalysis and ethnographic work by Gordon Macgregor on the Sioux, although they were somewhat critical of Erik Erikson's work.

3 These communities were part of the larger 'Values Project' undertaken by Harvard University (Kluckhohn and Strodtbeck 1961: 344).

4 The Spanish-American community selected for study contained only this number of adults, and hence this was used as the benchmark for the other communities as well.

5 Kluckhohn and Strodtbeck (1961: 105–6) provide a more detailed rationale for their use of such small samples.

6 Anthropologists did not completely vacate the field of ethics, values, and behaviours after the 1970s, however, as evident in the work of Green (1999), described below, but their interest in researching cultural values appeared to give way to the rote listing of assumed values for specific cultures as a contribution to the training of mental health and social service professionals.

7 Richardson is clearly the author of this chapter in Sue (1981), even though this is not stated at the beginning of the chapter itself.

8 But this is not the only example of such cognitive quantum leaping. Take, for instance, Still and Hodgins (1998) recent handbook chapter on the Navajo, in which they presented another of those all too common compara-

tive trait lists for the Pueblo Indians, Navajo, Apache, Pima, and Papago, lumped together and glossed as 'Indian culture.'

9 Note the use of capital letters in *Harmony Ethic*. This is common in so-called New Age literature pertaining to Aboriginal peoples, and represents another example of primitivist discourse. See Kehoe (1990).

10 Here, of course, I am taking the opposite stand to my argument in an earlier chapter that too many authors have simply assumed that colonization experiences were identical. My main point is that neither position has been empirically investigated, and assertions of one or the other are either the result of uninformed naivete or ideology.

11 The issue of therapist-client cultural affinity is relevant to many different cultural groups in North America. Sue (1998) discussed some recent research in this area and suggested that for some groups, such as 'Whites' and African Americans, ethnic matching did not appear to be related to better therapeutic outcomes than it is for other groups, such as Asian Americans and Mexican Americans.

12 Underutilization of mental health services is generally seen as problematic, but in a surprising twist Dinges, Trimble, Manson, & Pasquale (1981), along with LaFromboise and Rowe (1983) suggested that avoidance may well be a good thing, 'exposing fewer persons to the acculturative stress associated with traditional psychotherapy and avoiding large-scale exposure to the culturally biased attribution of problems that is inherent in the process' (LaFromboise & Rowe 1983: 589).

13 This caution went largely unheeded by subsequent researchers using Haviland, Horswill, O'Connell, & Dynneson's (1983) work; attention was concentrated on the finding of preference differences, as if these also meant differences in therapeutic outcome. Haviland et al., like Teft (1967), was a very specific, focused study whose substantial limitations were detailed by the authors. The cautious conclusions of both studies assumed new lives as substantiated scientific fact.

14 A careful reading of this chapter will have shown that at no point do I suggest that Aboriginal peoples do not share some values, or that their values and cultures are not different from those of non-Aboriginal peoples, or even that Aboriginal people should not be treated differently in psychotherapy. In critiquing various anthropological and psychological works on counselling and psychotherapy with Aboriginal peoples, I am not suggesting that conventional approaches are, in fact, unconditionally appropriate for this population. My concern here, and in this book as a whole, is with comprehending how the knowledge about Aboriginal peoples has been constructed and the need to grasp the meaning of contemporary Aboriginality.

Chapter 11. Healing the Traditional Aboriginal

1 According to Rogers (1944: 559, n2), Clements was building upon an even earlier foundation established by German scholar Max Bartels in 1893.

2 One must keep in mind that Clements's analysis, at least in part, was only as comprehensive as his data sources which, he noted, were inconsistent.

3 Consider the following recent comment by Spector (2000: 178): 'American Indians do not subscribe to the germ theory of modern medicine.' Where did Spector obtain such a ridiculous idea (setting aside the problems of generalizing across diverse cultural groups, as well as her suggestion that this view is a *current* one)? From a New Age style book about a shaman named 'Rolling Thunder,' healer to rock group the Grateful Dead.

4 Kroeber (1923; rpt 1948: 298) tantalized his readers by questioning if 'our discards, insane, and hypersuggestibles' were 'perhaps right and the rest of us wrong?' But he did not pursue this line of inquiry.

5 In DSM-IV (American Psychiatric Association 2000), references to the magical thinking of schizophrenics and primitive peoples were removed.

6 Csordas (1994: 7) also relates that Descartes saw the distinction between mind and body more as a methodological tool than a doctrine, and hence the notion of Cartesian dualism is really the handiwork of subsequent philosophers.

7 See the work of Richard De Mille (1976, 1990) on the controversy surrounding Carlos Castenada and his allegedly mythical Yaqui shaman teacher, Don Juan.

8 An 'invented tradition' is one that is modern in its development and seeks to achieve modern goals, yet uses as its authority a supposed connection to the past and historic continuity. For a good review of the issues surrounding indigenous peoples and invented tradition, see Babadzin (2000).

9 Only a few scholars have addressed this flip side to the Arcadian notion of shaman as noble healer; see, for example, Hallowell (1963), Kennedy (1984), Young, Ingram, and Swartz (1989), and Waldram (1997).

10 The expression 'medicine wheel' has two meanings. It refers to a stone structure, roughly like a wheel with spokes, that has been found throughout the northern plains in particular, the meaning of which is not readily apparent to either archeologists or contemporary Aboriginal peoples. It also refers to a pedagogical device, a drawing of a circle partitioned in various ways to represent Aboriginal philosophy and world-view. This latter form is commonly used in treatment programs and is viewed as a 'traditional' approach (e.g., Gray & Nye 2001). There is considerable doubt as to its authenticity as a strictly Aboriginal modality, however, and it has been

suggested that it was actually invented by New Age author Hyemeyohsts Storm, whose liberal use of Aboriginal symbolism was combined with suggestions that the author was Aboriginal (Kehoe 1990). Whether the Medicine Wheel is an effective tool is, of course, a separate issue. Its use is widespread, and those who employ it are often emphatic in their pronouncements of its effectiveness.

Chapter 12. Conclusion: The Windigo's Revenge

1 I am not suggesting that anthropologists no longer work with North American Aboriginal peoples; I am suggesting that this is no longer seen as significant to the contribution of theory or methodology in the discipline as it once was. Indeed, it is my view, echoed by many of my colleagues at conferences, that Aboriginal research is devalued in ways similar to local or urban work. 'Real' anthropology supposedly takes place somewhere else, among the decidedly exoticized and unfamiliar, and not in your own backyard. It would also be fair to suggest that some North American anthropologists have reacted to emerging Aboriginal criticisms of the discipline by abandoning Aboriginal research altogether, or else by eschewing their sense of scholarly privilege (and many years of specialized training) and turning over research to the 'community,' itself an essentialization.

References

Abbey, S., Hood, E., Young, T., & Malcolmson, S.A. (1993). Psychiatric consultation in the Eastern Canadian Arctic: III. Mental health issues in Inuit women in the Eastern Arctic. *Canadian Journal of Psychiatry, 38*(1), 32–5.

Abbott, P.J. (1996). American Indians and Alaska Native Aboriginal use of alcohol in the United States. *American Indian and Alaska Native Mental Health Research, 7*(2), 1–13.

Abbott, P.J. (1998). Traditional and Western healing practices for alcoholism in American Indian and Alaska Natives. *Substance Use and Misuse, 33*(13), 2605–46.

Abel, T., Metraux, R., & Roll, S. (1987). *Psychotherapy and culture.* Albuquerque, NM: University of New Mexico Press.

Aberle, D.F. (1951). The psychosocial analysis of a Hopi life-history. *Comparative Psychology Monographs, 21*(1), 80–138.

Aberle, D.F. (1966). *The peyote religion among the Navajo.* New York: Viking Fund Publication in Anthropology, No. 42.

Abu-Lughod, L. (1991). Writing against culture. In R. Fox (Ed.), *Recapturing anthropology: Working in the present.* Santa Fe: School of American Research Press.

Ackerknecht, E.H. (1943). Psychopathology, primitive medicine and primitive culture. *Bulletin of the History of Medicine, 14*(1), 30–67.

Ackerman, L.A. (1971). Marital instability and juvenile delinquency among the Nez Perces. *American Anthropologist, 73*(3), 595–603.

Ackerson, L.M., Dick, R.W., Manson, S.M., & Baron, A.E. (1990). Properties of the inventory to diagnose depression in American Indian adolescents. *Journal of the American Academy of Child and Adolescent Psychiatry, 29*, 601–7.

Adelson, N. (2000). *'Being alive well': Health and the politics of Cree well-being.* Toronto: University of Toronto Press.

Adelson, N. (2001). Towards a recuperation of souls and bodies: Community healing and the complex interplay of faith and history. In L. Kirmayer, M.E. Macdonald, & G. Brass (Eds.), *The mental health of Indigenous peoples* (pp. 120–34). (Culture and Mental Health Research Report No. 10). Montreal: Institute of Community and Family Psychiatry, Sir Mortimer B. Davis Jewish General Hospital, and Division of Social and Transcultural Psychiatry, McGill University.

Adrian, M., Layne, N., & Williams, R.T. (1991). Estimating the effect of Native Indian population on county alcohol consumption: The example of Ontario. *The International Journal of the Addictions, 25*(5A and 6A), 731–65.

Alarcón, R. (1995). Culture and psychiatric diagnosis: Impact on DSM-IV and ICD-10. *Psychiatric Annals of North America 18*(3), 449–65.

Alarcón, R.D. (2001). Hispanic psychiatry: From margin to mainstream. *Transcultural Psychiatry, 38*(1), 5–25.

Alarcón, R.D., Foulks, E.F., & Vakkur, M. (1998). *Personality disorders and culture. Clinical and conceptual interactions.* New York: John Wiley and Sons.

Alarcón, R., Westermeyer, J., Foulks, E., & Ruiz, P. (1999). Clinical relevance of contemporary cultural psychiatry. *Journal of Nervous and Mental Disease, 187*(8), 465–71.

Allen, J. (1998). Personality assessment with American Indians and Alaska Natives: Instrument considerations and service delivery style. *Journal of Personality Assessment, 70*(1), 17–42.

American Psychiatric Association. (1980). Diagnostic and statistical manual of mental disorders. (3rd ed.). Washington, DC: American Psychiatric Association.

American Psychiatric Association. (1987). Diagnostic and statistical manual of mental disorders. (3rd ed. Revised.). Washington, DC: American Psychiatric Association.

American Psychiatric Association. (1994). Diagnostic and statistical manual of mental disorders. (4th ed.). Washington, DC: American Psychiatric Association.

American Psychiatric Association. (2000). Diagnostic and statistical manual of mental disorders. (4th ed. Text Revision; DSM IV-TR). Washington, DC: American Psychiatric Association.

Anderson, E.N. (1992). A healing place: ethnographic notes on a treatment center. *Alcoholism Treatment Quarterly, 9*(3/4), 1–21.

Anderson, F. (1936). A mental-hygiene survey of problem Indian children in Oklahoma. *Mental Hygiene, 20*, 472–6.

Anderson, M.J., & Ellis, R. (1995). On the reservation. In N. Vacc, S. DeVaney,

& J. Wittmer (Eds.), *Experiencing and counseling multicultural and diverse populations* (pp. 179–97). Bristol, PA: Accelerated Development.

Angel, R., & Guarnaccia, P.J. (1989). Mind, body, and culture: Somatization among Hispanics. *Social Science and Medicine, 28*(12), 1229–38.

Antze, P., & Lambek, M. (1996). Preface. In P. Antze and M. Lambek (Eds.), *Tense past: Cultural essays in trauma and memory* (pp. vii–ix). New York: Routledge.

Archibald, Jr, C.W. (1974). Group psychotherapy with American Indians. In M. Rosenbaum (Ed.), *Group psychotherapy* (pp. 43–7). New York: Gordon and Breach Science Publishers.

Armstrong, H. (1993). Depression in Canadian Native Indians. In P. Cappeliez and R.J. Flynn (Eds.), *Depression and the social environment: Research and intervention with neglected populations* (pp. 218–34). Montreal: McGill-Queen's University Press.

Arthur, G. (1944). An experience in examining an Indian twelfth-grade group with the Multiphasic Personality Inventory. *Mental Hygiene, 28*, 243–50.

Ashby, M.R., Gilchrist, L.D., & Miramontez, A. (1987). Group treatment for sexually abused American Indian adolescents. *Social Work with Groups, 10*(4), 21–32.

Assembly of First Nations (AFN). (1994). *Breaking the silence: An interpretive study of residential school impact and healing as illustrated by the stories of First Nations individuals.* Ottawa: Assembly of First Nations.

Atkinson, D.R., Morten, G., & Sue, D.W. (1993). The American Indian client. In D.R. Atkinson, G. Morten, and D.W. Sue (Eds.), *Counseling American minorities: A cross-cultural perspective* (pp. 119–21). Madison, WI: Brown and Benchmark.

Attneave, C. (1969). Therapy in tribal settings and urban network intervention. *Family Process, 8*, 192–210.

Attneave, C. (1982). American Indians and Alaska Native Families: Emigrants in their own homeland. In M. McGoldrick, J. Pearce, and J. Giordano (Eds.), *Ethnicity and family therapy* (pp. 55–83). New York: Guilford Press.

Attneave, C. (1987). Practical counseling with American Indian and Alaska Native clients. In P. Pederson (Ed.), *Handbook of cross-cultural counseling and therapy* (pp. 135–40). Westport, CT: Greenwood Press.

Azar, B. (1999). Wider path to cultural understanding. Researchers move toward a multicultural, rather than a linear, model of acculturation. *APA Monitor [Online], 30*(3). Available: *www.apa.org/monitor/mar99/multi.html*.

Babadzin, A. (2000). Anthropology, nationalism and 'the invention of tradition.' *Anthropological Forum, 10*(20), 131–55.

Bachman, R. (1992). *Death and violence on the reservation: Homicide, family violence, and suicide in American Indian populations.* New York: Auburn House.

Bagley, C. (1991). Poverty and suicide among Native Canadians: A replication. *Psychological Reports, 69*(1), 149–50.

Bagley, C., Wood, M., & Khumar, H. (1990). Suicide and careless death in young males: Ecological study of an Aboriginal population in Canada. *Canadian Journal of Community Mental Health, 9*(1), 127–42.

Bailey, P. (1922). A contribution to the mental pathology of races in the United States. *Archives of Neurology and Psychiatry, 7*(2), 183–201.

Baker, J.L. (1959). Indians, alcohol, and homicide. *Journal of Social Therapy, 5,* 270–5.

Balikci, A. (1961). Suicidal behavior among the Netsiluk Eskimos. In B.R. Blishen, F.E. Jones, K.D. Naegele, and J. Porter (Eds.), *Canadian Society: Sociological Perspectives* (pp. 575–88). Toronto: Macmillan.

Balikci, A. (1968). Bad Friends. *Human Organization, 27*(3), 191–9.

Barger, W.K. (1977). Culture change and psychosocial adjustment. *American Ethnologist, 4*(1), 471–95.

Barker, J.C., & Kramer, B.J. (1996). Alcohol consumption among older urban American Indians. *Journal of Studies on Alcohol, 57*(2), 119–24.

Barnard, A. (2000). *History and theory in anthropology.* Cambridge: Cambridge University Press.

Barnouw, V. (1950). Acculturation and personality among the Wisconsin Chippewa. *American Anthropologist, 52* (4, Part 2), Memoir #72.

Barnouw, V. (1961). Chippewa social atomism. *American Anthropologist, 63*(5), 1006–13.

Barnouw, V. (1973). *Culture and personality.* (rev. ed.). Homewood, IL: Dorsey Press.

Baron, A.E., Manson, S.M., Ackerson, L.M., & Brenneman, D.L. (1990). Depressive symptomatology in older American Indians with chronic disease: Some psychometric considerations. In C.C. Attkisson and J.M. Zich (Eds.), *Depression in primary care: Screening and detection* (pp. 217–31). New York: Routledge, Chapman, and Hall.

Barrett, S. (1984). *The rebirth of anthropological theory.* Toronto: University of Toronto Press.

Beals, J., Manson, S.M., Keane, E.M., & Dick, R.W. (1991). Factorial structure of the Center for Epidemiologic Studies-Depression scale among American Indian college students. *Psychological Assessment, 3*(4), 623–7.

Beals, J., Piasecki, J., Nelson, S., Jones, M., Keane, E., Dauphinais, P., Red Shirt, R., Sack, W.H., & Manson, S.M. (1997). Psychiatric disorder among American Indian adolescents: Prevalence in Northern Plains youth. *Journal of the American Academy of Child and Adolescent Psychiatry, 36*(9), 1252–9.

Beauvais, F. (1998). American Indians and alcohol. *Alcohol Health and Research World, 22*(4), 253–9.

Beauvais, F., & LaBoueff, S. (1985). Drug and alcohol abuse intervention in American Indian communities. *International Journal of the Addictions, 20*(1), 139–71.

Bechtold, D.W. (1988). Cluster suicide in American Indian adolescents. *American Indian and Alaska Native Mental Health Research, 1*(3), 26–35.

Bechtold, D.W. (1994). Indian suicide: Clinical and developmental considerations. In C. Duclas and S. Manson (Eds.), *Calling from the rim: Suicidal behavior among American Indian and Alaska Native adolescents* (pp. 71–80). American Indian and Alaska Native Mental Health Research, 4. Denver: University Press of Colorado.

Bee, R.L. (1974). *Patterns and processes: An introduction to anthropological strategies for the study of sociocultural change.* New York: Free Press.

Beers, M.H., & Berkow, R. (1999). *The Merck manual of diagnosis and therapy* (17th ed.). Whitehorse Station, NJ: Merck Research Laboratories.

Begay, D., & Maryboy, N. (2000). The whole universe is my cathedral: A contemporary Navajo spiritual synthesis. *Medical Anthropology Quarterly, 14*(4), 498–520.

Beiser, M. (1981). Mental health of American Indian and Alaska Native children: Some epidemiological perspectives. *White Cloud Journal, 2*(2), 37–47.

Beiser, M. (1985). The grieving witch: A framework for applying principles of cultural psychiatry to clinical practice. *Canadian Journal of Psychiatry, 30,* 130–41.

Beiser, M., & Attneave, C. (1982). Mental disorders among Native American children: Rates and risk periods for entering treatment. *American Journal of Psychiatry, 139*(2), 192–8.

Beiser, M., & Gotowiec, A. (2000). Accounting for Native/Non-Native Differences in IQ scores. *Psychology in Schools, 37*(3), 237–52.

Beltrame, T., & McQueen, D.V. (1979). Urban and rural drinking patterns: The special case of the Lumbee. *International Journal of the Addictions, 14*(4), 533–48.

Benedict, R. (1922). The vision in Plains culture. *American Anthropologist, 24,* 1–23.

Benedict, R. (1923). *The concept of the guardian spirit in North America.* Memoirs of the American Anthropological Association No. 29. Washington, DC: American Anthropological Association.

Benedict, R. (1928). Psychological types in the cultures of the Southwest. *Proceedings of the 23rd International Congress of Americanists, USA,* 527–81.

Benedict, R. (1932). Configurations of culture in North America. *American Anthropologist, 34*(1), 1–27.

Benedict, R. (1934a). Anthropology and the abnormal. *Journal of General Psychology, 10*, 59–80.

Benedict, R. (1934b). *Patterns of culture.* Boston, MA: Houghton Mifflin.

Bennion, L.J., & Li, T. (1976). Alcohol metabolism in American Indians and Whites. *New England Journal of Medicine, 294*(1), 9–13.

Berkow, R., & Fletcher, A.J. (1992). *The Merck manual of diagnosis and therapy.* (16th ed.). Rahway, NJ: Merck Research Laboratories.

Berlin, I.N. (1985). Prevention of adolescent suicide among some Native American tribes. *Adolescent Psychiatry, 12*, 77–93.

Berlin, I.N. (1986). Psychopathology and its antecedents among American Indian adolescents. In B.B. Lahey and A.E. Kazdin (Eds.), *Advances in clinical child psychology, Vol. 9* (pp. 125–52). New York: Plenum Press.

Berlin, I.N. (1987). Suicide among American Indian adolescents: An overview. *Suicide and Life-Threatening Behavior, 17*(3), 218–32.

Berreman, Gerald D. (1956). Drinking patterns of the Aleuts. *Quarterly Journal of Studies on Alcohol, 17*, 503–14.

Berry, J.W. (1970). Marginality, stress and ethnic identification in an acculturated Aboriginal community. *Journal of Cross-Cultural Psychology, 1*(3), 239–52.

Berry, J.W. (1975). Ecology, cultural adaptation, and psychological stress: Traditional patterning and acculturative stress. In R.W. Brislin, S. Bochner, and W.J. Lonner (Eds.), *Cross-cultural perspectives on learning* (pp. 207–28). New York: John Wiley and Sons.

Berry, J.W. (1985). Acculturation among circumpolar peoples: Implications for health status. *Arctic Medical Research, 40*, 21–7.

Berry, J.W. (1991). Psychology of acculturation. *Nebraska Symposium on Motivation, 39*, 201–34.

Berry, J.W. (2003). Conceptual approaches to acculturation. In K. Chun, P. Organista, and G. Marín (Eds.), *Acculturation: Advances in theory, measurement, and applied research* (pp. 17–37). Washington, DC: American Psychological Association.

Berry, J.W., & Annis, R.C. (1974a). Acculturative stress: The role of ecology, culture and differentiation. *Journal of Cross-Cultural Psychology, 5*(4), 382–407.

Berry, J.W., & Annis, R.C. (1974b). Ecology, culture and psychological differentiation. *International Journal of Psychology, 9*(3), 173–93.

Berry, J.W., & Bennett, J.A. (1992). Cree conceptions of cognitive competence. *International Journal of Psychology, 27*(1), 73–88.

Berry, J.W., & Kim, U. (1988). Acculturation and mental health. In P. Dasen, J.

Berry, and N. Sartorius (Eds.), *Health and cross-cultural psychology: Toward applications* (pp. 207–36). Newbury Park, NJ: Sage Publications.

Berry, J.W., Kim, U., Minde, T., & Mok, D. (1987). Comparative studies of acculturative stress. *International Migration Review, 21,* 491–511.

Berry, J.W., Trimble, J.E., & Olmedo, E.L. (1986). Assessment of acculturation. In W.J. Lonner and J.W. Berry (Eds.), *Field methods in cross-cultural research* (pp. 291–349). Beverly Hills, CA: Sage Publications.

Berry, J.W., Wintrob, R.M., Sindell, P.S., & Mawhinney, T.A. (1982). Psychological adaptation to culture change among the James Bay Cree. *Le Naturaliste Canadien, 109*(1), 965–75.

Bertelson, A., Marks, P., & May, G. (1982). MMPI and race: A controlled study. *Journal of Counseling and Clinical Psychology, 50*(2), 316–18.

Bhabha, H. (1983). The other question – The stereotype and colonial discourse. *Screen 24,* 6–23.

Bhabha, H. (1991). Untitled conference presentation. In P. Mariani (Ed.), *Critical fictions: The politics of imaginative writing* (pp. 62–5). Seattle, WA: Bay Press.

Bhawuk, D.P.S. (in press). Evolution of culture assimilators: Toward theory-based assimilators. *International Journal of Intercultural Relations.*

Bibeau, G. (1997). Cultural psychiatry in a Creolizing world: Questions for a new research agenda. *Transcultural Psychiatry, 34*(1), 9–41.

Bieder, R.E. (1986). *Science encounters the Indian, 1820–1880: The early years of American ethnology.* Norman: University of Oklahoma Press.

Biolsi, T. (1997). The anthropological construction of 'Indians.' Haviland Scudder Mekeel and the search for the primitive in Lakota country. In T. Biolsi and L.J. Zimmerman (Eds.), *Indians and anthropologists: Vine Deloria, Jr. and the critique of anthropology* (pp. 133–59). Tucson: University of Arizona Press.

Bloom, J.D. (1980). Forensic psychiatric evaluation of Alaska Native homicide offenders. *International Journal of Law and Psychiatry, 3,* 163–71.

Boag, T.J. (1970). Mental health of Native peoples of the Arctic. *Canadian Psychiatric Association, 15*(2), 115–20.

Bock, P.K. (1988). *Rethinking psychological anthropology: Continuity and change in the study of human action.* New York: Freeman.

Bock, P.K. (1999). *Rethinking psychological anthropology: Continuity and change in the study of human action.* Prospect Heights, IL: Waveland Press.

Bock, P.K. (2000). Culture and personality revisited. *American Behavioral Scientist, 44*(1), 32–40.

Boehnlein, J.K., Kinzie, J.D., Leung, P.K., Matsunaga, D., Johnson, R., & Shore, J.H. (1993). The natural history of medical and psychiatric disorders in an American Indian community. *Culture, Medicine, and Psychiatry, 16,* 543–54.

Borofsky, R., Barth, F., Shweder, R., Rodseth, L., & Stolzenberg, N. (2001).
When: A conversation about culture. *American Anthropologist, 103*(2), 432–
46.

Boyer, L.B. (1961). Notes on the personality structure of a North American shaman. *Journal of the Hillside Hospital, 10*, 14–33.

Boyer, L.B. (1962). Remarks on the personality of shamans, with special references to the Apaches of the Mescalero Indian Reservation. *The Psychoanalytic
Study of Society, 2*, 233–54.

Boyer, L.B. (1964a). Folk psychiatry of the Apaches of the Mescalero Indian reservation. In A. Kiev (Ed.), *Magic, Faith, and Healing* (pp. 384–419). New York:
Free Press.

Boyer, L.B. (1964b). Psychological problems of a group of Apaches: Alcoholic
hallucinosis and latent homosexuality among typical men. *The Psychoanalytic
Study of Society, 3*, 203–77.

Boyer, L.B., & Boyer, R.M. (1972). Effects of acculturation on the vicissitudes of
the aggressive drive among the Apaches of the Mescalero Indian reservation. *Psychoanalytic Study of Society, 5*, 40–82.

Boyer, L.B., Boyer, R.M., Dithrich, C.W., Harned, H., Hippler, A.E., Stone, J.S.,
& Walt, A. (1989). The relation between psychological states and acculturation among the Tanaina and Upper Tanana Indians of Alaska: An ethnographic and Rorschach study. *Ethos, 17*(4), 450–79.

Boyer, L.B., Boyer, R.M., & Hippler, A.E. (1974). Ecology, socialization and personality development among Athabacans. *Journal of Comparative Family Studies, 5*(1), 61–73.

Boyer, L.B., De Vos, G., & Boyer, R.M. (1983). Longitudinal study of three
Apache brothers as reflected in their Rorschach protocols. *Journal of Psychoanalytic Anthropology, 6*, 125–61.

Boyer, L.B., Klopfer, B., Boyer, R., Brawer, F., & Kawai, H. (1965). Effects of
acculturation on the personality of the Mescalero and Chiricahua Apaches.
International Journal of Health Education, 8(2), 264–71.

Boyer, L.B., Klopfer, B., Brawer, F.B., & Kawai, H. (1964). Comparisons of the
shamans and pseudoshamans of the Apaches of the Mescalero Indian reservation: A rorschach study. *Journal of Projective Techniques and Personality
Assessment, 28*(4), 173–80.

Bracken, B., & McCallum, R. (2001). Assessing intelligence in a population that
speaks more that two hundred languages: A nonverbal solution. In L.
Suzuki, J. Ponterotto, and P. Meller (Eds.), *Handbook of Multicultural Assessment: Clinical, Psychological, and Educational Applications* (2nd ed.) (pp. 405–
31). San Francisco: Jossey-Bass.

Brady, M. (1995). Culture in treatment, culture as treatment: A critical appraisal of developments in addictions programs for indigenous North Americans and Australians. *Social Science and Medicine, 41*(11), 1487–98.

Brant, C.C. (1990). Native ethics and rules of behavior. *Canadian Journal of Psychiatry, 35,* 534–39.

Brant, C.C. (1993). Communications patterns in Indians: Verbal and non-verbal. *Annals of Sex Research, 6*(4), 259–69.

Brave Heart, M. (1998). The return to the sacred path: Healing the historical trauma and historical unresolved grief response among the Lakota through a psychoeducational group intervention. *Smith College Studies in Social Work, 68*(3), 288–305.

Brave Heart, M., & DeBruyn, L. (1998). The American Indian holocaust: Healing historical unresolved grief. *American Indian and Alaska Native Mental Health Research, 8*(2), 60–82.

Braveheart-Jordan, M., & DeBruyn, L. (1995). So she may walk in balance: Integrating the impact of historical trauma in the treatment of Native American Indian women. In J. Adleman and G.M. Enguidanos (Eds.), *Racism in the lives of women: Testimony, theory, and guides to antiracist practice* (pp. 345–68). New York: Hawthorn Press.

Briggs, J. (1970). *Never in anger: Portrait of an Eskimo family.* Cambridge: Harvard University Press.

Brill, A.A. (1913). Pibloktoq or hysteria among Peary's Eskimos. *Journal of Nervous and Mental Disease, 40,* 514–20.

Brod, T.M. (1975). Alcoholism as a mental health problem of Native Americans. *Archives of General Psychiatry, 32,* 1385–91.

Brown, G.L., Albaugh, B.J., Robin, R.W., Goodson, S.G., Trunzo, M., Wynne, D. K., & Goldman, D. (1993). Alcoholism and substance abuse among selected southern Cheyenne Indians. *Culture, Medicine, and Psychiatry, 16,* 534–42.

Brown, J.S.H. (1992). Preface. In A.I. Hallowell, *The Ojibwa of Berens River, Manitoba: Ethnography into history* (pp. xi–xviii). Fortworth: Harcourt Brace Jovanovich.

Browne, D.B. (1984). WISC-R scoring patterns among Native Americans of the Northern plains. *White Cloud Journal, 3*(2), 3–16.

Brucker, P.S., & Perry, B.J. (1998). American Indians: Presenting concerns and considerations for family therapists. *American Journal of Family Therapy, 26*(4), 307–19.

Bruner, F.G. (1912). The primitive races in America. *Psychological Bulletin, 9*(10), 380–90.

Bryde, J.F. (1971). *Modern Indian Psychology* (rev. ed.). Vermillion, SD: University of South Dakota.

Bunzel, R.L. (1933). *Zuni Texts*. Publications of the American Ethnological Society, Vol. XV. New York: G. Stechert and Co.

Butcher, J.N., Braswell, L., and Raney, D. (1983). A cross-cultural comparison of American Indian, Black, and White inpatients on the MMPI and presenting symptoms. *Journal of Consulting and Clinical Psychology, 51*(4), 587–94.

Butcher, J.N., Nezami, E., & Exner, J. (1998). Psychological assessment of people in diverse cultures. In S. Kazarian and D. Evans (Eds.), *Cultural clinical psychology: Theory, research, practice* (pp. 61–105). New York: Oxford University Press.

Caetano, R., Clark, C.L., & Tam, T. (1998). Alcohol consumption among racial minorities: Theory and research. *Alcohol Health and Research World, 22*(4), 233–41.

Carpenter, E.S. (1960). Alcohol in the Iroquois dream quest. *American Journal of Psychiatry, 116*, 148–51.

Caudill, W. (1949). Psychological characteristics of acculturated Wisconsin Ojibwa children. *American Anthropologist, 52*, 409–27.

Chance, N.A. (1965). Acculturation, self-identification and personality adjustment. *American Anthropologist, 6*, 372–93.

Chance, N.A., and Foster, D.A. (1962). Symptom formation and patterns of psychopathology in a rapidly changing Alaskan Eskimo society. *Anthropological Papers of the University of Alaska, 11*(1), 32–43.

Chandler, M.J., & Lalonde, C. (1998). Cultural continuity as a hedge against suicide in Canada's First Nations. *Transcultural Psychiatry, 35*(2), 191–219.

Chapleski, E.E., Lamphere, J.K., Kaczynski, R., Lichtenberg, P.A., & Dwyer, J.W. (1997). Structure of a depression measure among American Indian elders: Confirmatory factor analysis of the CES-D scale. *Research on Aging, 19*(4), 462–85.

Chief, E.H. (1940). An assimilation study of Indian girls. *Journal of Social Psychology, 11*, 19–30.

Choney, S.K., Berryhill-Paapke, E., & Robbins, R.R. (1995). The acculturation of American Indians: Developing frameworks for research and practice. In J.G. Ponterotto, J.M. Casas, L.A. Suzuki, and C.M. Alexander (Eds.), *Handbook of multicultural counseling* (pp. 73–92). Thousand Oaks, CA: Sage Publications.

Chrisjohn, R., & Young, S. (1997). *The circle game: Shadows and substance in the Indian residential school experience in Canada*. Penticton, BC: Theytus Books.

Chrisman, N.J., & Maretzki, T.W. (1982). Clinically applied anthropology: Anthropologists in health science settings. Dordrecht: D. Reidel.

Christopher, J.C. (1998). Placing culture at the center of multiculturalism: Moral visions and intercultural dialogue. *Dialogues in psychology* [Online] 1

(14 September 1998). Available: hubcap.clemson.edu/psych/Dialogues/
dialogues.html.

Churchill, W. (1994). *Indians are us? Culture and genocide in Native North America.* Toronto: Between the Lines.

Clements, F.E. (1932). Primitive concepts of disease. *University of California Publications in American Archaeology and Ethnology, 32*(2), 185–252.

Clifford, J. (1988). *The predicament of culture: 20th century ethnography, literature
and art.* Cambridge: Harvard University Press.

Cole, M. (1996). *Cultural psychology: A once and future discipline.* Cambridge:
Harvard University Press.

Collier, J. (1945). United States Indian administration as a laboratory of ethnic
relations. *Social Research, 12*(3), 265–303.

Collier, J. (1965). Foreword. In L. Thompson, and A. Joseph (Eds.), *The Hopi
Way* (pp. 5–10). New York: Russell and Russell.

Collier, J., & Thompson, L. (1946). The Indian education and administration
research. *Sociometry, 9*(2–3), 141–2.

Common, R.W., & Frost, L.G. (1988). The implications of the mismeasurement
of Native students' intelligence through the use of standardized intelligence
tests. *Canadian Journal of Native Education, 15*(1), 18–30.

Conrad, R.D., & Kahn, M.W. (1974). An epidemiological study of suicide and
attempted suicide among the Papago Indians. *American Journal of Psychiatry,
131*(1), 69–72.

Cooley, R. (1980). Community programs for Native Americans. In J.O. Wadell,
and M.W. Everett (Eds.), *Drinking behavior among southwestern Indians: An
anthropological perspective* (pp. 205–13). Tucson: University of Arizona Press.

Cooper, C.R., & Denner, J. (1998). Theories linking culture and psychology:
Universal and community-specific processes. *Annual Review of Psychology,
49,* 559–84.

Cooper, Rev. J.M. (1933). The Cree Witiko psychosis. *Primitive Man, 6*(1), 20–4.

Cooper, M., Corrado, R., Karlberg, A.M., & Pelletier Adams, L. (1992). Aboriginal suicide in British Columbia: An overview. *Canada's Mental Health,* September 1992: 19–23.

Cross, T., Bazron, B., Dennis, K., & Isaacs, M. (1989). *Towards a culturally competent system of care.* Washington, DC: CASSP Techical Assistance Center.

Csordas, T.J. (1994). Introduction: the body as representation and being-in-the-
world. In T.J. Csordas (Ed.), *Embodiment and experience: The existential ground
of culture and self* (pp. 1–24). Cambridge: Cambridge University Press.

Csordas, T.J. (2000). The Navajo healing project. *Medical Anthropology Quarterly, 14*(4), 463–75.

Cuellar, I., Harris, L.C., & Jasso, R. (1980). An acculturation scale for Mexican

American normal and clinical populations. *Hispanic Journal of Behavioral Science, 3*, 199–217.

Cundick, B.P. (1970). Measures of intelligence on Southwest Indian students. *Journal of Social Psychology, 81*, 151–6.

Curley, R.T. (1967). Drinking patterns of the Mescalero Apache. *Quarterly Journal of Studies on Alcohol, 28*, 116–31.

Curyto, K.J., Chapleski, E.E., Lichtenberg, P.A., Hodges, E., Kaczynski, R., & Sobeck, J. (1998). Prevalence and prediction of depression in American Indian elderly. *Clinical Gerontologist, 18*(3), 19–37.

Cushner, K., & Brislin, R. (1996). *Intercultural interactions: A practical guide* (2nd ed). Beverly Hills, CA: Sage Publications.

Dailey, R.C. (1968). The role of alcohol among North-American Indian tribes as reported in The Jesuit Relations. *Anthropologica n.s. II, 10*(1), 45–59.

Dana, R.H. (1984). Intelligence testing of American Indian children: Sidesteps in quest of ethical practice. *White Cloud Journal, 3*(3), 35–43.

Dana, R.H. (1986). Personality assessment and Native Americans. *Journal of Personality Assessment, 50*(3), 480–500.

Dana, R.H. (1993). *Multicultural assessment perspectives for professional psychology.* Needham Heights, MA: Allyn and Bacon.

Dana, R.H., Hornby, R., & Hoffman, T. (1984). Local norms for personality assessment of Rosebud Sioux. *White Cloud Journal, 3*(2), 17–25.

Danieli, Y. (1998). Introduction: History and conceptual foundations. In Y. Danieli (Ed.), *International handbook of multigenerational legacies of trauma* (pp. 1–17). New York: Plenum Press.

Darnell, R. (1998). *And along came Boas: Continuity and revolution in Americanist anthropology.* Amsterdam, The Netherlands: J. Benjamin.

Darnell, R. (2001). *Invisible genealogies: A history of Americanist anthropology.* Lincoln: University of Nebraska Press.

Darou, W.G. (1980). Experiencing Native American culture. *Counseling and Values, 25*(1), 3–17.

Darou, W.G. (1987). Counselling and the Northern Native. *Canadian Journal of Counselling, 21*(1), 33–41.

Dauphinais, P., & King, J. (1992). Psychological assessment with American Indian children. *Applied and Preventive Psychology, 1*(2), 97–110.

Davenport, J.A., & Davenport III, J. (1987). Native American suicides: A Durkheimian analysis. *Social Casework: The Journal of Contemporary Social Work, 68*(9), 533–539.

Davis, G.L., Hoffman, R.G., & Nelson, K.S. (1990). Differences between Native Americans and Whites on the California Psychological Inventory. *Psychological Assessment: A Journal of Consulting and Clinical Psychology, 2*(3), 238–42.

Dawson, J.L.M. (1969). Attitude change and conflict among Australian Aborigines. *Australian Journal of Psychology, 2*, 101–17.

Day, R., Boyer, L.B., & De Vos, G. (1989). Progressive restrictions in Apache youth. In G. DeVos and L.N. Boyer (Eds.), *Symbolic analysis cross-culturally: The rorschach test* (pp. 293–334). Berkeley: University of California Press.

Debo, A. (1940). *And still the waters run.* Princeton: Princeton University Press.

De Lacy, P.R. (1970). An index of contact for Aboriginal communities. *Australian Journal of Social Issues, 3*, 219–23.

Deloria, V. (1969). *Custer died for your sins.* London: Collier-Macmillan.

De Mille, R. (1976). *Castenada's journey: The power and the allegory.* Santa Barbara, CA: Capra Press.

De Mille, R. (1990). *The Don Juan papers: Further Castenada controversies.* Belmont, CA: Wadswirth.

Devereux, G. (1940). Primitive psychiatry. *Bulletin of the History of Medicine, 8*(8), 1194–1213.

Devereux, G. (1942). The mental hygiene of the American Indian. *Mental Hygiene, 26*, 71–84.

Devereux, G. (1948). The function of alcohol in Mohave society. *Quarterly Journal of Studies on Alcohol, 9*, 207–51.

Devereux, G. (1951). *Reality and dream: Psychotherapy of a Plains Indian.* New York: International Universities.

Devereux, G. (1969). *Mohave ethnopsychiatry: The psychic disturbances of an Indian tribe.* Washington, DC: Smithsonian Institution Press.

Devereux, G. (1971). Normal and abnormal: The key problem of psychiatric anthropology. In J. Casagrande and T. Goldwin (Eds.), *Some uses of anthropology: Theoretical and applied* (pp. 23–48). Washington, DC: The Anthropological Society of Washington.

De Vos, G.A., & Boyer, L.B. (1989). Conclusions: Transcultural assessment using psychological tests. In G.A. De Vos and L.B. Boyer (Eds.), *Symbolic analysis cross-culturally: The Rorschach Test* (pp. 439–66). Los Angeles: University of California Press.

Dick, L. (1995). 'Pibloktoq' (Arctic Hysteria): A construction of European-Inuit relations. *Arctic Anthropology 32*(2), 1–42.

Dick, R., Manson, S., & Beals, J. (1993). Alcohol use among American Indian adolescents: Patterns and correlates of students' drinking in a boarding school. *Journal of Studies on Alcohol, 54*, 172–7.

Dillard, D.A., & Manson, S.M. (2000). Assessing and treating American Indians and Alaska Natives. In I. Cuéllar and F.A. Paniagua (Eds.), *Handbook of multicultural health: Assessment and treatment of diverse populations* (pp. 225–48). San Diego, CA: Academic Press.

348   References

Dillard, J. (1983). *Multicultural counseling*. Chicago: Nelson-Hall.

Dinges, N.G., & Duong-Tran, Q. (1993). Stressful life events and co-occurring depression, substance abuse and suicidality among American Indian and Alaska Native adolescents. *Culture, Medicine, and Psychiatry, 16*, 487–502.

Dinges, N.G., Trimble, J.E., Manson, S.M., & Pasquale, F.L. (1981). Counseling and psychotherapy with American Indians and Alaskan Natives. In A.J. Marsella, and P.B. Pedersen (Eds.), *Cross-cultural counseling and psychotherapy* (pp. 243–76). New York: Pergamon Press.

Dizmang, L. (1967). Suicide among Cheyenne Indians. *Bulletin of Suicidology, 7*, 8–11.

Doob, L.W. (1967). Scales for assaying psychological modernization in Africa. *Public Opinion Quarterly, 31*, 415–21.

Dozier, E.P. (1966). Problem drinking among American Indians: The role of sociocultural deprivation. *Quarterly Journal of Studies on Alcohol, 27*, 72–87.

Driver, H. (1969). *Indians of North America*. 2nd ed. Chicago: University of Chicago Press.

DuBois, C. (1944). *The people of Alor: A social-psychological study of an East-Indian Island*. Minneapolis: University of Minnesota Press.

DuBray, W.H. (1985). American Indian values: Critical factor in casework. *Social Casework, 66*(1), 30–7.

Duckworth, J.C., & Anderson, W.P. (1994). *MMPI and MMPI-2: Interpretation manual for counselors and clinicians*, (4th ed.). Bristol, PA: Accelerated Development.

Duclos, C.W., Beals, J., Novins, D.K., Martin, C., Jewitt, C.S., & Manson, S.M. (1998). Prevalence of common psychiatric disorders among American Indian adolescent detainees. *Journal of the American Academy of Child and Adolescent Psychiatry, 37*(8), 866–73.

Dufrene, P.M., & Coleman, V.D. (1992). Counseling Native Americans: Guidelines for group process. *Journal for Specialists in Group Work, 17*(4), 229–34.

Duran, B.M., & Duran, E.F. (1999). Assessment, program planning, and evaluation in Indian country: Toward post-colonial practice. In R.M. Huff and M.V. Kline (Eds.), *Promoting health in multicultural populations: A handbook for practitioners* (pp. 291–311). Thousand Oaks, CA: Sage Publications, Inc.

Duran, E., & Duran, B. (1995). *Native American postcolonial psychology*. Albany: State University of New York Press.

Duran, E.F., Duran, B.M., Brave Heart, M., & Yellow Horse-Davis, S. (1998). Healing the American Indian soul wound. In Y. Danieli (Ed.), *International handbook of multigenerational legacies of trauma: The plenum series on coping* (pp. 341–54). New York: Plenum Press.

Edgerton, R.B. (1992). *Sick societies: challenging the myth of primitive harmony*. New York: Free Press.

Edwards, E.D., & Edwards, M.E. (1980). American Indians: Working with individuals and groups. *Social Casework* Oct: 499–506.

Edwards, E.D., & Edwards, M.E. (1984). Group work practice with American Indians. *Social Work With Groups, 7,* 7–21.

Eggan, D. (1943). The general problem of Hopi adjustment. *American Anthropologist, 45,* 357–73.

Eisenberg, L., & Kleinman, A. (1981). Clinical Social Science. In L. Eisenberg, and A. Kleinman (Eds.), *The relevance of social science for medicine* (pp. 1–23). Dordrecht: Reidel.

Erickson, P.E. & Murphy, L.D. (1998). *A history of anthropological theory.* Peterborough, ON: Broadview Press.

Erikson, E.H. (1950). *Childhood and society.* New York: W.W. Norton and Company.

Erikson, E.H. (1963). *Childhood and society* (2nd ed.). New York: W.W. Norton and Company.

Erikson, K.T. (1976). *Everything in its path: Destruction of community in the Buffalo Creek flood.* New York: Simon and Shuster.

Escalante, F. (1980). Group pressure and excessive drinking among Indians. In J.O. Waddell and M.W. Everett (Eds.), *Drinking behavior among Southwestern Indians: An anthropological perspective* (pp. 183–204). Tucson: University of Arizona Press.

Este, D. (1999). Social work and cultural competency. In G.-Y. Lie and D. Este (Eds.), *Professional social service delivery in a multicultural world* (pp. 27–45). Toronto: Canadian Scholars' Press.

Everett, M.W. (1970). Pathology in White Mountain Apache culture: A preliminary analysis. *Western Canadian Journal of Anthropology, 2*(1), 180–203.

Everett, M.W. (1973). American Indian 'social pathology': A re-examination. In T.R. Williams (Ed.), *Psychological anthropology* (pp. 249–85). The Hague: Mouton Publishers.

Fabrega Jr, H. (1982). Culture and psychiatric illness: biomedical and ethnomedical aspects. In A.J. Marsella and G.M. White (Eds.), *Cultural conceptions of mental health and therapy* (pp. 39–68). Dordrecht: D. Reidel Publishing Co.

Fadiman, A. (1997). *The spirit catches you and you fall down: A Hmong child, her American doctors, and the collision of two cultures.* New York: Noonday.

Farris, J.J., & Jones, B.M. (1978a). Ethanol metabolism in male American Indians and Whites. *Alcoholism: Clinical and Experimental Research, 2*(1), 77–81.

Farris, J.J., & Jones, B.M. (1978b). Ethanol metabolism and memory impairment in American Indian and White women social drinkers. *Journal of Studies on Alcohol, 39*(11), 1975–9.

Fathauer, G. (1951). The Mohave 'ghost doctor.' *American Anthropologist, 53,* 605–7.

Fenna, D., Mix, L., Schaefer, O., & Gilbert, J.A.L. (1971). Ethanol metabolism in various racial groups. *Canadian Medical Association Journal, 105,* 472–5.

Ferguson, F.N. (1962). Great Whale River Eskimo personality as revealed by Rorschach protocols. In J.J. Honigmann (Ed.), *Social networks in Great Whale River: Notes on an Eskimo, Montagnais-Naskapi, and Euro-Canadian community* (pp. 80–110). Ottawa: National Museum of Canada Bulletin No. 178.

Ferguson, F.N. (1968). Navajo drinking: Some tentative hypotheses. *Human Organization, 27*(2), 159–167.

Ferguson, F.N. (1970). A treatment program for Navaho alcoholics: Results after four years. *Quarterly Journal of Studies on Alcohol, 31*(4), 898–919.

Ferguson, F.N. (1976). Stake theory as an explanatory device in Navajo alcoholism treatment response. *Human Organization, 35*(1), 65–78.

Field, P.B. (1962). A new cross-cultural study of drunkenness. In D. Pittman and C. Snyder (Eds.), *Society, culture and drinking patterns* (pp. 48–74). New York: Wiley and Sons.

Fish, J.M. (2000). What anthropology can do for psychology: Facing physics envy, ethnocentrism, and a belief in 'Race.' *American Anthropologist, 102*(3), 552–63.

Fisher, A.D. (1987). Alcoholism and race: The misapplication of both concepts to North American Indians. *Canadian Review of Sociology and Anthropology, 24*(1), 81–98.

Fisher, G.L., & Harrison, T.C. (1997). *Substance abuse: Information for school counselors, social workers, therapists, and counselors.* Boston, MA: Allyn and Bacon.

Fitzgerald, J.A., & Ludeman, W.W. (1926). The intelligence of Indian children. *Journal of Comparative Psychology, 6,* 319–28.

Flanagan, J. (1954). The Critical Incident Technique. *Psychological Bulletin, 51,* 321–58.

Fleming, C.M. (1992). American Indians and Alaska Natives: Changing Societies Past and Present. In M. Orlandi (Ed.), *Cultural competence for evaluators* (pp. 147–71). Rockville, MD: US Department of Health and Human Services.

Fleming, C.M. (1996). Cultural formulation of psychiatric diagnosis: An American Indian woman suffering from depression, alcoholism, and childhood trauma. *Culture, Medicine, and Psychiatry, 20,* 145–54.

Flores, P.J. (1986). Alcoholism treatment and the relationship of Native American cultural values to recovery. *The International Journal of the Addictions, 20*(11/12), 1707–26.

Fogelson, R. (1999). Nationalism and the Americanist tradition. In L. Valentine and R. Darnell (Eds.), *Theorizing the Americanist tradition* (pp. 75–83). Toronto: University of Toronto Press.

Forbes, J. (1992). *Columbus and other cannibals: the Wetiko disease of exploitation, imperialism, and terrorism.* New York: Autonomedia.

Foster, G., & Anderson, B.G. (1978). *Medical Anthropology.* New York: John Wiley and Sons.

Foucault, M. (1973) *The birth of the clinic.* London: Oxford University Press.

Foulks, E.F. (1972). *The arctic hysterias of the North Alaskan Eskimo.* Washington, DC: American Anthropological Association.

Foulks, E.F. (1980). Psychological continuities: From dissociative states to alcohol use and suicide in Arctic populations. *Journal of Operational Psychiatry, 11*(2), 156–61.

Foulks, E.F. (1985). The transformation of arctic hysteria. In R.C. Simons, and C.C. Hughes (Eds.), *The Culture-bound syndromes: Folk illnesses of psychiatric and anthropological interest* (pp. 307–24). Dordrecht, Holland: D. Reidel Publishing Company.

Foulks, E.F., Freeman, D.M.A., & Freeman, P. (1979). Pre-oedipal dynamics in a case of Eskimo arctic hysteria. In W. Muensterberger and L.B. Boyer (Eds.), *The psychoanalytic study of society 8* (pp. 41–69). New Haven: Yale University Press.

Fournier, S., & Crey, E. (1997). *Stolen from our embrace: The abduction of First Nations children and the restoration of Aboriginal communities.* Vancouver: Douglas & McIntyre.

Fredericks, L., & Hodge, F.S. (1999). Traditional approaches to health care among American Indians and Alaska Natives: A case study. In R.M. Huff and M.V. Kline (Eds.), *Promoting Health in Multicultural Populations: A Handbook for Practitioners* (pp. 313–26). Thousand Oaks, CA: Sage Publications, Inc.

Freeman, D.M.A., Foulks, E.F., & Freeman, P.A. (1978). Child development and arctic hysteria in the North Alaskan Eskimo male. *Journal of Psychological Anthropology, 1*(10), 203–10.

French, L.A. (1979). Corrections and the Native American client. *Prison Journal, 59*(1), 49–60.

French, L.A. (1980). Anomie and violence among Native Americans. *International Journal of Comparative and Applied Criminal Justice, 4*(1), 75–84.

French, L.A. (1981). Counseling American Indians. *International Journal of Offender Therapy and Comparative Criminology, 25*(2), 139–55.

French, L.A. (1989). Native American alcoholism: A transcultural counseling perspective. *Counselling Psychology Quarterly, 2*(2), 153–66.

French, L.A. (1993). Adapting projective tests for minority children. *Psychological Reports, 72*(1), 15–18.

French, L.A. (1997). *Counseling American Indians.* Lanham, MD: University Press of America, Inc.

French, L.A., & Hornbuckle, J. (1972). An analysis of Indian violence: The Cherokee example. *American Indian Quarterly, 3,* 335–56.

French, L.A., & Hornbuckle, J. (1980). Alcoholism among Native Americans: An analysis. *Social Work, 25*(4), 275–80.

Freud, S. (1950). *Totem and taboo: Some points of agreement between the mental life of savages and neurotics.* London: Routledge and Kegan Paul.

Fritz, W.B. (1976). Psychiatric disorders among Natives and non-Natives in Saskatchewan. *Canadian Psychiatric Association Journal, 21,* 394–400.

Furniss, E. (1995). *Victims of benevolence: The dark legacy of the Williams Lake residential school.* Vancouver: Arsenal Pulp Press.

Gaddes, W.H., McKenzie, A., & Barnsley, R. (1968). Psychometric intelligence and spatial imagery in two Northwest Indian and two White groups of children. *The Journal of Social Psychology, 75,* 35–42.

Gagné, M.-A. (1998). The role of dependency and colonialism in generating trauma in First Nations citizens: The James Bay Cree. In Y. Danieli (Ed.), *International handbook of multigenerational legacies of trauma* (pp. 355–72). New York: Plenum Press.

Gaines, A.D. (1992a). Ethnopsychiatry: The cultural construction of psychiatries. In A.D. Gaines (Ed.), *Ethnopsychiatry: The cultural construction of professional and folk psychiatries* (3–49). Albany: State University of New York Press.

Gaines, A.D. (1992b). From DSM-I to III-R; Voices of self, mastery and the other: A cultural constructivist reading of U.S. psychiatric classification. *Social Science and Medicine, 35*(1), 3–24.

Garcia-Andrade, C., Wall, T.L., Ehlers, C.L. (1997). The firewater myth and response to alcohol in Mission Indians. *American Journal of Psychiatry, 154*(7), 983–8.

Garrett, J.T., & Garrett, M.W. (1994). The path of good medicine: Understanding and counseling Native American Indians. *Journal of Multicultural Counseling and Development, 22*(3), 134–44.

Garrett, M.T., & Pichette, E.F. (2000). Red as an apple: Native American acculturation and counseling with or without reservation. *Journal of Counseling and Development, 78*(1), 3–13.

Garro, L.C. (1988). Suicides by status Indians in Manitoba. *Arctic Medical Research, 47,* 590–2.

Garro, L.C. (1990). Continuity and change: The interpretation of illness in an Anishinaabe community. *Culture, Medicine and Psychiatry, 4,* 417–54.

Garth, T.R. (1921a). The results of some tests on full and mixed blood Indians. *Journal of Applied Psychology, 5,* 359–72.

Garth, T.R. (1921b). White, Indian and Negro work curves. *Journal of Applied Psychology, 5,* 14–25.

Garth, T.R. (1922). Mental fatigue of mixed and full blood Indians. *Journal of Applied Psychology, 6*, 331–41.

Garth, T.R. (1923). A comparison of the intelligence of mixed and full blood Indian children. *Psychological Review, 30*, 388–401.

Garth, T.R. (1925). The intelligence of full blood Indians. *Journal of Applied Psychology, 9*, 382–98.

Garth, T.R. (1927). The intelligence of mixed blood Indians. *Journal of Applied Psychology, 40*, 268–75.

Garth, T.R., Smith, H.W., & Abell, W. (1928). A study of the intelligence and achievement of full-blood Indians. *Journal of Applied Psychology, 12*, 511–16.

Geertz, C. (1973). *The interpretation of cultures.* New York: Basic Books.

Gillin, J., & Raimy, V. (1940). Acculturation and personality. *American Sociological Review, 5*, 371–80.

Goffman, E. (1961). *Asylums: Essays on the social situation of mental patients and other inmates.* New York: Anchor Books.

Gonzalez, C., & Griffith, E. (1996). Culture and the diagnosis of somatoform and dissociative disorders. In J. Mezzich, A. Kleinman, H. Fabregia, and D. Parron (Eds.), *Culture and psychiatric diagnosis: A DSM-IV perspective* (pp. 1374–9). Washington, DC: American Psychiatric Press Inc.

Good, B. (1996). Culture and DSM-IV: Diagnosis, knowledge and power. *Culture, Medicine and Psychiatry, 20*, 127–132.

Good, B. (1997). Studying mental illness in global context: Local, global, or universal? Ethos 25(2), 230–48.

Gould, S.J. (1996). *The mismeasure of man.* New York: W.W. Norton and Company.

Gracia, M.F. (1976). Analysis of incidence of excessive alcohol intake by the Indian population in Montana. In F.X. Grollig and H.B. Haley (Eds.), *Medical anthropology* (pp. 313–20). Paris: Mouton Publishers.

Graham, J.R. (1990). *MMPI-2: Assessing personality and psychopathology.* New York: Oxford University Press.

Graves, T.D. (1967a). Acculturation, access, and alcohol in a tri-ethnic community. *American Anthropologist, 69*, 306–21.

Graves, T.D. (1967b). Psychological acculturation in a tri-ethnic community. *Southwestern Journal of Anthropology, 23*, 337–50.

Gray, N. (1998). Addressing trauma in substance abuse treatment with American Indian adolescents. *Journal of Substance Abuse Treatment, 15*(5), 393–9.

Gray, N., & Nye, P. (2001). American Indian and Alaska Native substance abuse: Co- morbidity and cultural issues. *American Indian and Alaska Native Mental Health Research, 19*(2), 67–84.

Green, J.W. (1999). *Cultural awareness in the human services.* (3rd ed.). Boston, MA: Allyn and Bacon.

Greene, R.L. (1987). Ethnicity and MMPI performance: A review. *Journal of Counseling and Clinical Psychology, 55*(4), 497–512.

Greenfield, P.M. (2000). What psychology can do for anthropology, or why anthropology took postmodernism on the chin. *American Anthropologist, 102*(3), 564–76.

Grobsmith, E.S. (1989). The relationship between substance abuse and crime among Native American inmates in the Nebraska department of corrections. *Human Organization, 48*(4), 285–98.

Grobsmith, E.S., & Dam, J. (1990). The revolving door: Substance abuse treatment and criminal sanctions for Native American offenders. *Journal of Substance Abuse, 2,* 405–25.

Gussow, Z. (1960). Pibloktoq (hysteria) among the Polar Eskimo: An ethnopsychiatric study. *The Psycho-Analytic Study of Society, 1,* 218–36.

Gustafson, J. (1976). The group matrix of individual therapy with Plains Indian people. *Contemporary Psychoanalysis, 12*(2): 227–39.

Haggarty, J., Cernovsky, Z., Kermeen, P., & Merskey, H. (2000). Psychiatric disorders in an Arctic community. *Canadian Journal of Psychiatry, 45*(4), 357–62.

Hahn, R.A. (1978). Aboriginal American psychiatric theories. *Transcultural Psychiatric Research Review, 15,* 29–58.

Hahn, R.A. (1995). *Sickness and healing: An anthropological perspective.* New Haven: Yale University Press.

Haig-Brown, C. (1988). *Resistance and renewal: Surviving the Indian residential school.* Vancouver: Tillacum Library.

Hales, R.E., Yudofsky, S.C., & Talbott, J.A. (Eds.). (1999). *The American Psychiatric Press textbook of psychiatry.* Washington, DC: American Psychiatric Press.

Hall, G., & Phung, A. (2001). Minnesota Multiphasic Personality Inventory and Million Clinical Multiaxial Inventory. In L. Suzuki, J. Ponterotto, and P. Meller (Eds.), *Handbook of multicultural assessment: Clinical, psychological, and educational applications.* (2nd ed.) (pp. 307–30). San Francisco: Jossey-Bass.

Hall, R.L. (1985). Distribution of the sweat lodge in alcohol treatment programs. *Current Anthropology, 26*(1), 134–5.

Hall, R.L. (1986). Alcohol treatment in American Indian populations: An Indiginous treatment modality compared with traditional approaches. *Annals of the New York Academy of Sciences, 472,* 168–78.

Hallowell, A.I. (1934). Culture and mental disorder. *Journal of Abnormal and Social Psychology, 29,* 1–9.

Hallowell, A.I. (1935). Primitive concepts of disease. *American Anthropologist, 37,* 365–8.

Hallowell, A.I. (1936). Psychic stresses and culture patterns. *American Journal of Psychiatry, 92*, 1291–1310.

Hallowell, A.I. (1941a). The Rorschach method as an aid in the study of personalities in primitive society. *Character and Personality, 9*, 35–245.

Hallowell, A.I. (1941b). The social function of anxiety in a primitive society. *American Sociological Review, 6*, 69–881.

Hallowell, A.I. (1942). Acculturation processes and personality changes as indicated by the Rorschach technique. *Rorschach Research Exchange, 6*(1), 42–50.

Hallowell, A.I. (1945a). The Rorschach technique in the study of personality and culture. *Amercian Anthropologist, 47*(2), 195–210.

Hallowell, A.I. (1945b). Sociopsychological aspects of acculturation. In R. Linton (Ed.), *The science of man in the world crisis* (pp. 171–200). New York: Columbia University.

Hallowell, A.I. (1955). *Culture and experience.* New York: Schoken Books.

Hallowell, A.I. (1963). Ojibwa world view and disease. In I. Galdston (Ed.), *Man's image in medicine and anthropology* (pp. 258–315). New York: International Universities.

Hallowell, A.I. (1976). *Contributions to anthropology: Selected papers of A. Irving Hallowell.* Chicago: University of Chicago Press.

Hallpike, C.R. (1979). *The foundations of primitive thought.* Oxford: Clarendon Press.

Hamer, J.H. (1965). Acculturation stress and the functions of alcohol among the Forest Potawatomi. *Quarterly Journal of Studies on Alcohol, 26*(3), 285–302.

Hamer, J.H. (1969). Guardian spirits, alcohol and cultural defense mechanisms. *Anthropologica II, 2*, 215–41.

Hamer, J. H., & Steinbring, J. (1980). Alcohol and the North American Indian: Examples from the sub-Arctic. In J.H. Hamer and J. Steinbring (Eds.), *Alcohol and Native Peoples of the North* (pp. 1–29). Washington, DC: University Press of America.

Harris, M. (1968). *The Rise of Anthropological Theory.* New York: Cromwell.

Hathaway, S.R., & McKinley, J.C. (1989). *MMPI-2: Manual for administration and scoring.* Minneapolis: University of Minnesota Press.

Haught, B.F. (1934). Mental growth of the Southwestern Indian. *The Journal of Applied Psychology, 18*, 137–42.

Havighurst, R.J. (1957). Education among American Indians: Individual and cultural aspects. *The Annals of the American Academy of Political and Social Science, 311*, 105–15.

Havighurst, R.J. (1971). The extent and significance of suicide among American Indians today. *Mental Hygiene, 55*(2), 174–7.

Havighurst, R.J., & Hilkevitch, R.R. (1944). The intelligence of Indian children as measured by a performance scale. *The Journal of Abnormal and Social Psychology, 39*, 419–33.

Haviland, M.G., Horswill, R.K., O'Connell, J.J., & Dynneson, V.V. (1983). Native American college students' preference for counselor race and sex and the likelihood of their use of a counseling center. *Journal of Counseling Psychology, 30*(2), 267–70.

Hay, T.H. (1976). Personality and probability: The modal personality of the Tuscarora revisited. *Ethos, 4*(4), 509–24.

Heath, D.B. (1964). Prohibition and post-repeal drinking patterns among the Navaho. *Quarterly Journal of Studies on Alcohol, 25*(1), 119–35.

Heath, D.B. (1983). Alcohol use among Native American Indians: A cross-cultural survey of patterns and problems. In R. Smart et al. (Eds.), *Research Advances in Alcohol and Drug Problems, Vol. 7* (pp. 343–96). New York: Plenum Press.

Heath, D.B. (1987). Anthropology and alcohol studies: Current issues. *Annual Review of Anthropology, 16*, 99–120.

Heidenreich, C.A. (1976). Alcohol and drug use and abuse among Indian-Americans: A review of issues and sources. *Journal of Drug Issues, 6*(3), 256–72.

Heinrich, R.K., Corbine, J.L., & Thomas, K.R. (1990). Counseling Native Americans. *Journal of Counseling and Development, 69*, 128–33.

Helman, C.G. (2000). *Culture, health and illness* (4th ed.). Oxford: Butterworth/Heinemann.

Helms, J.E. (1981). Cultural identity in the treatment process. In P. Pedersen (Ed.), *Handbook of cross-cultural counseling and therapy* (pp. 240–5). Westport, CT: Greenwood Press.

Helms, J.E., & Richardson, T.Q. (1997). How 'multiculturalism' obscures race and culture as differential aspects of counseling competency. In D. Pope-Davis and H. Coleman (Eds.), *Multicultural counseling competencies: Assessment, education and training, and supervision* (pp. 60–79). Thousand Oaks, CA: Sage.

Hendrie, H.C., & Hanson, D. (1972). A comparative study of the psychiatric care of Indians and Metis. *American Journal of Orthopsychiatry, 42*, 480–9.

Henry, W.E. (1947). The thematic apperception technique in the study of culture-personality relations. *Genetic Psychology Monographs, 35*, 3–135.

Herman, J.L. (1992). *Trauma and recovery*. New York: Basic Books.

Hermans, H., & Kempen, H. (1998). Moving cultures: The perilous problems of cultural dichotomies in a globalizing society. *American Psychologist, 53*(10), 1111–20.

Herreid II, C.F., & Herreid, J.R. (1966). Differences in MMPI scores in Native and non-Native Alaskans. *The Journal of Social Psychology, 70,* 191–8.

Herring, R.D. (1989). The American Native family: Dissolution by coercion. *Journal of Multicultural Counseling and Development, 17,* 4–13.

Herring, R.D. (1990). Understanding Native-American values: Process and content concerns for counselors. *Counseling and Values, 34,* 134–7.

Herring, R.D. (1992). Seeking a new paradigm: Counseling Native Americans. *Journal of Multicultural Counseling and Development, 20,* 35–43.

Hickerson, H. (1960). The feast of the dead among the seventeenth century Algonkians of the Upper Great Lakes. *American Anthropologist, 62,* 81–107.

Hickerson, H. (1962). *The Southwestern Chippewa: An ethnohistorical study. American Anthropological Association, 64*(3), Part 2, Memoir no. 92.

Hickerson, H. (1967). Some implications of the theory of the particularity, or 'atomism,' of Northern Algonkians. *Current Anthropology, 8*(4), 313–43.

Hill, T.W. (1980). Life styles and drinking patterns of urban Indians. *Journal of Drug Issues, 10,* 257–72.

Hippler, A.E. (1975). Transcultural psychiatric and related research in the North American Arctic and Subarctic. *Transcultural Psychiatric Research Review, 12,* 103–15

Hippler, A.E. (1976). Shamans, curers, and personality: Suggestions toward a theoretical model. In W.P. Lebra (Ed.), *Culture-bound syndromes, ethnopsychiatry, and alternate therapies* (pp. 103–14). Honolulu: University of Hawaii Press.

Ho, M.K. (1987). *Family Therapy with Ethnic Minorities.* Beverly Hills, CA: Sage Publications.

Ho, M.K. (1992). *Minority Children and Adolescents in Therapy.* Newbury Park, NJ: Sage Publications.

Hochkirchen, B., & Jilek, W.G. (1985). Psychosocial dimensions of suicide and parasuicide in Amerindians of the Pacific NorthWest. *Journal of Operational Psychiatry, 16*(2), 24–8.

Hoffmann, T., Dana, R.H., & Bolton, B. (1985). Measured acculturation and MMPI-168 performance of Native American adults. *Journal of Cross-Cultural Psychology, 16*(2), 243–56.

Hoffman, H., & Jackson, D.N. (1973). Comparison of measured psychopathology in Indian and non-Indian alcoholics. *Psychological Reports, 33,* 793–4.

Hoffmann, H., & Noem, A.A. (1975). Alcoholism and abstinence among relatives of American Indian alcoholics. *Journal of Studies on Alcohol, 36*(1), 165.

Hollingshead, A., & Redlich, F. (1958). *Social class and mental illness.* New York: John Wiley and Sons.

Honigmann, J.J. (1946). *Ethnography and acculturation of the Fort Nelson Slave.*

Yale University Publications in Anthropology, No. 33. New Haven: Yale University Press.

Honigmann, J.J. (1949). *Culture and ethos of Kaska society.* Yale University Publications in Anthropology, No. 40. New Haven: Yale University Press.

Honigmann, J.J. (1961a). The interpretation of dreams in anthropological fieldwork: A case study. In B. Kaplan (Ed.), *Studying personality cross-culturally* (pp. 579–85). New York: Harper and Row.

Honigmann, J.J. (1961b). North America. In F.L.K. Hsu (Ed.), *Psychological anthropology: Approaches to culture and personality* (pp. 93–134). Homewood, IL: The Dorsey Press.

Honigmann, J.J. (1965). Social disintegration in five northern Canadian communities. *Canadian Review of Sociology and Anthropology, 2,* 199–214.

Honigmann, J.J. (1968). Interpersonal relations in atomistic communities. *Human Organization 27*(3), 220–9.

Honigmann, J.J., & Honigmann, I. (1945). Drinking in an Indian-White community. *Quarterly Journal of Studies On Alcohol, 5*(4), 575–619.

Honigmann, J.J., & Honigmann, I. (1965). How Baffin Island Eskimo have learned to use alcohol. *Social Forces, 44,* 73–83.

Honigmann, J.J., & Honigmann, I. (1970). *Arctic townsmen: Ethnic backgrounds and modernization.* Ottawa: Canadian Research Centre for Anthropology, Saint Paul University.

Hornby, R., & Dana, R.H. (1984). *Mni Wakan and the Sioux: Respite, release and recreation.* Brandon, MB: Justin Publishing.

Horton, D. (1943). The functions of alcohol in primitive societies: A cross-cultural study. *Quarterly Journal of Studies on Alcohol, 4,* 292–303.

Howard, M.O., Walker, R.D., Suchinsky, R.T., & Anderson, B. (1996). Substance-use and psychiatric disorders among American Indian veterans. *Substance Use and Misuse, 35*(5), 581–98.

Howell, R.J., Evans, L., & Downing, L.N. (1958). A comparison of test scores for the 16–17 year age group of Navajo Indians with standardized norms for the Weschler adult intelligence scale (Arizona and New Mexico). *The Journal of Social Psychology, 47,* 355–59.

Hrdlička, A. (1908). *Physiological and medical observations among the Indians of Southwestern United States and Northern Mexico.* Smithsonian Institution, Bureau of American Ethnology, Bulletin 34. Washington: Government Printing Office.

Hughes, C.C. (1985). Culture-bound or construct-bound? The syndromes and DSM-III. In R.C. Simons and C.C. Hughes (Eds.), *The culture bound syndromes: Folk illnesses of psychiatric and anthropological interest* (pp. 3–24). Dordrecht, Holland: D. Reidel Publishing Co.

Hughes, C.C. (1996). Ethnopsychiatry. In C.F. Sargent and T.M. Johnson (Eds.), *Medical anthropology: Contemporary theory and method* (Rev. ed.) (pp. 131–50). Westport, CT: Praeger.

Hughes, C., Simons, R., & Wintrob, R. (1997). The 'culture-bound syndromes' and DSM-IV. In T. Wideger, A. Francis, H. Pincus, R. Ross, M. First, and W. Davis (Eds.), *DSM-IV Sourcebook* (pp. 991–1000). Washington, DC: American Psychiatric Association.

Hughes, I., & Sasson, F. (1990). Cultural heritage as the cornerstone of a rehabilitation process: A single case study. *The Canadian Journal of Native Studies, 2,* 183–91.

Hummer, H.R. (1913). Insanity among the Indians. *American Journal of Insanity, 69,* 615–23.

Hunt, M. (1993). *The story of psychology.* New York: Anchor Books.

Hunter, W.S., & Sommermier, E. (1922). The relation of degree of Indian blood to score on the Otis Intelligence Test. *Journal of Comparative Psychology, 2,* 257–77.

Hurlburt, G., & Gade, E. (1984). Personality differences between Native American and Caucasian women alcoholics: Implications for alcoholism counseling. *White Cloud Journal, 3*(2), 35–9.

Hurlburt, G., Gade, E., & Fuqua, D. (1983). Sex and race as factors on locus of control scores with an alcoholic population. *Psychological Reports, 52*(2), 517–18.

Hurt, W.R., & Brown, R.M. (1965). Social drinking patterns of the Yankton Sioux. *Human Organization, 24,* 222–30.

Hynd, G.W., & Garcia, W.I. (1979). Intellectual assessment of the Native American student. *School Psychology Digest, 8*(4), 446–54.

Hynd, G.W., Quackenbush, R., Kramer, R., Conner, R., & Weed, W. (1979). Clinical utility of the WISC-R and the French Pictorial Test of intelligence with Native American primary grade children. *Perceptual and Motor Skills, 49,* 480–2.

Inkeles, A., & Smith, D.H. (1974). *Becoming modern: Individual change in six developing countries.* Cambridge: Harvard University Press.

Jackson, J. (1994). Chronic pain and the tension between the body as subject and object. In T. Csordas (Ed.), *Embodiement and experience: The existential ground of culture and self* (pp. 201–28). Cambridge: Cambridge University Press.

Jahoda, G. (1982). *Psychology and anthropology.* London: Academic Press.

Jahoda, G. (1999). *Images of savages: Ancient roots of modern prejudice in western culture.* London: Routledge.

James, B.J. (1954). Some critical observations concerning analysis of Chippewa 'atomism' and Chippewa personality. *American Anthropologist, 56*(2), 283–6.

James, B.J. (1961). Social-psychological dimensions of Ojibwa acculturation. *American Anthropologist, 63*(4), 721–46.

James, J.T.L. (1979). Toward a cultural understanding of the Native offender. *Canadian Journal of Criminology, 21,* 453–62.

Jarvis, G.K., & Boldt, M. (1982). Death styles among Canada's Indians. *Social Science and Medicine, 16*(14), 1345–52.

Jenness, D. (1933). An Indian method of treating hysteria. *Primitive Man, 6*(1), 13–20.

Jewell, D. (1952). The case of a 'psychotic' Navaho Indian male. *Human Organization, 11*(1), 32–6.

Jilek, W.G. (1971). From crazy witch doctor to auxiliary psychotherapist – the changing image of the Medicine Man. *Psychiatra Clinica, 4,* 200–20.

Jilek, W.G. (1978). Native renaissance: The survival and revival of indigenous therapeutic ceremonials among North American Indians. *Transcultural Psychiatric Research Review, 15,* 117–47.

Jilek, W.G. (1981). Anomic depression, alcoholism, and culture-congenial Indian response. *Journal on Studies on Alcohol, 9,* 159–70.

Jilek, W.G. (1982). *Indian healing: Shamanic ceremonialism in the Pacific Northwest Today.* Surrey, BC: Hancock House.

Jilek, W.G., & Jilek-Aall, L. (1971). A transcultural approach to psychotherapy with Canadian Indians: Experiences from the Fraser Valley of British Columbia. *Psychiatry (Part III),* Symposium 28, 1181–86.

Jilek, W.G., & Jilek-Aall, L. (1978). The psychiatrist and his Shaman colleague: Cross-cultural collaboration with traditional Amerindian therapists. *Journal of Operational Psychiatry, 9,* 32–9.

Jilek, W.G., & Jilek-Aall, L. (1985). The metamorphosis of 'culture-bound' syndromes. *Social Science and Medicine, 21*(2), 205–10.

Jilek, W.G., & Roy, C. (1976). Homicide committed by Canadian Indians and non-Indians. *International Journal of Offender Therapy and Criminology, 20*(3), 201–16.

Jilek, W.G., & Todd, N. (1974). Witch doctors succeed where doctors fail: Psychotherapy among Coast Salish Indians. *Canadian Psychiatric Association Journal, 19,* 351–5.

Jilek-Aall, L. (1974). Psychosocial aspects of drinking among Coast Salish Indians. *Canadian Psychiatric Association Journal, 19,* 357–61.

Jilek-Aall, L. (1976). The Western psychiatrist and his non-Western clientele. *Canadian Psychiatric Association Journal, 21*(6), 353–9.

Jilek-Aall, L. (1981). Acculturation, alcoholism and Indian-style Alcoholics Anonymous. *Journal of Studies on Alcohol,* Supplement No. 9, 143–58.

Jilek-Aall, L., Jilek, W.G., & Flynn, F. (1978). Sex role, culture and psychopathology: A comparative study of three ethnic groups in Western Canada. *Journal of Psychological Anthropology, 4,* 473–88.

Johnson, D. (1994). Stress, depression, substance abuse, and racism. *American Indian and Alaska Native Mental Health Research, 6*(1), 29–33.

Johnson, D.L., & Johnson, C.A. (1965). Totally discouraged: A depressive syndrome of the Dakota Sioux. *Transcultural Psychiatric Research Review, 2*(1), 141–3.

Johnson, M.E., & Lashley, K.H. (1989). Influence of Native-Americans' cultural commitment on preferences for counselor ethnicity and expectations about counseling. *Journal of Multicultural Counseling and Development, 17,* 115–22.

Jones, M.C., Dauphinais, P., Sack, W.H., & Somervell, P.D. (1997). Trauma-related symptomatology among American Indian adolescents. *Journal of Traumatic Stress, 10*(2), 163–73.

Jones-Saumty, D., Hochhaus, L., Dru, R., & Zeiner, A. (1983). Psychological factors of familial alcoholism in American Indians and Caucasians. *Journal of Clinical Psychology, 39*(5), 783–90.

Joseph, A., Spicer, R.B., & Chesky, J. (1949). *The Desert People.* Chicago: University of Chicago Press.

Kahn, M.W. (1982). Culture clash and psychopathology in three Aboriginal cultures. *Academic Psychology Bulletin, 4,* 553–61.

Kahn, M.W., Lewis, J., & Galvez, E. (1974). An evaluation of a group therapy procedure with reservation adolescent Indians. *Psychotherapy: Theory, Research and Practice, 11*(3), 239–42.

Kaplan, B. (1954). *A study of Rorschach responses in four cultures.* Papers of the Peabody Museum of American Archaeology and Ethnology, Harvard University, Vol. 42, No. 2.

Kaplan, B. (1961). Cross-cultural use of projective techniques. In F.L.K. Hsu (Ed.), *Psychological anthropology: Approaches to culture and personality* (pp. 235–54). Homewood, IL: Dorsey Press, Inc.

Kaplan, B., & Johnson, D. (1964). The social meaning of Navaho psychopathology and psychotherapy. In A. Kiev (Ed.), *Magic, faith, and healing: Studies in primitive psychiatry today* (pp. 203–29). New York: Free Press.

Kaplan, H.I., & Sadock, B.J. (1995). *Comprehensive textbook of psychiatry/V.* (6th ed.). Vol. 1. Baltimore: Williams and Wilkins.

Kaplan, H.I., & Sadock, B.J. (1996). *Concise textbook of clinical psychiatry.* Baltimore: Williams and Wilkins.

Kaplan, H.I., & Sadock, B.J. (1997). *Synopsis of psychiatry* (7th ed.). Baltimore: Williams and Wilkins.

Kaplan, H.I., & Sadock, B.J. (2000). *Synopsis of psychiatry* (8th ed.). Baltimore: Williams and Wilkins.

Kardiner, A. (1945). The concept of basic personality structure as an operational tool in the social sciences. In R. Linton (Ed.), *The science of man in the world crisis* (pp. 107–22). New York: Columbia University Press.

Kardiner, A., & Linton, R. (1939). *The individual and his society.* New York: Columbia University Press.

Katz, P. (1981). Psychotherapy with Native adolescents. *Canadian Journal of Psychiatry, 26,* 455–9.

Keane, E.M., Dick, R.W., Bechtold, D.W., & Manson, S.M. (1996). Predictive and concurrent validity of the suicidal ideation questionnaire among American Indian adolescents. *Journal of Abnormal Child Psychology, 24*(6), 735–47.

Keesing, R.M. (1990). Theories of culture revisited. *Canberra Anthropology, 13*(2), 46–60.

Kehoe, A.B. (1990). Primal Gaia: Primitivists and plastic medicine men. In J.A. Clifton (Ed.), *The invented Indian: cultural fictions and government policies* (pp. 193–209). New York: Transaction Publishers.

Kelso, D., & Attneave, C. (1981). *Bibliography of American Indian mental health.* Westport, CT: Greenwood.

Kemnitzer, L.S. (1972). The structure of country drinking parties on Pine Ridge reservation, South Dakota. *Plains Anthropologist, 17,* 134–42.

Kennedy, D. (1984). The quest for a cure: A case study in the use of health care alternatives. *Culture, 4*(2), 21–31.

Kerckhoff, A.C., & McCormick, T.C. (1955). Marginal status and marginal personality. *Social Forces, 34*(4), 48–55.

Kettl, P., & Bixler, E.O. (1993). Alcohol and suicide in Alaska Natives. *American Indian and Alaska Native Mental Health Research, 5*(2), 34–45.

Kiev, A. (1972). *Transcultural psychiatry.* New York: Free Press.

King, J., Beals, J., Manson, S., & Trimble, J. (1992). A structural equation model of factors related to substance abuse among American Indian adolescents. *Drugs and Society, 6*(3/4), 253–68.

Kinzie, J.D., Leung, P.K., Boehnlein, J.K., Matsunaga, D., Johnson, R., Manson, S., Shore, J.H., Heinz, J., & Williams, M. (1992). Psychiatric epidemiology of an Indian village: A 19-year replication study. *The Journal of Nervous and Mental Disease, 180*(1), 33–39.

Kirk, S.A., & Kutchins, H. (1992). *The selling of DSM: The rhetoric of science in psychiatry.* New York: Aldine de Gruyter.

Kirmayer, L.J. (1988). Mind and body as metaphors: Hidden values in biomedicine. In M. Lock and D. Gordon (Eds.), *Biomedicine Examined* (pp. 57–93). Dordrecht, Holland: Kluwer Academic Publishers.

Kirmayer, L.J. (1994). Suicide among Canadian Aboriginal people. *Transcultural Psychiatric Research Review, 31,* 3–58.

Kirmayer, L.J. (1996a). Confusion of the senses: Implications of cultural variations in somatoform and dissoociative disorders to PTSD. In A.J. Marsella,
M. Friedman, E. Gerrity, and R. Scurfield (Eds.), *Ethnocultural aspects of post-
traumatic stress disorders.* Washington, DC: American Psychiatric Press.

Kirmayer, L.J. (1996b). Landscapes of memory: Trauma, narrative, and dissoci-
ation. In P. Antze and M. Lambek (Eds.), *Tense past: Cultural essays in trauma
and memory* (pp. 173–98). New York: Routledge.

Kirmayer, L.J., Boothroyd, L.J., Tanner, A., Adelson, N., & Robinson, E. (2000).
Psychological Distress Among the Cree of James Bay. *Transcultural Psychiatry, 37*(1), 35–56.

Kirmayer, L.J., Brass, G.M., & Tait, C.L. (2000). The mental health of Aboriginal
peoples: Transformations of identity and community. *Canadian Journal of
Psychiatry, 45,* 607–16.

Kirmayer, L.J., Fletcher, C., & Boothroyd, L.J. (1998). Suicide among Inuit of
Canada. In A.A. Leenaars, S. Wenckstern, I. Sakinofsky, R.J. Dyck, M.J. Kral,
& R.C. Bland (Eds.), *Suicide in Canada* (pp. 189–211). Toronto: University of
Toronto Press.

Kirmayer, L.J., Fletcher, C.M., Corin, E., & Boothroyd, L.J. (1997). *Inuit concepts
of mental health and illness: An ethnographic study.* Culture and Mental Health
Research Unit, Report No. 4: Institute of Community and Family Psychiatry,
Sir Mortimer B. Davis-Jewish General Hospital and Division of Social and
Transcultural Psychiatry, Department of Psychiatry, McGill University.

Kirmayer, L.J., Gill, K., Fletcher, C., Ternar, Y., Boothroyd, L.J., Quesney, C.,
Smith, A., Ferrara, N., & Hayton, B. (1994). *Emerging trends in research on
mental health among Canadian Aboriginal peoples.* Culture and Mental Health
Research Unit, Report No. 2: Institute of Community and Family Psychiatry,
Sir Mortimer B. Davis-Jewish General Hospital and Division of Social and
Transcultural Psychiatry, Department of Psychiatry, McGill University.

Kirmayer, L.J., & Minas, H. (2000). The future of cultural psychiatry: An international perspective. *Canadian Journal of Psychiatry, 45,* 438–46.

Kirmayer, L.J. & Young, A. (1999). Culture and context in the evolutionary concept of mental disorder. *Journal of Abnormal Psychology, 108*(3), 446–52.

Kleinman, A. (1977). Depression, somatization and the 'new cross-cultural psychiatry.' *Social Science and Medicine, 11,* 3–10.

Kleinman, A. (1980). *Patients and healers in the context of culture: An exploration of
the borderland between anthropology, medicine and psychiatry.* Berkeley: University of California Press.

Kleinman, A. (1988). *Rethinking psychiatry: From cultural category to personal
experience.* New York: Free Press.

Kleinman, A. (1995). *Writing at the margin: Discourse between anthropology and
medicine.* Berkeley: University of California Press.

Kleinman, A. (1996). How is culture important for DSM-IV. In J. Mezzich, A. Kleinman, H. Fabrega, Jr., & D. Parron (Eds.), *Culture and psychiatric diagnosis: A DSM-IV perspective* (pp. 15–29). Washington, DC: American Psychiatric Press, Inc.

Kleinman, A., & Good, B. (1985). Introduction: Culture and Depression. In A. Kleinman and B. Good (Eds.), *Culture and depression* (pp. 1–23). Berkeley: University of California Press.

Kline, J.A., & Roberts, A.C. (1973). A residential alcoholism treatment program for American Indians. *Quarterly Journal of Studies on Alcohol, 34,* 860–8.

Kline, J.A., Rozynko, V.V., Flint, G., & Roberts, A.C. (1973). Personality characteristics of male Native American alcoholic patients. *International Journal of Addictions, 8*(4), 729–32.

Klopfer, B., & Boyer, B.L. (1961). Notes on the personality structure of a North American Indian Shaman: Rorschach interpretation. *Journal of Projective Assessment Techniques and Personality, 25,* 170–8.

Kluckhohn, C. (1943). Covert culture and administrative problems. *American Anthropologist, 45,* 213–27.

Kluckhohn, C., & Leighton, D. (1948). *Children of the people.* Cambridge: Harvard University Press.

Kluckhohn, F.R., & Strodtbeck, F.L. (1961). *Variations in value orientations.* Homewood, IL: Dorsey.

Konner, M. (1995). Anthropology and psychiatry. In H.I. Kaplan and B.J. Sadock (Eds.), *Comprehensive textbook of psychiatry/VI* (6th ed; Vol. 1) (pp. 337–56). Baltimore: Williams and Wilkins.

Koolage, W.W. (1975). Conceptual negativism in Chipewyan ethnology. *Anthropologica n.s. 17*(1), 45–60.

Koverola, C. (1992). Counseling Aboriginal people of North America, special issue: Multicultural counseling. *Journal of Psychology and Christianity, 11*(4), 345–57.

Kracke, W.H. (1987). A psychoanalyst in the field: Erikson's contributions to anthropology. In J. Rabow, G.M. Platt, & M.S. Goldman (Eds.), *Advances in psychoanalytic sociology* (pp. 35–69). Malabar, FL: Robert E. Krieger Publishing Co.

Kraus, R.F. (1971). Changing patterns of suicidal behavior in North Alaskan Eskimo. *Transcultural Psychiatry Research Review, 9,* 69–71.

Kraus, R.F. (1974). Suicidal behavior in Alaska Natives. *Alaska Medicine, 16*(1), 2–6.

Kraus, R.F. & Buffler, P.A. (1979). Sociocultural stress and the American Native in Alaska: An analysis of changing patterns of psychiatric illness and alcohol abuse among Alaska Natives. *Culture, Medicine and Psychiatry, 3*(2), 111–51.

Krause, I.-B. (1998). *Therapy Across Cultures*. London: Sage.

Kroeber, A.L. (1923; rpt 1948). *Anthropology*. New York: Harcourt and Brace.

Kroeber, A.L. (1939). Cultural and natural areas of Native North America. *University of California Publications in American Archaeology and Ethnology, 38,* 1–242.

Kunitz, S.J., & Levy, J.E. (1974). Changing ideas of alcohol use among Navaho Indians. *Quarterly Journal of Studies on Alcohol, 35,* 243–59.

Kunitz, S.J., & Levy, J.E. (1994). *Drinking careers: A twenty-five-year study of three Navajo populations.* New Haven: Yale University Press.

Kunitz, S., & Levy, J. (2000a). Conduct disorder, drinking, and the problem of prevention. In S. Kunitz and J. Levy (Eds.), *Drinking, conduct disorder, and social change: Navajo experiences* (pp. 1–13). New York: Oxford University Press.

Kunitz, S., & Levy, J. (2000b). Conclusions. In S. Kunitz and J. Levy (Eds.), *Drinking, conduct disorder, and social change: Navajo experiences* (pp. 155–78). New York: Oxford University Press.

Kuper, A. (1999). *Culture: The anthropologists' account.* Cambridge: Harvard University Press.

Kutchins, H., & Kirk, S. (1997). *Making us crazy: DSM: The psychiatric bible and the creation of mental disorders.* New York: Free Press.

Kuttner, R.E., & Lorincz, A.B. (1967). Alcoholism and addiction in urbanized Sioux Indians. *Mental Hygiene, 51,* 530–42.

LaFromboise, T.D. (1993). American Indian mental health policy. In D.R. Atkinson, G. Morten, and D. Wing Sue (Eds.), *Counseling American minorities: A cross-cultural perspective* (pp. 123–43). Madison, WI: Brown and Benchmark.

LaFromboise, T.D., Dauphinais, P., & Rowe, W. (1980). Indian student's perception of positive helper attributes. *Journal of American Indian Education, 19*(3), 11–16.

LaFromboise, T.D., & Jackson, M. (1996). MCT theory and Native-American populations. In D. Wing Sue, A. Ivey, and P.B. Pedersen (Eds.), *A theory of multicultural counseling* (pp. 192–203). Pacific Grove, CA: Brooks/Cole Publishing Co.

LaFromboise, T.D., & Rowe, W. (1983). Skills training for bicultural competence: Rationale and application. *Journal of Counseling Psychology, 39*(4), 589–95.

LaFromboise, T.D., Trimble, J.E., & Mohatt, G.V. (1990). Counseling intervention and American Indian tradition: An integrative approach. *Counselling Psychologist, 18*(4), 628–54.

LaFromboise, T.D., Trimble, J.E., & Mohatt, G.V. (1993). Counseling intervention and American Indian tradition: An integrative approach. In D.R. Atkinson, G. Morten, and D. Wing Sue (Eds.), *Counseling American minorities: A cross-cultural perspective* (pp. 145–70). Madison, WI: Brown and Benchmark Publishers.

Lamarine, R.J. (1988). Alcohol abuse among Native Americans. *Journal of Community Health, 13*(3), 143–55.

Landes, R. (1937). The personality of the Ojibwa. *Character and Personality, 6,* 51–60.

Landes, R. (1938). The abnormal among the Ojibwa Indians. *Journal of Abnormal and Social Psychology, 33,* 14–33.

Langness, L. (1976). Hysterical psychoses and possessions. In W.P. Lebra (Ed.), *Culture-bound syndromes, ethnopsychiatry, and alternate therapies* (pp. 56–67). Honolulu: University of Hawaii Press.

Lantz, H. (1948). Rorschach testing in pre-literate cultures. *American Journal of Orthopsychiatry, 18,* 287–91.

Legters, L. (1988). The American genocide. *Policy Studies Journal, 16*(4), 768–77.

Leighton, A.H. (1959a). Mental illness and acculturation. In I. Galdston (Ed.), *Medicine and Anthropology* (pp. 108–28). New York: International Universities Press.

Leighton, A.H. (1959b). *My name is legion.* Stirling County Study, Vol. 1. New York: Basic Books.

Leighton, A.H. (1968). The mental health of the American Indian. *American Journal of Psychiatry, 125*(2), 217–18.

Leighton, A.H., & Leighton, D. (1949). *Gregorio, the hand-trembler. A psychobiological personality study of a Navajo Indian.* Reports of the Ramah Project. Report No. 1. Peabody Museum of American Archaeology and Ethnology, Harvard University, Vol. 15, No.1. Cambridge: Peabody Museum.

Leighton, D., Harding, J., Macklin, D., Macmillan, A., & Leighton, A. (1963). *The character of danger.* Stirling County Study, Vol. 3. New York: Basic Books.

Leighton, D., & Adair, J. (1966). *People of the middle place: A study of the Zuni Indians.* New Haven: Human Relations Area Files.

Leighton, D., & Kluckhohn, C. (1969). *Children of the people.* New York: Octagon Books.

Leighton, A.H., & Hughes, C. (1955). Notes on Eskimo patterns of suicide. *Southwestern Journal of Anthropology, 11,* 327–38.

Leland, J. (1976). *Firewater myths: North American Indian drinking and alcohol addiction.* Brunswick, NJ: Rutgers Center of Alcohol Studies.

Leland, J. (1979a). Alcohol, anthropologists, and Native Americans. *Human Organization, 38*(1), 94–9.

Leland, J. (1979b). Comment on 'Psychocultural barriers to successful alcoholism therapy in an American Indian patient.' *Journal of Studies on Alcohol,* *40*(7), 737–42.

Lemert, E.M. (1954). *Alcohol and the Northwest Coast Indians.* Berkeley: University of California Press.

Lemert, E.M. (1958). The use of alcohol in three Salish Indian tribes. *Quarterly Journal of Studies on Alcohol, 19,* 90–107.

Levine, R.E., & Gaw, A.C. (1995). Culture-bound syndromes. *The Psychiatric Clinics of North America, 18*(3), 523–36.

Levy, J.E. (1965). Navajo suicide. *Human Organization, 24,* 308–18.

Levy, J.E., & Kunitz, S.J. (1971). Indian reservations, anomie, and social pathologies. *Southwestern Journal of Anthropology, 27*(2), 97–128.

Levy, J.E., & Kunitz, S.J. (1974). *Indian drinking: Navajo practices and Anglo-American theories.* New York: Wiley and Sons.

Levy, J.E., Neutra, R., & Parker, D. (1987). *Hand trembling, frenzy witchcraft, and moth madness: A study of Navajo seizure disorders.* Tucson: University of Arizona Press.

Lewis, G. (1993). Double standards of treatment evaluations. In S. Lindenbaum and M. Lock (Eds.), *Knowledge, power, and practice: The anthropology of medicine and everyday life* (pp. 189–218). Berkeley: University of California Press.

Lewis, R.G. (1980). Cultural perspectives on treatment modalities with Native Americans. In M. Bloom (Ed.), *Life span development: Bases for preventive and interventive healing* (pp. 458–64). New York: MacMillan Publishing Company.

Lewis, R.G. (1982). Alcoholism and the Native American: A review of the literature. In National Institute on Alcohol Abuse and Alcoholism. *Alcohol and Health Monograph 4 – Special Population Issues* (pp. 315–28). Rockville, MD: National Institute on Alcohol Abuse and Alcoholism.

Lewis, R.G., & Ho, M.K. (1975). Social work with Native Americans. *Social Work, 20*(5), 379–82.

Lewis, T.H. (1975). A syndrome of depression and mutism in the Oglala Sioux. *American Journal of Psychiatry, 132*(7), 753–55.

Lewton, E.L., & Bydone, V. (2000). Identity and healing in three Navajo religious traditions. *Medical Anthropology Quarterly, 14*(4), 476–97.

Leys, R. (2000). *Trauma: A genealogy.* Chicago: University of Chicago Press.

Liberman, D., & Frank, J. (1980). Individuals' perception of stressful life events: A comparison of Native American, rural, and urban samples using the Social Readjustment Rating Scale. *White Cloud Journal, 1*(4), 15–19.

Lieber, Charles S. (1972). Metabolism of ethanol and alcoholism: Racial and acquired factors. *Annals of Internal Medicine, 76*(2), 326–27.

Lindholm, C. (2001). *Culture and identity: The history, theory and practice of psychological anthropology.* Boston: McGraw Hill.

Linnekin, J. (1992). On the theory and politics of cultural construction in the Pacific. *Oceania, 62*(4), 249–63.

Littlewood, R. (2000). Psychiatry's Culture. In V. Skultans and J. Cox (Eds.), *Anthropological Approaches to Psychological Medicine: Crossing Bridges* (pp. 66–93). London: Jessica Kingsley.

Littlewood, R., & Lipsedge, M. (1985). Culture-bound syndromes. In K. Granville-Grossman (Ed.), *Recent advances in clinical psychiatry* (No. 5) (pp. 105–42). Edinburgh: Churchill Livingstone.

Littlewood, R., & Lipsedge, M. (1997). *Aliens and alienists: Ethnic minorities and psychiatry* (3rd ed.). London: Routledge.

Littman, G. (1970). Alcoholism, illness, and social pathology among American Indians in transition. *American Journal of Public Health, 60*(9), 1769–87.

Lock, M., & Scheper-Hughes, N. (1996). A critical-interpretive approach in medical anthropology: Rituals and routines of discipline and dissent. In S. Lindenbaum and M. Lock (Eds.), *The Anthropology of medicine and everyday life* (pp. 189–218). Berkeley: University of California Press.

Locke, D.C. (1992). *Increasing multicultural understanding: A comprehensive model*. Newbury Park, CA: Sage Publications.

Locust, C. (1988). Wounding the spirit: Discrimination and traditional American Indian belief systems. *Harvard Educational Review, 58*(3), 315–30.

Loney, M. (1995). Social problems, community trauma and hydro project impacts. *Canadian Journal of Native Studies, 15*(2), 231–54.

Long, K.A. (1983). The experience of repeated and traumatic loss among Crow Indian children: Response patterns and intervention strategies. *American Journal of Orthopsychiatry, 53*(1), 116–26.

Long, K.A., & Hamlin, C.M. (1988). Use of the Piers-Harris Self-Concept Scale with Indian children: Cultural considerations. *Nursing Research, 37*(1), 42–6.

Longclaws, L., Barnes, G.E., Grieve, L., & Dumoff, R. (1980). Alcohol and drug use among the Brokenhead Ojibwa. *Journal of Studies on Alcohol, 41*(1), 21–36.

Lowie, R. (1913). Crow military societies. *Societies of the Plains Indians*, C. Wissler (Ed.), *Anthropological Papers of the American Musuem of Natural History* 11.

Lucas, R.H., & Barrett, R.J. (1995). Interpreting culture and psychopathology: Primitivist themes in cross-cultural debate. *Culture, Medicine and Psychiatry, 19*(3), 287–326.

Luckert, K.W. (1972). Traditional Navaho theories of disease and healing. *Arizona Medicine, 29*, 571–3.

Lurie, N.O. (1971). The world's oldest on-going protest demonstration: North American Indian drinking patterns. *Pacific Historical Review, 40*(3), 311–32.

MacAndrew, C., & Edgerton, R.B. (1969). *Drunken comportment: A social explanation*. New York: Aldine Publishing Co.

MacAvoy, J., Orr, S., & Sidles, C. (1993). The Raven Matrices and Navajo children: Normative characteristics and culture fair application to issues of intelligence, giftedness, and academic proficiency. *Journal of American Indian Education, 33*(1), 32–43.

Macgregor, G. (1946). *Warriors without weapons*. Chicago: University of Chicago Press.

Mail, P.D. (1989). American Indians, stress, and alcohol. *American Indian and Alaska Native Mental Health Research, 3*(2), 7–26.

Mail, P.D., & Johnson, S. (1993). Boozing, sniffing, and toking: An overview of the past, present, and future of substance use by American Indians. *American Indian and Alaska Native Mental Health Research, 5*(2), 1–33.

Mail, P.D., & McDonald, D.R. (1980). *Tulapai to tokay: A bibliography of alcohol use and abuse among Native Americans in North America*. New Haven: Human Relations Area Files.

Mandelzys, N., & Lane, E. (1980). The validity of the MMPI as it pertains to Canadian Native inmates. *Canadian Journal of Criminology, 22*(2), 188–96.

Manson, S.M. (1986). Recent advances in American Indian mental health research: Implications for clinical research and training. In M. Miranda and M. Kitano (Eds.), *Mental health research and practice in minority communities: Development of culturally sensitive training programs* (pp. 51–89). Rockville, MD: US Dept. of Health and Human Services.

Manson, S.M. (1992). Depression and related mental illnesses among American Indian: The current state of the art in treatment. In E.E. Haller and L.P. Aitken (Eds.), *Mashkiki: Old medicine nourishing new* (pp. 81–91). Lanham, MD: University Press of America.

Manson, S.M. (1996). The wounded spirit: A cultural formulation of post-traumatic stress disorder. *Culture, Medicine and Psychiatry, 20*, 489–98.

Manson, S.M. (1997). Cross-cultural and multiethnic assessment of trauma. In J. Wilson and T. Keane (Eds.), *Assessing psychological trauma and PTSD* (pp. 239–66). New York: Guilford Press.

Manson, S.M. (2000). Mental health services for American Indians and Alaska Natives: Need, use, and barriers to effective care. *Canadian Journal of Psychiatry, 45*, 617–26.

Manson, S.M., Ackerson, L.M., Dick, R.W., Baron, A.E., & Fleming, C.M. (1990). Depressive symptoms among American Indian adolescents: Psychometric characteristics of the Center of Epidemiologic Studies depression scale (CES-D). *Psychological Assessment, 2*(3), 231–7.

Manson, S.M., Beals, J., O'Nell, T. Piasecki, J., Bechtold, D., Keane, E., & Jones,

M. (1996). Wounded spirits, ailing hearts: PTSD and related disorders among American Indians. In A.J. Marsella, M.J. Friedman, E.T. Gerrity, and R.M. Scurfield (Eds.), *Ethnocultural aspects of posttraumatic stress disorder: Issues, research, and clinical applications* (pp. 255–83). Washington, DC: American Psychological Association.

Manson, S.M., & Shore, J.H. (1981). Psychiatric epidemiological research among American Indians and Alaska Natives: Methodological issues. *White Cloud Journal, 2*(2), 48–56.

Manson, S.M., Shore, J. H., Baron, A.E., Ackerson, L., & Neligh, G. (1992). Alcohol abuse and dependence among American Indians. In J. Helzer and G. Canino (Eds.), *Alcoholism in North America, Europe, and Asia* (pp. 113–30). New York: Oxford University Press.

Manson, S.M., Shore, J.H. & Bloom, J.D. (1985). The depressive experience in American Indian communities: A challenge for psychiatric theory and diagnosis. In A. Klienman and B. Good (Eds.), *Culture and depression* (pp. 331–68). Berkeley, CA: University of California Press.

Manson, S.M., Walker, R.D., & Kivlahan, D.R. (1987). Psychiatric assessment and treatment of American Indians and Alaska Natives. *Hospital and Community Psychiatry, 38*(2), 165–73.

Manson, W.C. (1988). *The psychodyamics of culture: Abram Kardiner and Neo-Freudian anthropology.* Westport, CT: Greenwood Press.

Marano, L. (1982). Windigo psychosis: The anatomy of an emic-etic confusion. *Current Anthropology, 23,* 385–412.

Marano, L. (1985). Windigo psychosis: The anatomy of an emic-etic confusion. In R. Simons and C. Hughes (Eds.), *The culture-bound syndromes: Folk illnesses of psychiatric and anthropological interest* (pp. 411–48). Dordrecht, The Netherlands: D. Reidel Publishing Co.

Marcus, G., & Fischer, M.J. (1986). *Anthropology as cultural critique: An experimental moment in the human sciences.* Chicago: University of Chicago Press.

Margetts, E.L. (1975). Indian and Eskimo medicine, with notes on the early history of psychiatry among French and British colonists. In J.G. Howells (Ed.), *World History of Psychiatry* (pp. 400–31). NewYork: Brunner/Mazel Publishers.

Marín, G., & Gamba, R. (2003). Acculturation and changes in cultural values. In K. Chun, P. Organista, and G. Marín (Eds.), *Acculturation: Advances in theory, measurement, and applied research* (pp. 83–93). Washington, DC: American Psychological Association.

Marsella, A.J., Dubanoski, J., Hamada, W.C., & Morse, H. (2000). The measurement of personality across cultures. *American Behavioral Scientist, 44*(1), 41–62.

Martin, H.W., Smith Sutker, S., Leon, R.L., & Hales, W.M. (1968). Mental health of Eastern Oklahoma Indians: An exploration. *Human Organization, 27*(4), 308–15.

Martínez-Hernáez, A. (2000). *What's behind the symptom: On psychiatric observation and anthropological understanding.* Amsterdam, The Netherlands: Harwood Academic Publishers.

Mason, E.P. (1967). Comparison of personality characteristics of junior high students from American Indian, Mexican, and Caucasian ethnic backgrounds. *Journal of Social Psychology, 73*, 145–55.

Mason, E.P. (1968). Sex difference in personality characteristics of deprived adolescents. *Perceptual and Motor Skills, 27*, 934.

Mason, E.P. (1969). Cross-validation study of personality characteristics of junior high students from American Indian, Mexican, and Caucasian backgrounds. *Journal of Social Psychology, 77*, 15–24.

Mason, E.P. (1971). Stability of differences in personality characteristics of junior high students from American Indian, Mexican, and Anglo ethnic backgrounds. *Psychology in the Schools, 8*(1), 86–9.

May, P.A. (1977). Explanations of Native American drinking: A literature review. *Plains Anthropologist, 22*(77), 223–32.

May, P.A. (1982). Substance abuse and American Indians: Prevalence and susceptibility. *The International Journal of the Addictions, 17*(7), 1185–1209.

May, P.A. (1986). Alcohol and drug misuse prevention programs for American Indians: Needs and opportunities. *Journal of Studies on Alcohol, 47*(3), 187–5.

May, P.A. (1987). Suicide and self-destruction among American Indian youth. *American Indian and Alaska Native Mental Health, 1*(1), 52–69.

May, P.A. (1988). Mental health and alcohol abuse indicators in the Albuquerque area of Indian health service: An exploratory chart review. *American Indian and Alaska Native Mental Health Research, 2*(1), 33–46.

May, P.A. (1990). A bibliography on suicide and suicide attempts among American Indians and Alaska Natives. *Omega, Journal of Death and Dying, 21*(3), 199–214.

May, P.A. (1992a). Alcohol policy considerations for Indian reservations and bordertown communities. *American Indian and Alaska Native Mental Health Research, 4*(3), 5–59.

May, P.A. (1992b). Let the debate, study, and action continue: Response to twelve critiques. *American Indian and Alaska Native Mental Health Research, 4*(3), 126–2.

May, P.A. (1996). Overview of alcohol abuse epidemiology for American Indian populations. In G. Sandefur, R. Rindfuss, and B. Cohen (Eds.), *Changing numbers, changing needs: American Indian demography and public health* (pp. 235–61). Washington, DC: National Academy Press.

May, P.A. (1999). The epidemiology of alcohol abuse among American Indians: The mythical and real properties. In D. Champagne (Ed.), *Contemporary Native American cultural issues* (pp. 227–44). London: Altamira Press.

May, P.A., & Dizmang, L.H. (1981). Suicide and the American Indian. *Psychiatric Annals, 4*(9), 22–8.

Maynard, E. (1969). Drinking as part of an adjustment syndrome among the Oglala Sioux. *Pine Ridge Research Bulletin, 9*, 35–51.

McCormick, R.M. (1996). Culturally appropriate means and ends of counselling as described by the First Nations people of British Colombia. *International Journal for the Advancement of Counselling, 18*(3), 163–72.

McCormick, R.M. (1997). Healing through interdependence: The role of connecting in First Nations healing practices. *Canadian Journal of Counselling, 31*(3), 172–84.

McCullough, C.S., Walker, J.L., & Diessner, R. (1985). The use of Wechsler scales in the assessment of Native Americans of the Columbia River Basin. *Psychology in the Schools, 22*, 23–8.

McDonald, J.D., Morton, R., & Stewart, C. (1993). Clinical concerns with American Indian patients. In L. VandeCreek, S. Knapp et al. (Eds.), *Innovations in clinical practice: A source book, Vol. 12* (pp. 437–54). Sarasota, FL: Professional Resource Press/Professional Resource Exchange, Inc.

McDonald, T. (1975). Group therapy with Native American women. *International Journal of Group Psychotherapy, 25*, 410–20.

McIntosh, J.L. (1983). Suicide among Native Americans: Further tribal data and considerations. *Omega, Journal of Death and Dying, 14*(3), 215–29.

McIntosh, J.L., & Santos, J.F. (1981). Suicide among Native Americans: A compilation of findings. *Omega, Journal of Death and Dying, 11*(4), 303–16.

McMillan, A.D. (1995). Native peoples and cultures in Canada. (2nd ed.). Vancouver: Douglas & McIntyre.

McNickle, D. (1968). The sociocultural setting of Indian life. *American Journal of Psychiatry, 125*(2), 219–23.

McShane, D.A. (1980). A review of scores of American Indian children on the Wechsler Intelligence Scales. *White Cloud Journal, 1*(4), 3–10.

McShane, D.A., & Berry, J.W. (1988). Native North Americans: Indians and Inuit abilities. In S.H. Irvine and J.W. Berry (Eds.), *Human Abilities in Cultural Context* (pp. 385–426). New York: Cambridge University Press.

McShane, D.A., & Plas, J.M. (1982a). Weschler Scale performance patterns of American Indian children. *Psychology in the Schools, 19*(1), 8–17.

McShane, D.A., & Plas, J.M. (1982b). WISC-R factor structures for Ojibwa Indian children. *White Cloud Journal, 2*(4), 18–22.

McShane, D.A., & Plas, J.M. (1984). The cognitive functioning of American

Indian children: Moving from the WISC to the WISC-R. *School Psychology Review, 13*(1), 61–73.

Medicine, B. (1982). New roads to coping – Siouan sobriety. In S.P. Manson (Ed.), *New directions in prevention among American Indian and Alaska Native communities* (pp. 189–212). Portland: Oregon Health Services University.

Mezzich, J.E., Kirmayer, L.J., Kleinman, A., Fabrega Jr, H., Parron, D.L., Good, B.J., Lin, K.-M., & Manson, S.M. (1999). The place of culture in DSM-IV. *Journal of Nervous and Mental Disease, 187*(8), 457–64.

Mezzich, J., & Lin, K.-M. (1995). Acute and transient psychotic disorders and culture-bound syndromes. In H. Kaplan and B. Sadock (Eds.), *Comprehensive textbook of psychiatry/V* (6th ed.; Vol. 1) (pp. 1049–59). Baltimore: Williams and Wilkins.

Miles, J.E. (1967). The psychiatric aspects of the traditional medicine of the British Columbian Coast Indians. *Canadian Psychiatric Association Journal, 12*(4), 429–31.

Miller, J.R. (1996). *Shingwauk's vision: A history of Native residential schools.* Toronto: University of Toronto Press.

Milloy, J.S. (1999). *A national crime: The Canadian government and the residential school system, 1879 to 1986.* Winnipeg: University of Manitoba Press.

Milne, D., & Howard, W. (2000). Rethinking the role of diagnosis in Navajo religious healing. *Medical Anthropology Quarterly, 14*(4), 543–70.

Mishra, S.P. (1982). The WISC-R and evidence of item bias for Native-American Navajos. *Psychology in the Schools, 19,* 458–64.

Mishra, S.P., & Lord, J. (1982). Reliability and predictive validity of the WISC-R with Native-American Navajos. *The Journal of School Psychology, 20*(2), 150–4.

Mohatt, G. (1972). The sacred water: The quest for personal power through drinking among the Teton Sioux. In D.C. McClelland, W.N. Davis, R. Kalin, and E. Wanner (Eds.), *The Drinking Man* (pp. 261–75). New York: Free Press.

Mohatt, G., & Blue, A.W. (1982). Primary prevention as it relates to traditionality and empirical measures of social deviance. In S.P. Manson (Ed.), *New directions in prevention among American Indian and Alaska Native communities* (pp. 91–118). Portland: Oregon Health Services University.

Mohatt, G., & Varvin, S. (1998). Looking for 'A Good Doctor': A cultural-formulation of the treatment of a First Nations' woman using western and First Nations method. *American Indian and Alaska Native Mental Health Research, 8*(2), 83–100.

Morgan, W. (1936). *Human wolves among the Navajo.* New Haven: Yale University Press.

Morley, P. (1978). Culture and the cognitive world of traditional medical beliefs: Some preliminary considerations. In P. Morley and R. Wallis (Eds.),

Culture and curing: Anthropological perspectives on traditional medical beliefs and practices (pp. 1–18). London: Peter Owen.

Morris, C., Crowley, S., & Morris, C. (2002). A measure of traditionalism for American Indian children and families: Psychometric properties and factor structure. *American Indian and Alaska Native Mental Health Research, 10*(3), 33–55.

Morrison, R.B., & Wilson, R.C. (1995). *Native peoples: The Canadian experience* (2nd ed.). Toronto: McClelland & Stewart.

Morton, S.G. (1839). *Crania Americana, or, a comparative view of the skulls of various aboriginal nations of North and South America.* Philadelphia, PA: John Pennington.

Moss, F., Edwards, E.D., Edwards, M.E., Janzen, F.V., & Howell, G. (1985). Sobriety and American Indian problem drinkers. *Alcoholism Treatment Quarterly, 2*(2), 81–96.

Murdock, G.P. (1980). *Theories of illness: A world survey.* Pittsburgh: University of Pittsburgh Press.

Murphy, H.B.M. (1973). History and the evolution of syndromes: The striking case of Latah and Amok. In M. Hammer, K. Salzinger, and S. Sutton (Eds.), *Psychopathology: Contributions from the social, behavioral, and biological sciences* (pp. 33–55). New York: John Wiley and Sons.

Murphy, J.M. (1964). Psychotherapeutic aspects of Shamanism on St. Lawrence Island, Alaska. In A. Kiev (Ed.), *Magic, faith, and healing* (pp. 53–83). New York: Free Press.

Murphy, J.M., & Leighton, A.H. (1965). Native conceptions of psychiatric disorder. In J.M. Murphy, and A.H. Leighton (Eds.), *Approaches to cross-cultural psychiatry* (pp. 64–107). New York: Cornell University Press.

Murray, S.O. (1999). The non-eclipse of Americanist anthropology during the 1930s and 40s. In L. Valentine and R. Darnell (Eds.), *Theorizing the Americanist tradition* (pp. 52–74). Toronto: University of Toronto Press.

Navarro, J., Wilson, S., Berger, L.R., & Taylor, T. (1997). Substance abuse and spirituality: A program for Native American students. *American Journal of Health Behavior, 21*(1), 3–11.

Neligh, G. (1988). Major mental disorders and behavior among American Indians and Alaska Natives [Monograph]. In S. Manson and N. Dinges (Eds.), *Behavioral health issues among American Indians and Alaska Natives: Explorations on the frontiers of the behavioral sciences* (pp. 116–50). Denver, CO: American Indian and Alaska Native Mental Health Research.

Neligh, G., Baron, A.E., Braun, P., & Czarnecki, M. (1990). Panic disorder among American Indians: A descriptive study. *American Indian and Alaska Native Mental Health, 4*(2), 43–54.

Nichter, M. (1981). Idioms of distress: Alternatives in the expression of psychological distress: A case study from South India. *Culture, Medicine and Psychiatry 5*, 379–408.

Nofz, M.P. (1988). Alcohol abuse and culturally marginal American Indians. *Social Casework, 69*(1), 67–73.

Norton, I.M. (1999). American Indians and mental health: Issues in psychiatric assessment and diagnosis. In J.M. Herrera, W.B. Lawson, and J.J. Sramek (Eds.), *Cross-cultural psychiatry* (pp. 77–85). Chichester, England: John Wiley and Sons Ltd.

Norton, I.M., & Manson, S.M. (1996). Research in American Indian and Alaska Native Communities: Navigating the Cultural Universe of Values and Process. *Journal of Consulting and Clinical Psychology, 64*(5), 856–60.

Nuckolls, C.W. (1998). *Culture: A problem that cannot be solved.* Madison: University of Wisconsin Press.

Nuu-Chah-Nulth Tribal Council. (1996). *Indian residential schools: The Nuu-chah-nulth experience.* Vancouver: Nuu-chah-nulth Tribal Council.

Ogden, M., Spector, M.I., & Hill Jr, C.A. (1970). Suicides and homicides among Indians. *Public Health Reports, 85*(1), 75–80.

Oetting, E.R., & Beauvais, F. (1990). Adolescent drug use: Findings of national and local surveys. *Journal of Consulting and Clinical Psychology, 58*(4), 385–94.

Oetting, E.R., & Beauvais, F. (1991). Orthogonal cultural identification theory: The cultural identification of minority adolescents. *The International Journal of the Addictions, 25*, 655–85.

Olandi, M. (1992). Defining cultural competence: An organizing framework. In M. Olandi (Ed.), *Cultural competence for evaluators: A guide for alcohol and other drug abuse prevention practitioners working with ethnic/racial communities.* Rockville, MD: Dept of Health and Human Services.

Olmedo, E.L., Martinez Jr, J.L., & Martinez, S.R. (1978). Measure of acculturation for Chicano adolescents. *Psychological Reports, 42*, 159–70.

Olmedo, E.L., & Padilla, A.M. (1978). Empirical and construct validation of a measure of acculturation for Mexican Americans. *The Journal of Social Psychology, 105*, 179–87.

O'Nell, T.D. (1989). Psychiatric investigations among American Indians and Alaska Natives: A critical review. *Culture, Medicine and Psychiatry, 13*, 51–87.

O'Nell, T.D. (1993). 'Feeling worthless': An ethnographic investigation of depression and problem drinking at the Flathead reservation. *Culture, Medicine, and Psychiatry, 16*, 447–69.

O'Nell, T.D. (1996). *Disciplined hearts: History, identity and depression in an American Indian community.* Berkeley, CA: University of California Press.

O'Nell, T.D. (1998). Cultural formulation of psychiatric diagnosis: Psychotic depression and alcoholism in an American Indian man. *Culture, Medicine and Psychiatry, 22,* 123–36.

O'Nell, T.D., & Mitchell, C.K. (1996). Alcohol use among American Indian adolescents: The role of culture in pathological drinking. *Social Science and Medicine, 42*(4), 565–78.

Opler, M.E. (1936). An interpretation of ambivalence of two American Indian tribes. *Journal of Social Psychology, 7,* 82–116.

Opler, M.E. (1938). Further comparative anthropological data bearing on the solution of a psychological problem. *Journal of Social Psychology, 9,* 477–83.

Opler, M.E. (1945). The Lipan Apache death complex and its extensions. *Southwestern Journal of Anthropology, 1,* 122–44.

Opler, M.E. (1946). Reaction to death among the Mescalero Apache. *Southwestern Journal of Anthropology, 2,* 454–67.

Opler, M.E., & Bittle, W. (1961). The death practices and eschatology of Kiowa Apache. *Southwestern Journal of Anthropology, 17,* 383–94.

Orlansky, M.D., & Trap, J.J. (1987). Working with Native American persons: Issues in facilitating communications and providing culturally relevant services. *Journal of Visual Impairment and Blindness, 81*(4), 151–5.

Page, R.D., & Bozlee, S. (1982). A cross-cultural MMPI comparison of alcoholics. *Psychological Reports, 50,* 639–46.

Paniagua, F.A. (1994). *Assessing and treating culturally diverse clients: A practical guide.* Thousand Oaks, CA: Sage Publications.

Paniagua, F.A. (1998). *Assessing and treating culturally diverse clients: A practical guide* (2nd ed.). Thousand Oaks, CA: Sage Publications.

Parker, L. (1990). The missing component in substance abuse prevention efforts: A Native American example. *Contemporary Drug Problems, 17*(2), 251–70.

Parker, S. (1960). The Witiko psychosis in the context of Ojibwa personality and culture. *American Anthropologist, 62*(4), 603–23.

Parker, S. (1962). Eskimo psychopathology in the context of Eskimo personality and culture. *American Anthropologist, 64,* 76–94.

Parkin, M. (1974). Suicide and culture in Fairbanks: A comparison of three cultural groups in a small city of Interior Alaska. *Psychiatry, 37,* 60–7.

Parkman, F. (1909). *The old religion in Canada.* London, ON: MacMillan and Co.

Parsons, E.C. (1917; rpt 1964). *Notes on Zuni, Part I.* Memoirs of the American Anthropological Association, Vol. IV, No.3. New York: Kraus Reprint Co.

Pedersen, P. (1976). A model for training mental health workers in cross-cultural counseling. In J. Westermeyer (Ed.), *Anthropology and mental health* (pp. 83–99). Paris: Mouton Publishers.

Pedersen, P. (1994). *A handbook for developing multicultural awareness.* (2nd ed.). Alexandria, VA: American Counseling Association.

Pederson, P. (1997). *Culture-centered counseling interventions: Striving for accuracy.* Thousand Oaks, CA: Sage.

Pedigo, J. (1983). Finding the 'meaning' of Native American substance abuse: Implications for community prevention. *The Personnel and Guidance Journal, 61*(5), 273–7.

Peregoy, J.J. (1993). Transcultural counseling with American Indians and Alaskan Natives: Contemporary issues for consideration. In J. McFadden (Ed.), *Transcultural counseling: Bilateral and international perspectives* (pp. 163–91). Alexandria, VA: American Counseling Association.

Peters, R. (1981). Suicidal behavior among Native Americans: An annotated bibliography. *White Cloud Journal, 2,* 9–20.

Pfister, O. (1932). Instinctive psychoanalysis among the Navahos. *Journal of Nervous and Mental Disease, 76,* 209–54.

Phillips, M.R., & Inui, T.S. (1986). The interaction of mental illness, criminal behavior and culture: Native Alaskan mentally ill criminal offenders. *Culture, Medicine and Psychiatry, 10,* 123–49.

Pine, C.J. (1981). Suicide in American Indian and Alaska Native Tradition. *White Cloud Journal, 2*(3), 3–8.

Plank, G. (2001). Application of the cross battery approach in the assesment of American Indian children: A viable alternative. *American Indian and Alaska Native Mental Health Research, 10*(1), 21–33.

Pollack, D., & Shore, J.H. (1980). Validity of the MMPI with Native Americans. *American Journal of Psychiatry, 137*(8), 946–50.

Ponterotto, J.G., Casa, J.M., Suzuki, L.A., & Alexander, C. (1995). *Handbook of multicultural counseling.* Thousand Oaks, CA: Sage Publications.

Pope-Davis, D.B., & Dings, J.G. (1995). The Assessment of Multicultural Counseling Competencies. In J. Ponterotto, J. Casa, L. Suzuki, and C. Alexander (Eds.), *Handbook of multicultural counseling* (pp. 287–311). Thousand Oaks, CA: Sage Publications.

Popham, R.E. (1979). Psychocultural barriers to successful alcoholism therapy in an American Indian patient: The relevance of Hallowell's analysis. *Journal of Studies on Alcohol, 40*(7), 656–76.

Powers, W. (1990). When Black Elk speaks, everybody listens. In C. Vecsey (Ed.), *Religion in Native North America* (pp. 136–51). Moscow, ID: University of Idaho Press.

Preston, R.J. (1980). The Wiitiko: Algonqian knowledge and Whiteman knowledge. In M. Halpin and M. Ames (Eds.), *Manlike monsters on trial: Early records and modern evidence* (pp. 111–31). Vancouver: UBC Press.

Price, B.K., & McNeill, B.W. (1992). Cultural commitment and attitudes toward seeking counseling services in American Indian college students. *Professional Psychology: Research and Practice, 23*(5), 376–81.

Price, J.A. (1975). An applied analysis of North American Indian drinking patterns. *Human Organization, 34*(1), 17–26.

Price-Williams, D. (1975). *Explorations in cross-cultural psychology.* San Francisco, CA: Chandler and Shay.

Prince, R., & Tcheng-Laroche, F. (1987). Culture-bound syndromes and international disease classifications. *Culture, Medicine and Psychiatry, 11,* 3–19.

Prince, R.H. (1993). Psychiatry among the James Bay Cree: A focus on pathological grief reactions. *Transcultural Psychiatric Research Review, 30*(1), 3–50.

Prince, R. (2000). Transcultural psychiatry: Personal experiences and Canadian perspective. *Canadian Journal of Psychiatry, 45*(5), 431–7.

Puri, B., Laking, P., & Treasaden, I. (2002). *Textbook of Psychiatry.* New York: Elsevier.

Putsch, R.W. (1988). Ghost illness: A cross-cultural experience with the expression of a non-Western tradition in clinical practice. *American Indian and Alaska Native Mental Health Research, 2*(2), 6–26.

Red Horse, J. (1980). Family structure and value orientation in American Indians. *Social Casework* Oct: 462– 467.

Redfield, R., Linton, R., & Herskovits, M. (1936). Memorandum on the study of acculturation. *American Anthropologist, 38,* 149–52.

Reed, T.E. (1978). Racial comparisons of alcohol metabolism: Background, problems, and results. *Alcoholism: Clinical and Experimental Research, 2*(1), 83–7.

Reed, T.E., Kalant, H., Gibbins, R.J., Kapur, B.M., & Rankin, J.G. (1976). Alcohol and acetaldehyde metabolism in Caucasians, Chinese and Amerinds. *Canadian Medical Association Journal, 115*(9), 851–5.

Reimer, C.S. (1999). *Counseling the Inupiat Eskimo.* Westport, CT: Greenwood Press.

Renfrey, G.S. (1992). Cognitive-behavior therapy and the Native American client. *Behavior Therapy, 23,* 321–40.

Resnik, H.L.P., & Dizmang, L.H. (1971). Observations on suicidal behavior among American Indians. *American Journal of Psychiatry, 127*(7), 882–7.

Rex, D.K., Bosron, W.F., Smialek, J.E., & Li, T.-K. (1985). Alcohol and aldehyde dehydrogenase isoenzymes in North American Indians. *Alcoholism: Clinical and Experimental Research, 9*(2), 147–52.

Richardson, B. (1975). *Strangers devour the land.* Toronto: Macmillan.

Richardson, E.H. (1977, August). The role of the medicine man as part of the modern therapeutic team in psychotherapy for Indians. Paper presented at the Sixth International Congress of Group Psychotherapy and the University of Pennsylvania, Philadelphia.

Richardson, E.H. (1981). Cultural and historical perspectives in counseling

American Indians. In D. Wing Sue (Ed.), *Counseling the culturally different* (pp. 216–55). New York: John Wiley and Sons.

Ridley, C.R., Espelage, D.L., & Rubinstein, K.J. (1997). Course development in multicultural counseling. In D. Pope-Davis and H. Coleman (Eds.), *Multicultural counseling competencies: Assessment, education and training, and supervision* (pp. 131–58). Thousand Oaks, CA: Sage.

Ridley, C.R., Mendoza, D.W., & Kanitz, B.E. (1994). Multicultural training: Reexamination, operationalization, and integration. *The Counseling Psychologist, 22*(2), 227–89.

Ritzler, B. (2001). Multicultural use of the Rorschach. In L. Suzuki, J. Ponterotto, and P. Meller (Eds.), *Handbook of Multicultural Assessment: Clinical, Psychological, and Educational Applications* (2nd ed.) (pp. 237–52). San Francisco: Jossey-Bass.

Robbins, R.H. (1973). Alcohol and the identity struggle: Some effects of economic change on interpersonal relations. *American Anthropologist, 75,* 99–122.

Robin, R.W., Chester, B., & Goldman, D. (1996). Cumulative trauma and PTSD in American Indian communities. In A.J. Marsella, M.J. Friedman, E.T. Gerrity, and R.M. Scurfield (Eds.), *Ethnocultural aspects of Posttraumatic Stress Disorder: Issues, research, and clinical applications* (pp. 239–53). Washington, DC: American Psychological Association.

Robin, R.W., Chester, B., & Rasmussen, J.K. (1998). Intimate violence in a Southwestern American Indian tribal community. *Cultural Diversity and Mental Health, 4*(4), 335–44.

Robin, R.W., Chester, B., Rasmussen, J.K., Jaranson, J.M., & Goldman, D. (1997a). Prevalence and characteristics of trauma and posttraumatic stress disorder in a Southwestern American Indian community. *American Journal of Psychiatry, 154*(11), 1582–8.

Robin, R.W., Chester, B., Rasmussen, J.K., Jaranson, J.M., & Goldman, D. (1997b). Prevalence, characteristics, and impact of childhood sexual abuse in a Southwestern American Indian tribe. *Child Abuse and Neglect, 21*(8), 769–87.

Robin, R.W., Long, J.C., Rasmussen, J.K., Albaugh, B., & Goldman, D. (1998). Relationship of binge drinking to alcohol dependence, other psychiatric disorders, and behavioral problems in an American Indian tribe. *Alcohol: Clinical and Experimental Research, 22*(2), 518–23.

Rodgers, D.D. (1974). Incidence of psychopathology and instability of eco-systems in two Northern communities. *Canadian Psychiatric Association Journal, 19*(4), 369–73.

Rodseth, L. (1998). Distributive models of culture: A Sapirian alternative to essentialism. *American Anthropologist, 100*(1), 55–69.

Rogers, S.L. (1944). Disease concepts in North America. *American Anthropologist, 46*(4), 559–64.

Rogler, L.H. (1996). Framing research on culture in psychiatric diagnosis: The case of the DSM-IV. *Psychiatry, 59*(2), 145–55.

Rohner, R.P. (1969). *The ethnography of Franz Boas.* Chicago: University of Chicago Press.

Rohrer, J.H. (1942). The test intelligence of Osage Indians. *The Journal of Social Psychology, 16,* 99–105.

Romney, A.K., Weller, S.C., & Batchelder, W.H. (1986). Culture as consensus: A theory of culture and informant accuracy. *American Anthropologist, 88,* 313–38.

Ronnau, J. (1994). Teaching cultural competence: Practical ideas for social work educators. *Journal of Multicultural Social Work, 3*(1), 29–42.

Root, D. (1996). *Cannibal culture: Art, appropriation, and the commodification of difference.* Boulder, CO: Westview Press.

Ross, C.A., & Davis, B. (1986). Suicide and parasuicide in a Northern Canadian Native community. *Canadian Journal Of Psychiatry, 31*(4), 331–4.

Roy, C., Choudhuri, A., & Irvine, D. (1970). The prevalence of mental disorders among Saskatchewan Indians. *Journal of Cross-Cultural Psychology, 1*(4), 383–92.

Rubel, A., & Kupferer, H. (1968). Perspectives on the atomistic-type society. *Human Organization, 27*(3), 189–90.

Sachs, D.A. (1974). The WISC and the Mescalero Apache. *Journal of Social Psychology, 92,* 303–4.

Sack, W.H., Beiser, M., Baker-Brown, G., & Redshirt, R. (1994). Depressive and suicidal symptoms in Indian children: Findings from the Flower of Two Soils. In *Calling from the rim: Suicidal behavior among American Indian and Alaska Native Adolescents* (pp. 81–94). American Indian and Alaska Native Mental Health Research Monograph 4. Denver: University of Colorado Press.

Sack, W.H., Beiser, M., Clarke, G., & Redshirt, R. (1987). The high achieving Sioux Indian child: Some preliminary findings from the Flower of the Two Soils project. *American Indian and Alaska Native Mental Health Research, 1*(1), 37–51.

Sack, W.H., Beiser, M., Phillips, N., & Baker-Brown, G. (1993). Co-morbid symptoms of depression and conduct disorder in First Nations children: Some findings from the Flower of Two Soils project. *Culture, Medicine, and Psychiatry, 16,* 471–86.

Sage, G.P. (1997). Counseling American Indian adults. In C.C. Lee (Ed.), *Multicultural issues in counseling: New approaches to diversity* (pp. 35–52). Alexandria, VA: American Counseling Association.

Saindon, Rev. J.E. (1933). Mental disorders among the James Bay Cree. *Primitive Man, 6*(1), 1–12.

Sampath, H.M. (1974). Prevalence of psychiatric disorders in a Southern Baffin Island Eskimo settlement. *Canadian Psychiatric Association Journal, 19*(4), 363–7.

Sampath, H.M. (1976). Modernity, social structure, and mental health of Eskimos in the Canadian eastern arctic. In R.J. Shepard and S. Ioh (Eds.), *Circumpolar health* (pp. 479–97). Toronto: University of Toronto Press.

Sapir, E. (1924). Culture, genuine and spurious. *American Journal of Sociology, 29*, 401–29.

Sapir, E. (1932). Cultural anthropology and psychiatry. In D. Mandelbaum (Ed.), *Selected Writings of Edward Sapir* (pp. 509–21). Berkeley: University of California Press.

Savishinsky, J.S. (1991). The ambiguities of alcohol: Deviance, drinking, and meaning in a Canadian Native community. *Anthropologica, 33*(1–2), 81–98.

Scheper-Hughes, N. (1987). The best of two worlds, the worst of two worlds: Reflections on culture and field work among the rural Irish and Pueblo Indians. *Comparative Studies in Society and History, 29*(1), 56–75.

Scurfield, R.M. (1995). Healing the warrior: Admission of two American Indian war-veteran cohort groups to a specialized inpatient PTSD unit. *American Indian and Alaska Native Mental Health Research, 6*(3), 1–22.

Seltzer, A. (1980). Acculturation and mental disorders in the Inuit. *Canadian Journal of Psychiatry, 25*, 173–81.

Shore, B. (1996). *Culture in mind: Cognition, culture and the problem of meaning.* New York: Oxford University Press.

Shore, J.H. (1974). Psychiatric epidemiology among American Indians. *Psychiatric Annals, 4*(9), 56–66.

Shore, J.H. (1975). American Indian suicide: Fact or fantasy. *Psychiatry, 38*, 86–91.

Shore, J.H., Kinzie, D.J., Hampson, J.L., & Pattison, E.M. (1973). Psychiatric epidemiology of an Indian village. *Psychiatry, 36*, 70–81.

Shore, J.H., & Manson, S.M. (1981). Cross-cultural studies of depression among American Indians and Alaska Natives. *White Cloud Journal, 2*(2), 5–12.

Shore, J.H., Manson, S.M., Bloom, J.D., Keepers, G., & Neligh, G. (1987). A pilot study of depression among American Indian patients with research diagnostic criteria. *American Indian and Alaska Native Mental Health Research, 1*(2), 1–15.

Shore, J. H., & von Fumetti, B. (1972). Three alcohol programs for American Indians. *American Journal of Psychiatry, 128*, 1450–4.

Shorter, E. (1997). *A history of psychiatry.* New York: John Wiley and Sons.

Shweder, R.A. (1982). On savages and other children. *American Anthropologist, 84*(2), 354–66.

Silk-Walker, P., Walker, R.D., & Kivlahan, D. (1988). Alcoholism, alcohol abuse, and health in American Indians and Alaska Natives. *American Indian and Alaska Native Mental Health*, Monograph No. 1, 65–93.

Silver, S.M., & Wilson, J.P. (1988). Native American healing and purification for war stress. In J.P. Wilson, Z. Harel, and B. Kahana (Eds.), *Human adaptation to extreme stress: From the holocaust to Vietnam* (pp. 337–55). New York: Plenum Press.

Simons, R., & Hughes, C. (Eds.). (1985). *The culture-bound syndromes: folk illnesses of psychiatric and anthropological interest*. Dordrecht: D. Reidel Publishing Company.

Slotkin, J.S. (1953). Social psychiatry of a Menomini community. *The Journal of Abnormal and Social Psychiatry*, *48*(1), 10–16.

Smith, D.H., & Hackathorn, L. (1982). Some special and psychological factors related to suicide in primitive societies: A cross-cultural comparative study. *Suicide and Life Threatening Behavior*, *12*(4), 195–211.

Smith, J.G.E. (1976). Notes on Wittiko. In W. Cowan (Ed.), *Papers of the Seventh Algonquian Conference, 1975* (pp. 18–28). Ottawa: Carleton University Press.

Snidecor, J.C. (1947). Why the Indian does not stutter. *Quarterly Journal of Speech*, *33*, 493–5.

Snider, J.G., & Coladarci, A.P. (1960). Intelligence test performance of acculturated Indian children. *California Journal of Educational Research II*, *11*, 34–6, 48.

Snipp, C.M. (1997). Some observations about racial boundaries and the experiences of American Indians. *Ethnic and Racial Studies*, *20*(4), 667–89.

Somervell, P.D., Beals, J., Kinzie, D.J., Boehnlein, J., Leung, P., & Manson, S.M. (1993a). Criterion validity of the Center for Epidemiologic Studies Depression Scale in a population sample from an American Indian village. *Psychiatry Research*, *47*(3), 255–66.

Somervell, P.D., Beals, J., Kinzie, D.J., Boehnlein, J., Leung, P., & Manson, S.M. (1993b). Use of the CES-D in an American Indian village. *Culture, Medicine, and Psychiatry*, *16*, 503–17.

Somervell, P.D., Manson, S.M., & Shore, J.H. (1995). Mental illness among American Indians and Alaska Natives. In I. Al-Issa (Ed.), *Handbook of culture and mental illness: An international perspective* (pp. 315–29). Madison, CT: International Universities Press.

Spang, A. (1965). Counseling the Indian. *Journal of American Indian Education, 5*, 10–15.

Spaulding, J.M. (1986). The Canton asylum for insane Indians: An example of institutional neglect. *Hospital and Community Psychiatry*, *37*(10), 1007–11.

Spector, R.E. (2000). *Cultural diversity in health and illness* (5th ed.). Upper Saddle River, NB: Prentice Hall Health.

Spicer, P. (1997). Toward a (dys)functional anthropology of drinking: Ambivalence and the American Indian experience with alcohol. *Medical Anthropology Quarterly, 11*(3), 306–23.

Spindler, G. (1955). *Sociocultural and psychological processes in Menomini acculturation.* Berkeley: University of California Press.

Spindler, G. (1978). Introduction to Part One. In G. Spindler (Ed.), *The making of psychological anthropology* (pp. 7–38). Berkeley: University of California Press.

Spindler, G.D., & Spindler, L.S. (1957). American Indian personality types and their sociocultural roots. *Annals of the American Academy of Political and Social Science, 311*, 147–57.

Spindler, G.D., & Spindler, L.S. (1972). American Indian personality types and their sociocultural roots. In D.E. Walker, Jr (Ed.), *The emergent Native Americans: A reader in culture contact* (pp. 502–13). Boston, MA: Little, Brown and Company.

Spindler, L. (1962). *Menomini women and culture change.* American Anthropological Association Memoir 91. Volume 64(1), Part 2. Washington, DC: American Anthropological Association.

Stern, P. (1999). Learning to be Smart: An Exploration of the Culture of Intelligence in a Canadian Inuit Community. *American Anthropologist, 101*(3), 502–14.

Stevens, S.M. (1981). Alcohol and world view: A study of Passamaquoddy alcohol use. *Journal of Studies on Alcohol,* Suppl. 9, 122–42.

Stevenson, M.C. (1904). *The Zuni Indians: Their mythology, esoteric fraternities, and ceremonies.* 23rd Annual report of the Bureau of American Ethnology (pp. 13–634). Washington, DC: Bureau of American Ethnology.

Still, O., & Hodgins, D. (1998). Navajo Indians. In L. Purnell and B. Paulanka (Eds.), *Transcultural health care: A culturally competent approach* (pp. 423–8). Philadelphia, PA: F. A. Davis Company.

Stonequist, E.V. (1937). The marginal man. New York: Charles Scribner and Sons.

Storck, M., Csordas, T.J., & Strauss, M. (2000). Depressive illness and Navajo healing. *Medical Anthropology Quarterly, 14*(4), 571–97.

Stratton, R., Zeiner, A., & Paredes, A. (1978). Tribal affiliation and prevalence of alcohol problems. *Journal of Studies on Alcohol, 39*(7), 1166–77.

Streit, F., & Nicolich, M.J. (1977). Myths versus data on American Indian drug abuse. *Journal of Drug Education, 7*(2), 117–22.

Strickland, C.J. (1997). Suicide among American Indian, Alaskan Native, and Canadian Aboriginal youth: Advancing the research agenda. *International Journal of Mental Health, 24*(4), 11–32.

Sue, D.W. (1981). *Counseling the culturally-different: Theory and practice.* New York: John Wiley and Sons.

Sue, D.W., & Sue, S. (1977). Barriers to effective cross-cultural counseling. *Journal of Counseling Psychology, 2,* 11–17.

Sue, D.W., & Sue, D. (1990). *Counseling the culturally different* (2nd ed.). New York: John Wiley and Sons.

Sue, D.W., & Sue, D. (2003). *Counseling the culturally diverse.* New York: John Wiley and Sons.

Sue, D.W., Arrendondo, P., & McDavis, R.J. (1992). Multicultural counseling competencies and standards: A call to the profession. *Journal of Counseling and Development, 70,* 477–86.

Sue, D.W., Bernier, J.E., Durran, A., Feinberg, L., Pedersen, P., Smith, E.J., & Vasquez-Nuttall, E. (1982). Position paper: Cross-cultural counseling competencies. *The Counseling Psychologist, 10,* 45–52.

Sue, S. (1998). In search of cultural competence in psychotherapy and counseling. *AmericanPsychologist, 53*(4), 440–8.

Sue, S., Allen, D.B., & Conaway, L. (1978). The responsiveness and equality of mental health care to Chicanos and Native Americans. *American Journal of Community Psychology 6,* 137–46.

Summer Seminar on Acculturation (including H.G. Barnett, L. Broom, B.J. Siegel, E.Z. Vogt, & J.B. Watson). (1954). Acculturation: An exploratory formulation. *American Anthropologist, 56,* 973–1002.

Sutker, P., & Adams, H. (1993). *Comprehensive handbook of psychotherapy* (2nd ed.). New York: Plenum Publishing.

Sutton, C., Etta T., & Broken Nose, M.A. (1996). American Indian families: An overview. In M. McGoldrick, J. Giordano, and J. Pearce (Eds.), *Ethnicity and family therapy* (2nd ed.) (pp. 31–54). New York: Guilford Press.

Szathmary, E.J., & Reed, T.E. (1972). Caucasian Admixture in Two Ojibwa Indian Communities in Ontario. *Human Biology, 44,* 655–71.

Tafoya, T. (1989). Circles and cedar: Native Americans and family therapy. *Journal of Psychotherapy and the Family, 6* (1/2), 71–98.

Tasman, A., Kay, J., & Lieberman, J. (Eds). (1997). *Psychiatry.* Philadelphia: Saunders.

Taussig, M. (1999). *Defacement: Public secrecy and the labor of the negative.* Stanford: Stanford University Press.

Taylor, D.H. (2000). How Native is Native if you're Native? In R. Laliberte, P. Settee, J. Waldram, R. Innes, B. Macdougall, L. McBain, and F.L. Barron (Eds.), *Expressions in Canadian Native studies* (pp. 60–2). Saskatoon: University of Saskatchewan Extension Press.

Tefft, S.K. (1967). Anomie, values and culture change among teen-age Indians: An exploration. *Sociology of Education, 40*(2), 145–57.

Tempest, P. (1998). Local Navajo norms for the Wechsler Itelligence Scale for Children – Third Edition. *Journal of American Indian Education, 37*(3), 18–30.

Tempest, P., & Skipper, B. (1988). Norms for the Weschler Intelligence Scale for Children – Revised for Navajo Indians. *Diagnostique, 13*, 123–9.

Terman, L.W. (1916). *The measurement of intelligence.* Boston, MA: Houghton-Mifflin.

Thomas, R.K. (1981). The history of North American Indian alcohol use as a community-based phenomenon. *Journal of Studies on Alcohol Supplement, 9*, 29–39.

Thomason, T.C. (1991). Counseling Native Americans: An introduction for non-Native American counselors. *Journal of Counseling and Development, 69*(4), 321–7.

Thompson, J.W. (1994). Issues in the psychiatric care of American Indian and Alaska Native elders. In *Ethnic minority elderly: A task force report of the American Psychiatric Association* (pp. 91–113). Washington, DC: American Psychiatric Association.

Thompson, J.W., Walker, R.D., & Silk-Walker, P. (1993). Psychiatric care of American Indians and Alaska Natives. In A.C. Gaw (Ed.), *Culture, ethnicity, and mental illness* (pp. 189–243). Washington, DC: American Psychiatric Press.

Thompson, L. (1946). *The Hopi crisis: A report to Administration.* Washington, DC: United States Office of Indian Affairs.

Thompson, L. (1950). *Culture in crisis: A study of the Hopi Indians.* New York: Harper and Brothers Publishers.

Thompson, L. (1951). *Personality and government: Findings and recommendations of the Indian administration research.* Mexico City: Ediciones del Instituto Indigenista Interamericano.

Thompson, L., & Joseph, A. (1965). *The Hopi Way.* New York: Russell and Russell.

Thornton, R. (1987). *American Indian holocaust and survival: A population history since 1492.* Norman: University of Oklahoma Press.

Timpson, J.B., McKay, S., Kakegamic, S., Roundhead, D., Cohen, C., & Matewapit, G. (1988). Depression in a Native Canadian in Northwestern Ontario: Sadness, grief or spiritual illness? *Canada's Mental Health, 2/3*, 5–7.

Topper, M.D. (1974). Drinking patterns, culture change, sociability, and Navajo 'adolescents.' *Addictive Diseases, 1*(1), 97–116.

Topper, M.D. (1981). The drinker's story: an important but often forgotten source of data. In D. Heath, J. Waddell, and M. Topper (Eds.), *Cultural factors in alcohol research and treatment of alcohol problems.* Journal of Studies on Alcohol Supplement 9 (pp. 7773–86). New Brunswick, NJ.

Topper, M.D. (1985). Navajo 'alcoholism': Drinking, alcohol abuse, and treatment in a changing cultural environment. In L.A. Bennett and G.M. Ames (Eds.), *The American experience with alcohol: Contrasting cultural perspectives* (pp. 227–51). New York: Plenum Press.

Topper, M.D. (1992). Multidimensional therapy: A case study of a Navajo adolescent with multiple problems. In L.A. Vargas and J.D. Koss-Chioino (Eds.), *Working with culture: Psychotherapeutic interventions with ethnic minority children and adolescents* (pp. 225–45). San Francisco, CA: Jossey-Bass Publishers.

Topper, M.D., & Curtis, J. (1987). Extended family therapy: A clinical approach to the treatment of synergistic dual anomic depression among Navajo agency-town adolescents. *Journal of Community Psychology, 15*(3), 334–48.

Torgovnick, M. (1990). *Gone primitive: Savage intellects, modern lives.* Chicago: University of Chicago Press.

Torgovnick, M. (1996). *Primitive passions: Men, women, and the quest for ecstasy.* Chicago: University of Chicago Press.

Townsley, H.C., & Goldstien, G.S. (1977). One view of the etiology of depression in the American Indian. *Public Health Report, 92*(5), 458–61.

Triandis, H.C. (1996). The psychological measurement of cultural syndromes. *American Psychologist, 51*, 407–15.

Trigger, B., & Washburn, W. (1996). *The Cambridge history of the Native peoples of the Americas.* Vol 1. Cambridge: Cambridge University Press.

Trimble, J.E. (1975). The intrusion of Western psychological thought on Native American ethos: Divergence and conflict among the Lakota. In J.W. Berry and W.J. Lonner (Eds.), *Applied cross-cultural psychology: Selected papers from the Second International Conference of the International Association for Cross-Cultural Psychology* (pp. 303–8). Amsterdam: Swets and Zeitlinger.

Trimble, J.E. (1976). Value differentials and their importance in counseling American Indians. In P.B. Pedersen, J.G. Draguns, W.J. Lonner, and J.E. Trimble (Eds.), *Counseling across cultures* (pp. 203–26). Honolulu: University Press of Hawaii.

Trimble, J.E. (1981). Value differentials and their importance in counseling American Indians. In P.B. Pedersen, W.J. Lonner, and J.G. Draguns (Eds.), *Counseling across cultures* (pp. 203–26). Honolulu: University Press of Hawaii.

Trimble, J.E. (1990). Application of psychological knowledge for American Indians and Alaska Natives. *The Journal of Training and Practice in Professional Psychology, 4*(1), 45–63.

Trimble, J.E. (1992). A cognitive-behavioral approach to drug abuse prevention and intervention with American Indian youth. In L.A. Vargas and J.D. Koss-Chioino (Eds.), *Working with culture: Psychotherapeutic interventions with ethnic minority children and adolescents* (pp. 246–75). San Francisco, CA: Jossey-Bass Publishers.

Trimble, J.E. (2003). Introduction: Social change and acculturation. In K. Chun, P. Organista, and G. Marín (Eds.), *Acculturation: Advances in theory, measurement, and applied research* (pp. 3–13). Washington, DC: American Psychological Association.

Trimble, J.E., & Fleming, C.M. (1989). Providing counseling services for Native American Indians: Client, counselor, and community characteristics. In P.B. Pedersen, J.G. Draguns, W.J. Lonner, and J.E. Trimble (Eds.), *Counseling across cultures* (3rd ed.) (pp. 177–204). Honolulu: University of Hawaii Press.

Trimble, J.E., Fleming, C.M., Beauvais, F., & Jumper-Thurman, P. (1996). Essential cultural and social strategies for counseling Native American Indians. In P.B. Pedersen, J.G. Draguns, W.J. Lonner, and J.E. Trimble (Eds.), *Counseling across cultures* (pp. 177–209). Thousand Oaks, CA: Sage Publications.

Trimble, J.E., & Hayes, S.A. (1984). Mental health intervention in the psychosocial contexts of American Indian communities. In W.A. O'Connor and B. Lubin (Eds.), *Ecological approaches to clinical and community psychology* (pp. 293–321). New York: John Wiley and Sons.

Trimble, J.E., & LaFromboise, T. (1987). American Indians and counseling process: Culture, adaptation and style. In P. Pedersen (Ed.), *Handbook of cross-cultural counseling and therapy* (pp. 127–33). Westport, CT: Greenwood Press.

Trimble, J.E., Manson, S.M., Dinges, N.G., & Medicine, B. (1984). American Indian concepts of mental health: Reflections and directions. In P.B. Pedersen, N. Sartorius, and A.J. Marsella (Eds.), *Mental health services: The cross cultural context* (pp. 199–220). Beverly Hills, CA: Sage Publications.

Trimble, J.E., and Medicine, B. (1993). Diversification of American Indians: Forming an Indigenous perspective. In U. Kim and J.W. Berry (Eds.), *Indigenous psychologies: Research and experience in cultural context* (pp. 133–51). Newbury Park, CA: Sage Publications, Inc.

Uecker, A.E., Boutilier, L.R., and Richardson, E.H. (1980). 'Indianism' and MMPI scores of men alcoholics. *Journal of Studies on Alcohol, 41*(3), 357–62.

Vallee, F.G. (1966). Eskimo theories of mental illness in the Hudson Bay Region. *Anthropologica, 8,* 53–83.

Vallee, F.G. (1968). Stresses of change and mental health among the Canadian Eskimos. *Arch Environmental Health, 17,* 565–70.

van Winkle, N., & May, P.A. (1986). Native American suicide in New Mexico, 1957–79: A comparative study. *Human Organization, 45*(5), 296–309.

van Winkle, N., & May, P.A. (1993). An update on American Indian suicide in New Mexico, 1980–1987. *Human Organization, 52*(3), 304–15.

Vayda, A. (1994). Actions, variations, and change: The emerging anti-essentialist view in anthropology. In R. Borofsky (Ed.), *Assessing cultural anthropology* (pp. 320–8). New York: McGraw-Hill.

Vizenor, G. (1990). Firewater and phrenology. In G. Vizenor (Ed.), *Crossbloods, bone courts, bingo, and other reports* (pp. 300–19). Minneapolis: University of Minnesota Press.

Vizenor, G. (1994). Manifest manners: Postindian warriors of survivance. Hanover, NH: University Press of New England.

Vogt, E.Z. (1951). *Navajo veterans: a study of changing values.* Cambridge: Peabody Museum.

Waddell, J.O. (1980). Drinking as a means of articulating social and cultural values: Papagos in an urban setting. In J.O. Waddell, and M.W. Everett (Eds.), *Drinking behavior among Southwestern Indians: An anthropological perspective* (pp. 37–82). Tucson: University of Arizona Press.

Wade, A. (1995). Resistance knowledges: Therapy with Aboriginal persons who have experienced violence. In P.H. Stephenson, S.J. Elliot, L.T. Foster, and J. Harris (Eds.), *A persistant spirit: Towards understanding in Aboriginal health in British Columbia* (pp. 167–206). Victoria, BC: University of Victoria.

Waldram, J.B. (1997). *The way of the pipe: Aboriginal spirituality and symbolic healing Canadian prisons.* Peterborough, ON: Broadview Press.

Waldram, J.B. (2000). The efficacy of traditional medicine: Current theoretical and methodological issues. *Medical Anthropology Quarterley, 14*(4), 603–25.

Waldram, J.B., Herring, D.A., & Young, T.K. (1995). *Aboriginal health in Canada: Historical, cultural and epidemiological perspectives.* Toronto: University of Toronto Press.

Waldram, J.B., & Wong, S. (1995). Group therapy of Aboriginal offenders in a Canadian forensic psychiatric facility. *American Indian and Alaska Native Mental Health Research, 6*(2), 34–56.

Wallace, A.F.C. (1952). *The modal personality structure of the Tuscarora Indians, as revealed by the Rorschach Test.* Bureau of American Ethnology Bulletin, 150. Washington, DC: Smithsonian Institution.

Wallace, A.F.C. (1961). Mental illness, biology and culture. In F.L.K. Hsu (Ed.), *Psychological anthropology: Approaches to culture and personality* (pp. 255–95). Homewood, IL: Dorsey Press, Inc.

Walters, K.L., & Simoni, J.M. (1999). Trauma, substance use, and HIV risk among urban American Indian women. *Cultural Diversity and Ethnic Minority Psychology, 5*(3), 236–48.

Ward, J.A., & Fox, J. (1977). A suicide on an Indian reserve. *Canadian Psychiatric Association Journal, 22*, 423–6.

Washburn, W.E. (1975). *The Indian in America.* New York: Harper Colophon Books.

Watts, L.K., & Gutierres, S.E. (1997). A Native-American-based cultural model of dependency and recovery. *Human Organization, 56*(1), 9–18.

Wax, R.H., & Thomas, R.K. (1961). American Indians and White people. *Phylon, 22*(4), 305–17.

Webb, J.P., & Willard, W. (1975). Six American Indian patterns of suicide. In N.L. Farberow (Ed.), *Suicide in Different Cultures* (pp. 17–33). Baltimore: University Park Press

Weibel-Orlando, J.C. (1984). Indian alcoholism treatment programs as flawed rites of passage. *Medical Anthropology Quarterly, 15*(3), 62–7.

Weibel-Orlando, J.C. (1987). Culture specific treatment modalities: Assessing client-to-treatment fit in Indian alcoholism programs. In W.M. Cox (Ed.), *Treatment and prevention of alcohol problems* (pp. 261–83). Orlando, FL: Academic Press.

Weibel-Orlando, J.C. (1989). Hooked on healing: Anthropologists, alcohol and intervention. *Human Organization, 48*(2), 148–55.

Weisner, T.S., Weibel-Orlando, J.C., & Long, J. (1984). 'Serious drinking,' 'white man's drinking' and 'teetotaling': Drinking levels and styles in an urban American Indian population. *Journal of Studies on Alcohol, 45*(3), 237–50.

West, L.W., & MacArthur, R.S. (1964). An evaluation of selected intelligence tests for two samples of Metis and Indian children. *Alberta Journal of Educational Research, 10*(1), 17–27.

Westermeyer, J.J. (1972a). Chippewa and majority alcoholism in the Twin Cities: A comparison. *Journal of Nervous and Mental Disorders, 155*(5), 322–7.

Westermeyer, J.J. (1972b). Options regarding alcohol use among the Chippewa. *American Journal of Orthopsychiatry, 42*(3), 398–403.

Westermeyer, J.J. (1974a). Alcoholism from cross cultural perspectives: A review and critique of clinical studies. *American Journal of Drug and Alcohol Abuse, 1*, 89–105.

Westermeyer, J.J. (1974b). The drunken Indian: Myths and realities. *Psychiatric Annals, 4*(9), 29–36.

Westermeyer, J.J. (1979). The apple syndrome in Minnesota: A complication of racial-ethnic discontinuity. *Journal of Operational Psychiatry, 10*(2), 134–40.

Westermeyer, J.J. (1996). Alcoholism among New World peoples: A critique of history, methods, and findings. *American Journal on Addictions, 5*(2), 110–23.

Westermeyer, J.J., & Baker, J.M. (1986). Alcoholism and the American Indian. In N.J. Estes and M.E. Heinemann (Eds.), *Alcoholism: development, consequences, and interventions* (3rd ed.) (pp. 273–82). St Louis, MO: C.V. Mosby Company.

Westermeyer, J.J., & Neider, J. (1985). Cultural affiliation among American Indian alcoholics: Correlations and change over a ten year period. *Journal of Operational Psychiatry, 16*(2), 17–23.

Westermeyer, J.J., Neider, J., & Westermeyer, M. (1993). Substance use and other psychiatric disorders among 100 American Indian patients. *Culture, Medicine, and Psychiatry, 16*, 519–29.

Whittaker, J.O. (1962). Alcohol and the Standing Rock Sioux Tribe. I. The patterns of drinking. *Quarterly Journal of Studies on Alcohol, 23*(3), 468–79.

Whittaker, J.O. (1963). Alcohol and the Standing Rock Sioux Tribe. II. Psychodynamic and cultural factors in drinking. *Quarterly Journal of Studies on Alcohol, 24*, 80–90.

Whorton, J.E., & Morgan, R.L. (1990). Comparison of the test of nonverbal intelligence and Wechsler Intelligence Scale for Children-Revised in rural Native American and white children. *Perceptual and Motor Skills, 70*, 12–14.

Wikan, U. (1999). Culture: A new concept of race. *Social Anthropology, 7*(1), 57–64.

Wilgosh, L., Mulcahy, R., & Watters, B. (1986). Assessing intellectual performance of culturally different, Inuit children with the WISC-R. *Canadian Journal of Behavioural Science, 18*(3), 270–7.

Willms, D.G., Lange, P., Bayfield, D., Beardy, M., Lindsay, E.A., Cole, D.C., & Arbuthnot Johnson, N. (1992). A lament by women for 'the people, the land' (Nishnabi-Aski Nation): An experience of loss. *Canadian Journal of Public Health, 5*, 331–4.

Wilson, C., Civic, D., & Glass, D. (1995). Prevalence and correlates of depressive syndromes among adults visiting an Indian health service primary care clinic. *American Indian and Alaska Native Mental Health Research, 6*(2), 1–12.

Wiltshire, E.B., & Gray, J.E. (1969). Draw-a-Man and Raven's progressive matrices (1938) intelligence test performance of reserve Indian children. *Canadian Journal of Behavioural Science, 1*(2), 119–22.

Wolf, E. (1982). *Europe and the people without history*. Berkeley: University of California Press.

Wolff, P.H. (1973). Vasomotor sensitivity to alcohol in diverse Mongoloid populations. *American Journal of Human Genetics, 25*, 193–9.

Wolman, C. (1970). Group therapy in two languages, English and Navajo. *American Journal of Psychotherapy, 24*, 677–85.

World Health Organization (WHO). (1993). The ICD-10 Classification of Mental and Behavioural Disorders: Diagnostic criteria for research. Geneva, Switzerland: World Health Organization.

Wrenn, G. (1962). The culturally encapsulated counselor. *Harvard Educational Review, 32*, 444–9.

Wyman, L.C., & Thorne, B. (1945). Notes on Navaho suicide. *American Anthropologist, 47*, 278–88.

Yap, P.M. (1967). Classification of the culture-bound reactive syndromes. *Australia and New Zealand Journal of Psychiatry, 1*, 172–9.

Young, A. (1995). *The harmony of illusions: Inventing post-traumatic stress disorder.* Princeton, NJ: Princeton University Press.

Young, A. (1996). Bodily memory and traumatic memory. In P. Antze and M. Lambek (Eds.), *Tense past: Cultural essays in trauma and memory* (pp. 89–102). New York: Routledge.

Young, D., Ingram, G., & Swartz, L. (1989). *Cry of the eagle: Encounters with a Cree healer.* Toronto: University of Toronto Press.

Young, T.J. (1989). Alcohol use and misuse among Native Americans. *Social Pharmacology, 3*, 271–96.

Young, T.J. (1990). Poverty, suicide, and homicide among Native Americans. *Psychological Reports, 67*, 1153–4.

Young, T.J. (1991). Suicide and homicide among Native Americans: Anomie or social learning. *Psychological Reports, 68*, 1137–8.

Young, T.J. (1993). Alcohol misuse and criminal violence among Native Americans. *The Psychiatric Forum, 16*(1), 20–6.

Youngman, G., & Sadongei, M. (1974). Counseling the American Indian child. *Elementary School Guidance and Counseling, 8*(4), 273–7.

Zane, N., & Mak, W. (2003). Major approaches to the measurement of acculturation among ethnic minority populations: A content analysis and an alternative empirical strategy. In K. Chun, P. Organista, and G. Marín (Eds.), *Acculturation: Advances in the measurement, and applied research* (pp. 39–60). Washington, DC: American Psychological Association.

Zintz, M.V. (1969). *Education across cultures* (2nd ed.). Dubuque, RA: Kendall/ Hunt.

Zitzow, D. & Estes, G. (1981). The heritage consistency continuum in counseling Native American children. In *Spring Conference on Contemporary American Issues in Higher Education* (pp. 133–9). No publisher.

Index

Note: Pages numbers ending with '*t*' denote a Table.

Abbott, P.J., 164

Abel, T., 197

Aberle, D.F., 240

Aboriginal drinking, 25, 134–42, 154–5, 304; adjustment syndrome, 145; binge drinking, 158; as boundary-maintaining mechanism, 156; and caught-between-two-worlds paradigm, 146; death styles, 327n. 10; disinhibition theory of use of, 147–9; dreaming and visioning, 156–7; drinking patterns, 146; Flores comparative study of, 255–6; how and why of, 142–57; Indian Culturalization Test, 79–80; *mni wakan* (Sioux), 157; patterns and consequences of drinking, 142; post-contact learned behaviours, 147, 150; pre-contact, 147, 149; problem or not, 162–3; prohibitions against, 157; social function of, 144; and sociocultural behaviours, 148–50, 154–5; spirituality and power and, 156; treatment approach, 265–6; and white man's drinking, 87, 157–61

Aboriginal Healing Foundation (AHF): intergenerational trauma and, 233–4; website, 331n. 8

Aboriginal peoples: client/therapist relationship, 261–3; contemporary understanding of, 186, 300; cultural continuity/integration paradigm, 147–57; cultures of, 6–9, 49–50; defining, 16–17, 312–16; distinction between 'Whiteman' sickness and, 281–2; identity and culture problems, 76, 162, 291–2; intellectual traditions of, 4; intra-ethnic diversity of, 98; pathological construct of, 105; personality and psychopathology of, 67–8; psychiatric disorders among, 133; residential schools impact, 231–2; skills of, 95; social definition of, 126–7; 'talking circle,' 287; and trauma, 215–21

Aboriginal variable: in comparative

research, 95–101; psychiatric epidemiological study, 97

acculturation: affect on MMPI-168
scores, 88; and alcohol consumption, 153; as anthropological issue,
29–30, 41, 70, 118; Barnouw on, 57;
as cause of alcohol abuse, 145; and
conceptualization of Aboriginality, 69–76; index, 77; individual,
71, 76; measuring, 303; multicultural model, 123; to non-Aboriginal values, 250; orthogonal model
of, 123; Rorschach testing of, 51;
theory, 117, 172

acculturative stress, 14, 15, 105, 117,
118–24; and Aboriginal drinking,
139–40; caught-between-two-
worlds paradigm, 52, 250, 303; and
historical trauma, 225; James Bay,
121; and pre-contact cultures, 122–
3; of Vietnamese refugees, 122

Ackerknecht, E.H., 275

Ackerman, L.A., 157

Acoma people, witchcraft and, 112–
13

Adair, John, 39, 60

Adelson, N., 259, 282, 290, 292, 296

Adrian, M., 159

Alarcón, R., 206, 317, 319

Albaugh, B., 160

alcohol. *See* Aboriginal drinking

Alcoholics Anonymous, 288, 293

alcoholism, 14; and alcohol abuse
compared, 164–5; definition of,
151–2; in Minnesota, 162–3; Pacific
Northwest community, 129–30;
Western assumptions of, 153, 166.
See also Aboriginal drinking

Aleuts, 144; University of Alaska,
85–6

Algonkians: values research, 240;
windigo mythology, 5, 193–5

Allen, J., 89

American Indian Depression Scale,
180–1

Americanist tradition, in anthropology, 22, 32

amok, culture-bound syndromes,
207

Anderson, E.N., 293

Anderson, F., 110

Anderson, M.J., 260, 263

Anglican Church, residential
schools, 230

Anishinaabe (Ojibwa), 281–2, 290

Annis, Robert C., 77–8, 81, 120–1

Anomie, 143, 166

anthropology, 4, 319; Aboriginal culture and, 306–7; Aboriginal mental
health and, 7; and Aboriginal values, 240–1; anachronisms of, 306–
8; changes in discipline of, 319;
constructivist framework in, 12;
critical-interpretive framework in,
12; depression defined in, 168,
188–9; ethnographic truth issue,
10; as primitivist discipline, 11–12;
and roots of Aboriginal values
research, 239–49; and the Rorschach, 44–8

Antze, P., 215

Apache, 101; alcohol use, 152–3;
Chiricahua, 64, 199; ghost sickness, 199, 201–2; Jicarilla, 199;
Kiowa, 199; Lipan, 199; Mescalero, 62–6, 144, 199, 201–2; sociocultural integration levels of, 152;
White Mountain, 202

Apollonian societies, 23

Arapaho, 256

Arcadian and Barbarian models, 11, 122–3, 300, 309–10, 321n. 12; and Aboriginal drinking, 136; and alcohol, 134; and contact with the West, 143; and cultural change, 114–18; depression and suicide, 167, 170; therapeutic model in, 286; and trauma, 235

Arctic hysteria. See *pibloktoq*

Arensberg, Conrad, 32

Armstrong, H., 175

Arthur, Grace, 32, 85

Asian populations, compared with Aboriginal populations, 138–9

Assembly of First Nations: residential schools study, 229, 231; and 'truth' of residential schools, 232

assimilation: American Indian population, 30; education as key to, 229–30

Athapaskan peoples, 149; values research, 240

atomism: concept of, 302; and the Northern Indian, 55–60

Attneave, C., 7, 258, 264, 268

Bailey, Pearce, 90–1

Baker, James, 111, 135, 147–9, 164

Balikci, Asen, 59

Barbarian model. *See* Arcadian and Barbarian models

Barnouw, Victor, 25, 26, 56–8, 304–5

Barnsley, R., 93

Baron, A.E., 265

Barrett, R.J., 11, 12, 112, 207, 286

basic personality structure, 62; Northern Athapascans, 66

Beals, J., 223

Beauvais, F., 123, 141–2, 164

Bechtold, D.W., 178, 223

Beck, Samuel J., 45

Bee, R.L., 78

Begay, D., 278

behaviours, 239–40, 244, 249–56, 269–70, 311; relevant for psychotherapy, 251–3. *See also* ethics; values

Beiser, M., 80, 82, 94, 97, 282

Benedict, Ruth, 9, 32, 45, 52, 112, 254; and the Boasian tradition, 22–7; culture and personality theory, 15, 27–8, 42, 278–9, 278–9; social atomism, 57

Bennett, J.A., 282

Bennion, L.J., 137

Berens, Chief, 46

Berger, L.R., 286

Bering Strait theory, 226–7; of population movement, 138–9

Berreman, Gerald D., 144

Berry, John, 77–8, 81, 97, 118–24, 225, 282; integration/biculturalism, 124

Berryhill-Paapke, E., 75

Bhabha, Homi, 10

Bibeau, Gilles, 13, 319

Biolsi, Thomas, 40, 41

biomedicine: and Aboriginal healing, 293; psychotherapeutic component, 296

Bittle, W., 199

Black Elk (Lakota), 284

blood quantum: and Aboriginal drinking, 139–40; in Aboriginal research, 96; contradictions in studies of, 141; intelligence and race in, 91–2; as measure of culture, 69, 162–3, 314

Blue, A.W., 81–2

Boag, T.J., 197, 203

boarding schools: American Indian,

177–8; mental health issues, 217–18. *See also* residential schools

Boas, Franz, 9, 22, 25, 26–7, 28, 44–5

Boasian anthropologists, 9, 22, 25, 240; idea of culture areas from, 96

Boldt, M., death styles, 327n. 10

Bolton, B., 80

Boothroyd, L.J., 131–2, 198

Boyer, L. Bryce, 62–7, 112, 160, 199, 202

Bozlee, S., 87

Brady, M., 298

Brant, Clare C., 172, 256

Brass, G.M., 13, 259, 263, 288

Braun, P., 265

Brave Heart, M., soul wound, 225, 227

Briggs, Jean, 280–1

Brill, A.A., 195–6

Brod, T.M., review of Wolff's work, 138–9

Brown, Jennifer, 46

Browne, D.B., 92–3

Bruner, F.G., 109

Bryde, John F., 244–5, 247–9, 254; value conflict, 260

Buffler, P.A., 115, 144

Bunzel, Ruth, 25, 254

Butcher, J.N., 87

Bydone, V., 295

Caetano, R., 141

California Psychological Inventory (CPI), 100–1

cannibalism, windigo mythology, 192–5

Cannibal society, 26, 29

Canton Asylum for Insane Indians, 107–8

Carpenter, E.S., 157

Carrier people, 119, 157–8

Cartesian dualism, 283-4

Catholic Church, residential schools, 230

Caudill, William, 50–1

caught-between-two-worlds paradigm: and anomic depression, 172; marginality and, 114–18, 123

Center for Epidemiologic Studies Depression Scale (CES-D). *See* CES-D

Cernovsky, Z., 184

CES-D, 177–9, 179; acculturation issue, 179–80; research population, 177–8, 183–4

Chance, Norman, 77, 124–5

Chandler, Michael J., 174–5

Chapleski, E.E., 183

Cherokee, 248; ethanol metabolization issue, 138

Chester, B., 216, 217, 222

Chickasaw, 248

children: Oklahoma Indian, 110; Wisconsin Chippewa, 116

Chippewa, 99, 116, 162; drinking patterns, 158; Lac du Flambeau, Wisconsin, 49–50, 51–2, 57; and social atomism, 58

Choctaw, 248

Choney, S.K., 75

Choudhuri, A., 125

Chrisjohn, R., 232, 234

Civic, D., 180

Clark, C.L., 141

Clarke, G., 80

class. *See* socio-economic status

Clements, Forrest, schema of, 272–3, 280

CMI. *See* Cornell Medical Index (CMI)

Coast Salish, 145, 157, 172, 277;
anomic depression among, 172;
drinking patterns, 157; ghost sickness, 203; holism thesis, 276; spirit
dancing, 156, 209, 292; spirit sickness among, 281; WISC performance scores of, 93
cognitive anthropology, 22
Cohen, C., 169
collective/individual dichotomy,
163, 263, 266–8
Collier, John, 30–1, 37–8, 40, 42, 109
colonization: anomie and sociocultural disorganization from, 143–7;
and collapse of Aboriginal societies, 223; effects of on Aboriginal
cultures, 303; and 'Whiteman's
sickness,' 282
Committee on Human Development, University of Chicago, 31–4
'Configurations of Culture in North
America' (Benedict), 23
constructivism, 12
Cooper, John M., 193
Corin, E., 198
Cornell Medical Index (CMI), 325n.
6, 124–5; gender differences in,
124–5
counselling: client/therapist relationship, 261–3; ethics, values, and
behaviour in, 251–3, 259–60. *See
also* psychotherapy
Crania Americana (Morton), 90
Creek, 248
Cree, 5; Attawapiskat, Ontario, 56–7;
culture of, 119, 120–1; psychiatric
cases, 125–6; spirit intrusion as
cause of insanity, 272; values, 255.
See also James Bay Cree
creolization, 13–14, 316–20

critical-interpretivism, 12
cross-cultural studies: Alaska Native
groups and non-Aboriginal students, 85–6; concept of depression,
175–6; research, 308, 312; treatment literature, 247
Crow children, traumatic loss
among, 221
Crowley, S., 82
Csordas, T.J., 169, 283, 290; holism
thesis, 276
cultural affinity: in therapy, 261–3
cultural change: adaptation to, 301,
324–5n. 3; and Arcadian Aboriginals, 114–18; and colonial experiences, 311–12; role of individual in
society in, 122; theory, 78
cultural continuity/integration paradigm, 147–57, 174–5, 309
cultural continuity, and suicide, 174–
5
cultural discontinuity, 117, 309
cultural diversity, 98, 249–50, 256
cultural epidemiology, 189
cultural evolutionists, 152
cultural heterogeneity, 89, 256, 309–
10, 312–13
cultural homogeneity, 178, 250;
assumption of, 99, 101, 178, 309–
11, 312–13; in MMPI-2, 89
cultural integration paradigm, 149,
154–6, 161
cultural orientation, measuring, 76–
84
culture: authenticity of, 74, 80, 260,
295–6, 312–13; comparative study
of, 87, 89; conceptualizing of, 317;
confused with race, 85; definition
of, 22–3; and history, 306–12;
magic as pathology of, 109; opera-

tionalization of, 69–70; and personality theory, 27, 42, 60–1, 67; of science, 318; two-cultures model of North America, 83
culture and personality theory, 32–3, 301; of Benedict, 15, 26–9, 42, 278–9; Trimble criticism of, 246–9
culture areas: in anthropological research, 97; as sampling frames, 69, 96–7
culture-bound syndromes, 190–1, 203–11, 273; depression, 169; DSM definition of, 191; and Inuit, 195; windigo psychosis, 205
Cundick, B.P., 93
Curley, R.T, 144
Curtis, J., 116, 172, 265
Czarnecki, M., 265

Dailey, R.C., 156
Dakota, and social atomism, 58
Dam, J., 293
Dana, R.H., 80, 93, 253, 279
Darnell, R., 49, 295
Darou, W.G., 253, 261
Dauphinais, P., 101, 218–19, 263
Davis, G.L., 100
Debo, Angie, 107
deculturation, of Northwest Coast Indians, 143–4
Deloria, Vine, Jr, 146
depression: affective symptoms of, 186–7; among Indian elderly, 183, 184–5; among the Flathead, 76, 169, 186–9; anomic, 116, 172; biological factors, 175; colonization and, 169–70; concepts of, 168, 309; culture-bound syndrome, 169; as Inuit mental problem, 281; measuring and treating, 176–85;

Navajo term for, 169; Nishnawbe (Ojibwa) language, 169; treatment for, 184–5
Devereux, George, 111–13, 115, 169, 170, 317; Mohave 'ethnopsychiatry,' 279; on therapist affinity, 262–3
De Vos, George, 67
Diagnostic and Statistical Manual (DSM). See DSM
Diagnostic Interview Schedule (DIS), 181
Diagnostic Interview Schedule for Children (DISC), 217–18
Dick, L., critique of pibloktoq, 197–9, 204
Diessner, R., 93
Dillard, D.A., 253, 258, 269
Dillard, John, 254, 267
Dinges, N.G., 199, 256, 263; on Aboriginal sickness, 273
Dionysian societies, 23–4
disease causation, Clements's theories of, 272–3
disorganization theory, 143–7, 171–3, 175; and alcohol assumptions, 160–1; and social integration, 171–2
Dobu Islanders, 23
Dogrib people, drinking patterns, 156
Dozier, Edward, 254; disorganization thesis of, 145
Driver, Harold, 96
Dru, R., 161
drugs, 24; cultural education and, 290–1. See also Aboriginal drinking
DSM, 7, 206; culture-bound syndromes, 191, 206, 208; depression criteria, 185; Eskimo community

mental status examination, 127–8; ghost sickness defined in, 204–5; 'heartbreak' as sign of depression, 182; idioms of distress, 209; 'magical thinking' as sign of mental disorder, 109, 274; O'Nell's critique of, 187; *pibloktoq* defined in, 204–5, 206; PTSD, 213–14, 218, 222, 236; Traumatic Events Booklet, 216

dualism/holism: debate, 283–4, 285, 299, 305. *See also* holism

DuBois, Cora, 52

DuBray, Wynne Hanson, 254–5

Duran, B., 224–6, 228, 276

Duran, Eduardo F., 223–6, 228, 276, 297

Durkheim, Émile, 114, 116, 171

Dwyer, J.W., 183

Dynneson, V.V., 262

dysfunction, assumptions of, 304

Edgerton, Robert, 149–50, 154

Edmonton, alcohol experiment in, 136–7

education: assimilation as key to, 229–30; cultural, 290–1

Edwards, E.D., 265, 267

Edwards, M.E., 265, 267

Eggan, Dorothy, 322n. 6

Eggan, Fred, 32, 254

Ehlers, C.L., 139

Ellis, R., 260, 263

epidemiology: community-based studies, 124–32; and definition of cultural groups, 125; emerging issues, 161–5; population health, 308; psychiatric, 114, 128. *See also* psychopathology

Erasmus, Georges, 232–3

Erikson, Erik, 9, 32, 40, 41, 62, 65–6

Erikson, Kai, 222

Escalante, F., 155

Eskimos: Alaskan, 77, 124; Baffin Island, 197; Briggs's linguistic analysis, 280–1; and cultural change, 324–5n. 3; culture contact damage to, 115; eastern Arctic, 127–8, 280; Greenlandic, 90, 195; Inuvik and Edmonton alcohol study, 136–7; *pibloktoq*, 195–7; spirit intrusion as cause of insanity, 280; University of Alaska, 85–6; use of physicians for physical problems, 280. *See also* Inuit

essentialism: of Aboriginal/non-Aboriginal dichotomy, 256–9; bloodedness, 314

Estes, G., on Aboriginal acculturation, 74–5

ethanol metabolization issue: American Indians and whites, 137–8; reviews of, 140–1

ethics, 239–40, 244, 249–56, 269–70, 311; relevance for psychotherapy, 251–3. *See also* behaviours; values

ethnic matching: in therapy, 261–3

ethnography: and Aboriginal depression, 185–8; alcohol in Aboriginal societies, 142–3; culture experts in, 82; role of, 38–42

ethnopsychiatry, of Devereux, 111–12

Everett, M.W., 101, 202–3

evolutionary theory, and Aboriginal drinking, 136

family therapy. *See* psychotherapy

Farris, J.J., 137–8

Fathauer, G., 199, 200–2

Fenna, D., 136–7, 142

Ferguson, Francis, 47–8

Field, P.B., 148

Fish, J.M., 12

Fisher, A.D., 140

Fitzgerald, J.A., 91

Flathead: depression among, 76; drinking, 146–7; and DSM criteria for depression, 187–8; research of O'Nell among, 185–9

Fleming, Candace M., 172, 263; acculturation schema of, 72; family therapy, 264; holism mantra, 276; value conflict, 261

Fletcher, C.M., 198

Flint, G., 86

Flores, P.J., 255

Flower of Two Soils project, 82, 97–8; and English-language ability, 94

Flower of Two Soils Reinterview project, 217–18

Fogelson, R., 22

Fontaine, Phil, 232

Forbes, Jack, 207

Foster, D.A., 124–5

Foster, Nancy, 77

Foucault, Michel, 12, 224

Foulks, E.F., 196–7, 198, 317

Foundations of Indian Teens project, 218

Fredericks, L., 287

Free Drawing Test, Indian Education Research Project, 33

Freeman, D.M.A., 196

Freeman, P.A., 196

French, Laurence A., 146, 159, 160–1; ethics, values, and behaviours, 253, 258, 260; on marginal Indians, 115, 117; race and cultural authenticity, 74

Freud, Anna, 41

Freud, Sigmund, 9, 22, 109; psychological anthropology, 27

Fritz, W.B., 127

Fromm, Erich, 34, 62

Gaddes, W.H., 93

Gaines, Attwood, 12–13

Garcia, W.I., 94

Garcia-Andrade, C., 139

Garrett, J.T., 117, 253, 258

Garrett, M.W., 117, 253, 258

Garro, Linda, 281–2; traditional healers, 289–90

Gaw, A.C., 205

Geertz, Clifford, 12

genetic traits, of individuals, 142

ghost sickness, 199–211, 273; culture-bound syndrome, 203

Gibbons, R.J., 141

Gilbert, J.A.L., 136–7

Glass, D., 180

globalization, 319; and concept of cultures, 13; cultural fact of, 315

Goffman, E., 229–30

Goldman, D., 160, 216, 222

Goldstein, G.S., 172

Good, B., 168, 189

Goodenough Draw-A-Man Test, Indian Education Research Project, 33–5, 36

Gotowiec, A., 94, 97

Grace Arthur Point Performance Scale, Indian Education Research Project, 33, 34–5, 36

Graves, Theodore D., 77, 118, 145, 255

Gray, Norma, 227

Great Whale River Eskimos, 47–8

Green, James W., 97, 253–4, 257–8

Grobsmith, E.S., 292, 293

group therapy. *See* psychotherapy
Gussow, Zachary, 196
Gustafson, J., 265
Gutierres, S.E., 287–8

HADS. *See* Hospital Anxiety and
Depression Scale (HADS)
Haggerty, J., 184
Hahn, R.A., 282, 283
Haig-Brown, C., 231
Hales, W.M., 125
Hall, G., 89
Hall, R.L., 293
Hallowell, A. Irving, 62, 110, 241,
304–5; on Aboriginal drinking,
147–9; critique of Clements's
schema, 272–3; cultural change
issues, 49–52; on Ojibwa culture
contact, 114–15; Saulteaux Ror-
schach protocols, 9, 44–6; social
atomism, 57–9; values research,
240; windigo psychosis, 192–3
Hallpike, C.R., 277–8
Hamer, J.H., 144–5, 156, 157–8
Hanson, D., 126–7, 130
Hare, 160
Harris, Marvin, 25, 27, 29
Harvard Psychological Clinic, 34
Harvard Value Study Questionnaire,
256
Hassrick, Royal, 39
Havighurst, Robert, 32, 93
Haviland, M.G., 262
Hay, Thomas, criticisms of, 54
Health Opinion Survey (HOS),
Eskimo community mental status
examination, 127–8
'heartbreak': among the Mohave,
169–70, 279; as depression symp-
tom, 182

Heath, D.B., 141, 161, 163
Heinrich, R.K., 253
Helman, C.G., 206
Hendrie, H.C., 126–7, 130
Henry, William E., 32, 34, 38, 39, 60
Herman, Judith Lewis, 222
Hermans, H., 319
Herreid, J.R., 85
Herreid II, C.F., 85
Herring, R.D., 74–5, 253, 267
Herscovits, Melville, 30
Highwater, Jamake, 89
Hippler, Arthur E., 65, 67, 114, 197–8
historical particularism, 22
history: memory as, 224, 228–9; in
therapy, 226
Hmong, ghost sickness, 203
Ho, M.K., 262, 263, 267
Hobbes, Thomas, 11
Hochhaus, L., 161
Hodge, F.S., 287
Hoffman, R.G., 100
Hoffmann, T., 80, 87–8
holism, 271–2, 275, 282; and Aborigi-
nal peoples, 271–2, 275–8; as heal-
ing, 296; and mind/body dualism,
283; as a post-1960s Aboriginal
concept, 282–3
holocaust, North American, 223
Honigmann, I., on the atomistic society, 149
Honigmann, John, 70, 144, 240, 304–
5; on the atomistic society, 56–7,
59, 149, 322–3n. 10; psychological
homogeneity of American Indians,
255, 258; Slave culture (Fort Nelson, BC), 47
Hopi, 32, 34; affective nosology, 181;
alcohol use, 152–3; Eggan on, 322n.
6; ethnosemantic interviewing of,

181; Oraibi community, 35–8; personality of, 36; sociocultural integration levels of, 152; testing the, 35–8; values, 240, 255; Walpi (First Mesa) community, 35–8

Hornbuckle, J., 146, 160–1; drinking patterns, 159; race and cultural authenticity, 74

Horse-Davis, S., 225

Horswill, R.K., 262

Horton, Donald, 148–9

HOS. *See* Health Opinion Survey (HOS)

Hospital Anxiety and Depression Scale (HADS), translation concerns, 184

Howard, W., 295

Howell, R.J., 92

Hrdlicka, Aleš, 107

Hughes, C., 208, 275–6

Hughes, I., 291

Human Relations Area Files, 273

Hummer, H.R., 108–9

Hunter, W.S., 91

Huron, 106

Hynd, G.W., 94

hysteria, 198, 201, 208

ICQ. *See* Indian Culture Quotient (ICQ)

ihuma, 281

Indian Administration Research Project. *See* Indian Education Research Project

Indian Culturalization Test, 87; MMPI study, 79; Northern Plains peoples, 79; Sioux, 5–6, 79

Indian Culture Quotient (ICQ), 79–80, 87

Indian Culture Scale, 80

Indian Depression Scale, 181

Indian Education Research Project, 15, 22, 29–42, 85, 254, 301; battery of tests, 32–5; project staff, 32; tribes selected for, 32

Indian Health Services, 180

Indian peoples, and Western psychiatric diagnosis, 112

Indian Personality Research Project. *See* Indian Education Research Project

Indians: basic personality structure concept, 27–9; Chicago, 144; cultural integration paradigm, 155–6; Eastern Oklahoma, 125; ethanol metabolization issue, 137–8; Inuvik and Edmonton alcohol study, 136–7; Lake Winnipeg region, 49–50; Northwest Coastal, 143; University of Alaska, 85–6. *See also* Aboriginal peoples

individual: acculturation and, 76; and collective dichotomy, 163, 263, 266–8; as culture-bound, 315; genetic traits, 142; in society, 122

individual therapy. *See* psychotherapy

intelligence, confusion of race and culture in measurement of, 89–95

intelligence tests (IQ). *See* Wechsler intelligence tests

'Inter-cultural contact scale,' North Alaskan Eskimos, 77

International Classification of Mental and Behaviourial Disorders (WHO), 206–7

Internet, 207

Inui, T.S., 115; acculturative stress, 117–18

Inuit: children, 94; and cultural

change, 324–5; and culture-bound syndromes, 195; Inuktitut terms for mental problems, 281; northern Quebec, 198; spirit intrusion as cause of insanity, 280. *See also* Eskimos

Inuktitut language, 94; glosses for mental illness terms, 280–1; word 'psychiatry,' 280

Inuvik, alcohol experiment in, 136–7

Inventory to Diagnose Depression (IDD), 178, 180

inverted 'U' pattern, of Indian ancestry, 139

Irvine, D., 125

Jackson, M., 264, 267

James, Bernard J., 115; critic of atomism, 58–9

James Bay Cree, 78, 109, 121, 131, 138–9, 192, 205, 259, 282, 292; Christian and traditionalists disagreements, 290; healing in community context, 296; ownership scale, 78. *See also* Cree

Jaranson, J.M., 216

Jarvis, G.K., death styles, 327n. 10

Jenness, Diamond, 109

Jesuit Relations, 106, 156

Jewell, D., 113

Jewish Holocaust, 223–5

Jilek, W.G., 172, 209, 292; Coast Salish healing, 296; Coast Salish spirit dancing, 294; spirit sickness as an 'Indian sickness,' 281

Jilek-Aall, L., 145, 157, 209, 277*t*; holism thesis, 276

Johnson, C.A., 169

Johnson, D., 279

Johnson, Dale L., 169, 172, 199, 202–3

Johnson, M.E., 262

Johnson, S., 161

Jones, B.M., 137–8

Jones, M.C., 218, 223

Jones-Saumty, D., 161

Joseph, Alice, 33–4, 37, 61

Jung, Carl, 26

Kaczynski, R., 183

Kahn, M.W., 266

Kakegamic, S., 169

Kalant, H., 141

Kaplan, Bert, 32–3, 60–2, 199, 202–3, 206, 279

Kaplan, H.I., 205

Kapur, B.M., 141

Kardiner, Abram, 9, 27–9, 38, 41, 52, 57, 62

Kaska, 47

Katz, P., 259

Keane, E.M., 178, 223

Keesing, Roger, 11–12, 314

Kehoe, A.B.: critique of New Age 'Indian' healing, 284–5; cultural primitivist debate, 285

Kelso, D., 7

Kemnitzer, L.S., 156–7

Kempen, H., 319

Kerckhoff, A.C., 116

Kermeen, P., 184

Kiev, K., 194

Kim, U., 119, 122

Kimball, Solon T., 32

King, J., 101

Kinzie, J.D., 131

Kirmayer, L.J., 205, 263; and Aboriginal alcoholism data, 164; concept of culture, 317–19; cultural critique of psychiatry, 14; Inuktitut terms for mental problems, 281; 'inverted

U' pattern, 173; landscape of memory, 228; *pibloktoq* cases, 198; and PTSD, 213–14; Santé Québec health survey data, 131–2; syndrome definition, 329–30n. 12; traditional healing practices, 288; trauma and collective memory, 232–3; values, 259

Kivlanhan, D.R., 86

Kleinman, Arthur, 168, 181, 186, 189, 214–15

Kline, J.A., 86, 267

Klopfer, Bruno, 45; examination of the Sioux of Pine Ridge, 39–40; Indian Education Research Project, 33–4; Mescalero Apache, 62–3; research on Indian tribes, 32; Rorschach analyst, 46, 48, 57

Kluckhohn, Clyde, 32, 38, 246; Indian Education Research Project, 60; on Indian policy development, 31; Navajo study, 35, 39, 113; values orientation, 240, 241, 249, 254–6

Kluckhohn, Florence, 241–3

Konner, M., 205

Koverola, C., 253, 267

Kraus, R.F., 115, 144

Kroeber, Alfred L., 9, 25, 41, 96, 105, 109; characterizations of societies, 274; values research, 240

Kunitz, Stephen J., 123, 151–4, 162, 174, 285, 293

Kupferer, Harriet, 59

Kutchin, 59

Kuttner, R.E., 161

Kwakiutl, 23–6, 29; WISC performance scores of, 93

LaBoueff, S., 164

LaFromboise, T.D., 263, 267; acculturation schema of, 73–4; family therapy, 264; on marginal Indians, 115

Lake Winnipeg region, 49–50

Lakota people: culture of, 41, 79, 80, 81–2; F scale, 323n. 5, 88; *tiospaye* concept, 81; traumatic grief of, 227; values, 255

Lakota Sioux Reservation (Rosebud), 80

Lalonde, Christopher, 174–5

Lambek, M., 215

Lamphere, J.K., 183

Landes, Ruth, 55–6, 110; and social atomism, 57; windigo psychosis, 192–3

Lane, E., 86

Langness, Lewis, 208

language: acculturation index, 77; and Native American acculturation, 80; translation in cross-cultural settings, 184

Lantz, Herman, 61, 62

Lashley, K.H., 262

Layne, N., 159

Leavenworth penitentiary, Kansas, 148

Leighton, Alexander H., 9, 32, 128–9, 144, 280

Leighton, Dorothea, 32, 34–5, 39, 113, 128–9

Leland, J., 135

Lemert, Edwin M., 143, 156, 157

Leon, R.L., 125

Levine, R.E., 205

Levy, Jerrold E., 123; on Aboriginal drinking, 151–4, 162; biomedicine and Aboriginal healing, 293; cultural continuity/integration paradigm, 174; holism and New Age ideas, 285; 'moth madness,' 280

Lewis, Gilbert, 298
Lewis, Ronald G., 140, 263, 267, 275
Lewis, T.H., 169
Lewton, E.L., 295
Li, T., 137
Lichtenberg, P.A., 183
Lin, K.-M., 205
Linnekin, J., 295
Linton, Ralph, 9, 27–9, 30
Lipsedge, M., 106
Littlewood, R., 106
Littman, G., 144
Lock, M., 12
Locke, D.C., 74–5
Long, J.C., 139, 160
Long, K.A., 221
Lorincz, A.B., 161
Lowie, Robert, 25
Lucas, R.H., 11, 12, 112, 207, 286
Luckert, K.W., 279–80
Ludeman, W.W., 91
Lummi Nation, 179
Lurie, Nancy O., 155–6

MacAndrew, Craig, 149–50, 154
Macgregor, Gordon, 58, 144; on the
  Sioux, 39–42
McCormick, T.C., 116, 296
McCullough, C.S., 93
McDonald, D.R., 7, 259
McGaa, Ed (Eagle Man), 287
McKay, S., 169
McKenzie, A., 93
McNeill, B.W., 262
McNickle, D'Arcy, 31; caught-
  between-two-worlds paradigm,
  116
McShane, D.A., 93, 95, 97, 99
Mail, P.D., 7, 141, 144, 161
Mandelzys, N., 86

Manson, Spero M., 86; and Aboriginal drinking, 162, 164; Aboriginal
  lexicons for emotional states, 282;
  on Aboriginal sickness, 273; and
  the American Indian Depression
  Scale, 180–2, 185; bibliographic
  material on Aboriginal mental
  health, 7; culture areas, 97–8; culture-bound syndromes, 204, 205;
  depression and suicide, 168, 176,
  177–8; ethics, values, and behaviours, 253, 258; ghost sickness, 199;
  gourd society, 223; group therapy,
  265–6; on healing ceremonies, 297;
  on Indian subcultures, 188–9; population studies review, 130–1;
  trauma and PTSD, 216–21; treatment approach, 269
Marano, Lou, 207; on windigo psychosis, 5, 17–18, 193–5, 204, 205
Margetts, E.L., 106–7, 279
marginality: apple syndrome, 115–
  16; caught-between-two-worlds
  paradigm, 114–18, 119
Marsella, A.J., 76
Martin, H.W., 125
Martínez-Hernáez, A., 206
Maryboy, N., 278
Matewapit, G., 169
May, Philip A.: Aboriginal and non-
  Aboriginal drinking patterns, 161–
  2; alcohol abuse problems, 141;
  anomie perspective, 166; assumption of biological factors in drinking, 135; binge drinking pattern,
  158; caught-between-two-worlds
  paradigm, 146; issues of alcoholism and alcohol abuse, 164; white
  people's patterns of drinking, 159
Maynard, E., 145

Mead, Margaret, 9, 23, 32, 52, 254
measurement: of acculturation to
   non-Aboriginal society, 79; of cultural orientation, 76–84; intelligence and personality, 90
Medicine, B., 160, 199, 273
medicine wheel, 286, 333–4n. 10
medico-legal systems, and Aboriginal healing, 294
Megalomaniac societies, 23
Mekeel, Scudder, 40; critical review
   of, 40–1
'Memorandum on the Study of
   Acculturation' (Redfield, Linton,
   and Herscovits [1936]), 29–30, 70,
   77, 240
memory, 215, 223, 224, 226, 228–33,
   236
Menominee: adaptation of to Western culture, 71; psychopathology
   of, 110–11; religion among the, 71
mental health issues, 3–4; and
   Aboriginal supernatural beliefs,
   109; Aboriginal theories of, 272–5;
   alcohol and, 304; blood quantum,
   108; boarding school survey, 217–
   18; and contemporary Aboriginality, 300; contradictory reports of,
   305–6; environmental stress, 110;
   insanity, 107; role of culture in, 76–
   84; sensationalist reports of, 109;
   suicide, 107
*Merck Manual of Diagnosis and Ther-
   apy*, spirit disease in, 206
Merskey, H., 184
Merton, Robert, 116
Métis, defined as Aboriginal population, 126–7
Metraux, R., 197
Mezzich, J., 205

Miller, J.R., 231
Milne, D., 295
Minas, H., 205, 317–19
mind/body dualism, 276, 278–85,
   283; of Westerners, 271–2. *See also*
   dualism/holism
Minde, T., 120–1
Minnesota Multiphasic Personality
   Inventory (MMPI), 15, 69; cultural
   appropriateness of, 84–5, 302; and
   cultural influence, 86–7; educa-
   tion/occupation and, 88; funda-
   mental flaw in comparisons in, 96;
   and Indian Culturalization Test, 79
Mishra, S.P., 95
Mission (Indians), 139–40
Mitchell, C.K., 155
Mix, L., 136–7
MMPI. *See* Minnesota Multiphasic
   Personality Inventory (MMPI)
MMPI-168, 80
modal personality structure, 52–3;
   Northern Athabascans, 66
Mohatt, G., 81–2, 144, 157, 290, 297
Mohave: ghost sickness, 199, 201–2;
   psychopathology, 112; suicide
   among, 112, 115
Mohawk values, 255, 256–7
Mok, D., 120–1
Moral Ideology Test, Indian Educa-
   tion Research Project, 33
Morgan, William, on ghost sickness,
   199–200
Morley, P., 275
Mormon culture, 60
Morris, C., 82
Morton, S.G., 90
Mosaic Minds, 207
'moth craziness' (brother-sister
   incest), 279, 280

Mulcahy, R., 94
Murdock, George, 273
Murphy, J.M., 280
Murray, Henry, 33–4

Narragansett: cultural education of adolescents, 290–1; Rhode Island, 290–1
Naskapi, 154
National Center for American Indian and Alaska Native Mental Health, 176
'Native American,' contrasted with 'White American,' 257t
Native American Church, 290; peyote use in, 294
Navaho. See Navajo
Navajo, 32, 34–5, 39, 60–1, 99, 254; alcohol use, 152–3; amok, 207, 328n. 5; and anomic depression, 172; cultural trauma among, 222–3; cures for anti-social tendencies, 279–80; and depression, 185; drinking patterns, 153–4, 159, 161; Enemy Way ceremony, 223; ethanol metabolization issue, 138; Evilway ceremony, 280; ghost sickness, 199, 199–200, 203; healing traditions of, 290; holism thesis, 276; item bias in WISC-R, 95; Mountainway healing ceremony, 280; personality traits of, 113; precontact society and drinking, 151; psychiatric sophistication of, 279; sociocultural integration levels of, 152; traditional medical treatments, 279; trauma and, 221; value orientations, 242, 243t; WAIS performance scores, 92–3
Navajo Christian faith healing, 290

Navajo Healing Project, 295
Navarro, J., 286
Neligh, G., 265–6
Nelson, K.S., 100
neo-Freudians, 27
Neutra, R., 280
New Age movement: Aboriginal traditions and, 287; and holism thesis, 284–5; 'Indian' healing, 284–5; pan-Indian sentiment, 97
Nez Perce people, 157
Nichter, M., 209
noble savage, 149
Nofz, M.P., 146
Nooksack Tribe, 179
Northern Woodlands, Flower of Two Soils project, 97
Northwest Coastal Indians, 179; Flower of Two Soils project, 97; validity of MMPI for, 86
Norton, I.M., 97–8, 259
Norway House, 177
Nuckolls, Charles, 269–70

O'Connell, J.J., 262
Oetting, E.R., 123
Ogden, M., 167, 168, 173–4
Oglala (Sioux), 41
Ojibwa, 5, 119; personality of, 55–6; and social atomism, 57; southern Ontario, 110; windigo psychosis, 192
Oklahoma Indian, value orientations study, 248–9
O'Nell, Theresa D., 75, 146–7, 155, 169, 185–9; and the Flathead of Montana, 185–9; on trauma of warriors, 223
Opler, Morris E., 32, 199; on ghost sickness, 201–2

oppression, history of, 228
Orlansky, M.D., 253

Page, R.D., 87
Paniagua, F.A., 253, 258, 260, 264–5, 267
Papago, 32, 39
Paranoid societies, 23
Parker, D., 280
Parker, L., 290
Parker, Seymour, 110, 192–4, 196–7
Parsons, Elsie Clews, 25–6, 254
Parsons, Talcott, 240
Passamaquoddy, 157
Patterns of Culture (Benedict), 23, 25, 26–7; criticism of, 25
Peary, Admiral Robert, 195
Pedigo, J., 144
Peron, François de, 106
personality: Aboriginal portraits, 48–60; alcohol acceptance or rejection of, 147; basic personality structure concept, 27–8; construction of the Aboriginal, 21–43; disorders issue, 62, 206; of the Hopi, 36; measuring, 84–9; psychometric approaches to, 101. *See also* basic personality structure concept
Phillips, M.R., 115; acculturative stress, 117–18
Phoenix alcohol study, American Indians and whites, 137
phrenology, 90
Phung, A., 89
Piasecki, J., 223
pibloktoq, 195–9, 203–11, 273; culture-bound syndrome, 203; Eskimo community, 128; hysteric acts, 195–6
Pine, C.J., 170

Pine Ridge Dakota (Sioux), 39–40
Plains Indians, 23–5, 86, 265; Flower of Two Soils project, 97; Northern Plains, 155, 218–19; psychopathology among, 176–7
Plank, G., 92, 94–5
Plas, J.M., 99
Plateau Indians, validity of MMPI for, 86
politics: race and biology, 314–15; of traditional healing, 288–9, 292, 299
Pollack, D., 86
post-colonialism, 315; of Duran and Duran, 224; ideas of, 10, 30–1; and scientific hegemony, 318–19
post-contact cultural convergence, 98
post-traumatic stress disorder. *See* PTSD
potlatching, 24
Pottawotami, 144, 156
pre-contact Aboriginal populations, 311; Hallowell on, 49–50
Preston, Richard, 192, 194
Price, B.K., 262
Price, J.A., 161
Price-Williams, D., 275
primitive peoples, 28, 109, 148, 211, 274
primitive thought, Hallpike on, 277–8
primitivism, 10, 30, 53, 316; Aboriginal peoples and, 10–11, 133, 300; and alcohol, 165; Erikson and, 41
Prince, R.H., 205
prisons, 5, 86; and Aboriginal Elders, 226; bureaucratizing of Aboriginal healing in, 293–4; identity and culture problems in, 292; and MMPI use in, 86; payment issue for heal-

ers, 294; politics of traditional healing, 292; traditional healing in, 289–90

psychiatry, 4; Aboriginal culture and, 306–8; Aboriginal mental health and, 7; case studies in Winnipeg, 126–7; colonial, 106; depression defined in, 168, 188–9

psychoanalytical anthropology, 302; dream analysis, 56–7; emergence of, 27–9

psychological acculturation, 118

'Psychological Analysis of Primitive Cultures' seminar, 57

psychological anthropology, 39; and social atomism, 56–7; values research, 240

psychological distress instrument, Santé Québec, 131–2

psychology, 4; Aboriginal culture and, 306–8; Aboriginal mental health and, 7; and anthropology, 243–4; approach to Aboriginal values, 243–9; Indian compared to 'white people,' 241; and intergenerational trauma, 224

psychopathology, 11, 14, 15; construction of the Aboriginal, 105–33; culture contact and change in, 118; epidemiology studies in Aboriginal communities, 124–32, 303–4; latent schizophrenics and primitive people, 105–14; Mohave, 112; personality and, 106; and Plains Indians, 176–7; rates of, 303–4; research in, 106–9

psycho-social nomadism, 267

psychotherapy, 15–16; client/therapist relationship, 261–3, 266; ethics, values, and behaviour in, 251–

3, 259–60; family therapy, 264; group, 263–9; individual, 263–9

PTSD: and Aboriginal peoples, 216–21, 236; cultural level of, 222; cumulative, 222; Detroit study, 219; heritable component of, 214; and individuals, 236; intergenerational, 221–2, 225; low rates of, 217–21; medicalization of, 214–15; politics of traditional healing, 288–9; trauma and, 212–15, 235–6. See also DSM; trauma

Pueblo peoples, 23, 25, 28; and Anglo values, 254

Putsch, R.W., 203

race: and cultural authenticity, 74, 80, 312–13; and culture confused, 89–95

racial polygenism, 90

racism, scientific, 22

Rankin, J.G., 141

Rasmussen, J.K., 160, 216, 217

RCAP. See Royal Commission on Aboriginal Peoples (RCAP)

Redfield, Robert, 30, 171

Red Horse, J., 264

Redshirt, R., 80, 82

Reed, T.E., 141

Renfrey, G.S., 253, 256

research base, validity of, 253–6

residential schools: abuses, 230–1; disclosure of abuse at, 232; lawsuits from abuse at, 232, 234; perpetrators, 230–1; as total institutions, 229–30

residential school syndrome, 236; origins of, 233–4; trauma and, 228–34

Richardson, Edwin H., 79, 82, 247–8,

253, 262, 268; comparison of Indian and White Values, 244–6, 257–8

Robbins, R.H., 75, 154

Roberts, A.C., 86, 267

Robin, R.W., 160, 216, 217, 222–3

Rogers, S.L., critique of Clements's schema, 273

Rogler, L.H., 208

Rohner, R.P., 26

Roll, S., 197

Rolling Thunder, 284

Rorschach, 28, 33, 44–8, 302; Aboriginal populations, 15; administration and interpretation of, 45–6, 51; criticism of, 47–8, 61–2; cultural change issues, 48–9; Hallowell's assessment of, 45–6; Indian Education Research Project, 33, 36; intracultural issues, 48–9; persistence of, 60–7; problems with, 47–8; Saulteaux protocols, 9, 45, 49–50, 51

Rorschach, Hermann, 33

Rorschach Psychodiagnostic (Inkblot) Test. See Rorschach

Rosebud Lakota Sioux Reservation, 80

Roundhead, D., 169

Rousseau, Jean Jacques, 11

Rowe, W., 263

Roy, C., 125

Royal Commission on Aboriginal Peoples (RCAP), 232–3

Rozynko, V.V., 86

Rubel, Arthur J., 59

Sack, W.H., 80, 82, 93, 219

Sadock, B.J., 205, 206

SADS-L. See Schedule for Affective Disorders and Schizophrenia - Lifetime Version (SADS-L)

Sage, G.P., 117, 253

Saindon, J.E., 109, 190; windigo psychosis, 192–3, 203

Salish. See Coast Salish

Sampath, H.M., 127–8, 129

Santé Québec health survey, James Bay Cree, 131

Sapir, Edward, 44, 96; genuine and spurious culture of, 40, 114–15, 117–18, 119

Sapirstein, Milton, 57

Saskatchewan: Fritz's study of psychiatric patients, 127; psychiatric hospital admission statistics, 125–6

Sasson, S., 291

Saulteaux: psychiatric cases, 125–6; Rorschach protocols, 9, 45, 49–50, 51; and social atomism, 57; spirit intrusion as cause of insanity, 272; values research, 240

Saulteaux/Ojibwa/Chippewa, personality analysis of, 49–50

Savishinsky, J.S., 160

Schaefer, O., 136–7

Schedule for Affective Disorders and Schizophrenia - Lifetime Version (SADS-L), 130, 176–7, 179, 181–2

Scheper-Hughes, N., 12

science, culture of, 318

Scurfield, R.M., 226; on traditional healing practices, 288–9

Seltzer, A., 133

Seminole, 248

Service, Elman, 152

shamans: in Arcadian images, 286; Mescalero, 62–4; personality of, 112; and psychiatric problems, 280

Shore, Bradd, 269–70, 316

Shore, James H., 86, 128, 130–1, 168, 176–7, 178, 180–1; culture-bound syndromes, 205; on Indian subcultures, 188–9
Shoshone, 256
Silk, Samuel, 108–9
Silk-Walker, P., 205
Silver, S.M., 275
Simons, R., 208
Sioux, 32, 39–42, 87, 99; aggression, 40; drinking patterns, 161; ethanol metabolization issue, 138; Northern Plains, 79–80; Oglala, 145, 169; reservation system, 40; WISC-R performance scores of, 93
Sitting Bull, 227
Skipper, B., 93
Slave (Fort Nelson, BC), 47
Slotkin, J.S., 110–11
Smith, James G.E., 192
Smith-Sutker, S., 125
Snidecor, J.C., 107
Snipp, C.M., 140
sobriety, 160
social atomism, 55–60, 149
social class, 129–30
Social Darwinism, 90
social disintegration concept, 144
social disorganization theory, 143–7; and alcohol assumptions, 160–1; and social integration, 171–2
social organization, and drinking practices, 151–2
social pathology, justice system and, 146
Society for Applied Anthropology, 32
socio-economic status: and class, 251, 325n. 9; depression and suicide and, 173

Somervell, P.D., 219
Sommermier, E., 91
soul loss, 273
soul wound, 225–7
South Dakota, Canton Asylum for Insane Indians, 107–8
Spang, A., 253, 260, 267
Spanish-American culture, 60
Spaulding, J.M., 108
Spector, R.E., 206
Spicer, Edward H., 32
Spider-Man comic book series, 208
Spindler, George, 62, 71–2, 115, 246; ethics, values, and behaviours, 240–1
Spindler, Louise, 71–2, 115, 246; ethics, values, and behaviours, 240–1
spirit dancing, 156, 209, 294
spirit intrusion, 273
Steinbring, J., 156, 157–8
Stevens, S.M., 157
Stevenson, Matilda Coxe, 25–6
Steward, Julian, 152
Stewart, Omer C., 32, 39
Stirling County, Nova Scotia, psychiatric epidemiology study in, 128–9
Stonequist, E.V., 116
Storck, M., 169, 185
Storm, Hyemeyohsts, 284, 287
Strauss, M., 169
Strodtbeck, Fred L., 241–3, 249, 254–6
Sue, D., 261, 268
Sue, D.W., 261, 268
suicide, 167–76, 309, 327n. 4; among the Kwakiutl, 24; cultural continuity and, 167–8; colonization and, 169–70; in the Cree and Métis community, 177; cultural continuity and, 167–8; Hopi, Navajo, and Apache rates, 152–3; 'inverted U'

pattern of traditionalism and, 173;
measuring and treating, 176–85;
and traditionalism, 173
Suicide Ideational Questionnaire, 178
Sun Bear, 284
Sun Dance, Erikson and, 41–2
sweatlodge ceremonies, 286–8; in
Aboriginal healing, 293; schisms
within, 226

taboo breaking, 273
Tafoya, T., 267
Tait, C.L., 13, 259, 263, 288
talking circles, 287–8
Tam, T., 141
Tanaina, 65–6
Taylor, Drew Hayden, 70
Taylor, T., 286
Tefft, Stanton, 256
Tempest, P., 93–4
Terman, Lewis, 107
Texans, value orientations, 242, 243t
Thematic Apperception Test (TAT),
33–4, 61; Indian Education
Research Project, 33, 36, 38
Thomas, Robert, 241
Thompson, J.W., 205
Thompson, Laura, 31, 32, 33–4, 35–8
Timpson, J.B., 169, 172
Todd, N., 296
Tönnies, Ferdinand, 171
Topper, M.D., 116, 154–5, 172, 265;
Aboriginal drinking patterns, 159,
161
Totem and Taboo (Freud), 27
Townsley, H.C., 172
traditional Aboriginal healing, 305;
ambiguities in, 297, 299; authentic-
ity of healers, 295–6; defining, 294–
8; importance of cultural heritage,

297; Navajo, 279, 295; political
dimension in, 299; in prisons, 289–
90, 292; and PTSD, 288–9
'Traditional Cultural Value Preferences for U.S. Middle-Class'/
'American Indian/Alaska Native
Populations,' 268–9
traditionalism, and suicide, 173
traditionality scale, and Native
American acculturation, 80–1
Trap, J.J., 253
trauma: and Aboriginal peoples,
215–21, 234–6; cumulative and collective, 221–8, 235–6; and history,
223–4, 235; individual, 214–15, 222;
and PTSD, 212–15; of relocation,
223. See also PTSD
treatment: approach to alcohol, 265–
6; cross-cultural studies literature,
247; culture and tradition in, 286–
94; for depression, 184–5; Navajo
traditional medical, 279; non-
Aboriginal modalities, 305; and
values, 259–69
Treaty Indians, Saskatchewan, 125
tribal membership, in Aboriginal
research, 96
Trimble, Joseph E., 117, 123–4, 247,
253–4, 256, 263, 267, 276; on
Aboriginal sickness, 273; acculturation schema of, 72; concept of the
Aboriginal, 308; criticism of the
culture and personality anthropologists, 246–9; culture-bound syndromes, 199, 202, 205, 211; family
therapy, 264; value conflict, 260,
261
Tsimshian, food accumulation of,
119–20
Tuscarora, 46–7, 52–4

Uecker, A.E., 79, 87
Underhill, Ruth, 32
United Church, residential schools, 230
United States census 1970, WAIS and Aboriginal peoples, 92
United States census 1980, target subjects from, 89
United States Indian Bureau, 31
United States Indian Reorganization Act, 30
United States National Museum, 107
University of Alaska, 85
University of Chicago, 31–2
University of Colorado, 176
Upper Tanana, 65–6

Vallee, Frank G., 114, 116, 197, 210, 280
value orientations, 241–3; in American southwest, 242; selected comparison of, 243t
values, 239–40, 244, 269–70, 311; counselling Native Americans, 246; comparison of Indian and White, 245t; Cultural Contrasts table, 257t; relevant for psychotherapy, 251–3; and treatment, 259–69. See also behaviours; ethics
Varvin, S., 290, 297
Vietnamese refugees, acculturative stress levels of, 122
Vietnam veterans project, trauma and PTSD, 217–18
Vietnam war, 226–7, 236; PTSD and, 213–15
Vizenor, Gerald, 285
Vogt, Evan, 32

'wacinko syndrome,' among the Oglala Sioux, 169
Wade, Allan, 228, 231
Waldram, James B., 292; traditional healing in prisons, 226, 289–90; trauma, 222
Walker, J.L., 93
Walker, R.D., 86, 205
Wall, T.L., 139
Wallace, Anthony F.C., 46–7, 246; on group personality differences, 52–4
Warm Springs Indian Reservation, 179
Warner, W. Lloyd, 32, 38
Washburn, Wilcomb, 241
Washington State (Tacoma), sample from, 89
Watters, B., 94
Watts, L.K., 287–8
Wax, Rosalie, 241
Wechsler intelligence tests, 15, 69; criticism of, 93–4; cultural appropriateness of, 302; and culture fairness, 95; and English-language ability, 93–4, 98–9; fundamental flaw in comparisons in, 96; and hearing loss among Indian children, 94; race and culture confusion in, 92; urban or rural students and, 94; WAIS (adults), 92; WISC (school children), 92, 95; WPPSI (pre-schoolers), 92
Weibel-Orlando, J.C., 139, 291, 292
Weisner, T.S., 139, 159; drinking patterns, 158–9
West, concept of, 12
Westermeyer, Joseph, 135, 141, 159, 162, 164, 317; apple syndrome, 115–16; drinking patterns, 158; Indian Culture Scale, 80

'Western Identification Scale,' North Alaskan Eskimos, 77
white people: caught-between-two-worlds paradigm, 116; and drinking, 157–60; ethanol metabolization issue, 137–8; Inuvik and Edmonton alcohol study, 136–7; in mental health literature, 315–16
Whiting, Alfred, 38
Whorf, Benjamin, 241
Wikan, U., 314–15
Wilgosh, L., 94
Williams, R.T., 159
Williams Lake (BC), study of, 231
Wilson, C., 180
Wilson, J.P., 275
Wilson, S., 286
windigo, 5, 17–18
windigo psychosis, 5, 17–18, 192–5, 203–11, 273, 320
Winnebago, drinking patterns, 156

Winnipeg, psychiatric case studies in, 126–7
Wissler, Clark, 25, 96
witchcraft, Acoma people and, 112–13
Wolff, P.H., 138–9
Wounded Knee massacre, 227

Yakima Indian Nation, 179
Yap, Pow Meng, 191
Young, Alan, 213, 215
Young, S., 232, 234
Young, T.J., 141

Zeiner, A., 161
Zia, 32
Zintz, Miles, Pueblo/Anglo values, 254
Zitzow, D., on Aboriginal acculturation, 74–5
Zuni, 23, 25–6, 28–9, 32, 38–9, 60–1, 254; value orientations, 242, 243t

ANTHROPOLOGICAL HORIZONS

Editor: Michael Lambek, University of Toronto

Published to date:

1 *The Varieties of Sensory Experience: A Sourcebook in the Anthropology of the Senses*
   Edited by David Howes
2 *Arctic Homeland: Kinship, Community, and Development in Northwest Greenland*
   Mark Nuttall
3 *Knowledge and Practice in Mayotte: Local Discourses of Islam, Sorcery, and Spirit Possession*
   Michael Lambek
4 *Deathly Waters and Hungry Mountains: Agrarian Ritual and Class Formation in an Andean Town*
   Peter Gose
5 *Paradise: Class, Commuters, and Ethnicity in Rural Ontario*
   Stanley R. Barrett
6 *The Cultural World in Beowulf*
   John M. Hill
7 *Making It Their Own: Severn Ojibwe Communicative Practices*
   Lisa Philips Valentine
8 *Merchants and Shopkeepers: A Historical Anthropology of an Irish Market Town, 1200–1991*
   Philip Gulliver and Marilyn Silverman
9 *Tournaments of Value: Sociability and Hierarchy in a Yemeni Town*
   Ann Meneley
10 *Mal'uocchiu: Ambiguity, Evil Eye, and the Language of Distress*
   Sam Migliore
11 *Between History and Histories: The Production of Silences and Commemorations*
   Edited by Gerald Sider & Gavin Smith
12 *Eh, Paesan!: Being Italian in Toronto*
   Nicholas DeMaria Harney
13 *Theorizing the Americanist Tradition*
   Edited by Lisa Philips Valentine and Regna Darnell
14 *Colonial 'Reformation' in the Highlands of Central Sualwesi, Indonesia, 1892–1995*
   Albert Schrauwers

15 *The Rock Where We Stand: An Ethnography of Women's Activism in Newfoundland*
Glynis George

16 *Being Alive Well: Health and the Politics of Cree Well-Being*
Naomi Adelson

17 *Irish Travellers: Racism and the Politics of Culture*
Jane Helleiner

18 *Writing and Colonialism in Northern Ghana: The Encounter between the LoDagaa and the 'World on Paper,' 1892–1991*
Sean Hawkins

19 *An Irish Working Class: Explorations in Political Economy and Hegemony, 1800–1950*
Marilyn Silverman

20 *The Double Twist: From Ethnography to Morphodynamics*
Edited by Pierre Maranda

21 *Of Property and Propriety: The Role of Gender and Class in Imperialism and Nationalism*
Edited by Himani Bannerji, Shahrzad Mojab, and Judith Whitehead

22 *Guardians of the Transcendent: An Ethnography of a Jain Ascetic Community*
Anne Vallely

23 *The House of Difference: Cultural Politics and National Identity in Canada*
Eva Mackey

24 *The Hot and the Cold: Ills of Humans and Maize in Native Mexico*
Jacques M. Chevalier and Andrés Sánchez Bain

25 *Figured Worlds: Ontological Obstacles in Intercultural Relations*
Edited by John Clammer, Sylvie Poirier, and Eric Schwimmer

26 *Revenge of the Windigo: The Construction of the Mind and Mental Health of North American Aboriginal Peoples*
James B. Waldram